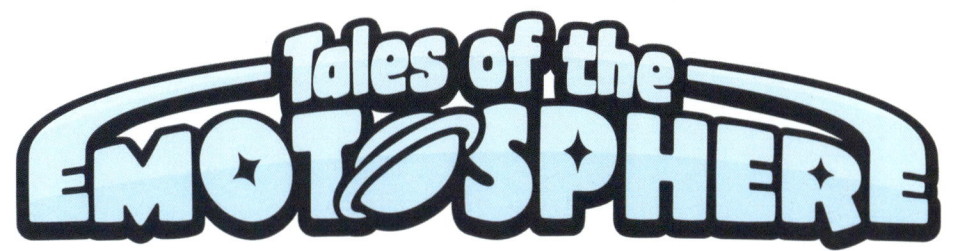

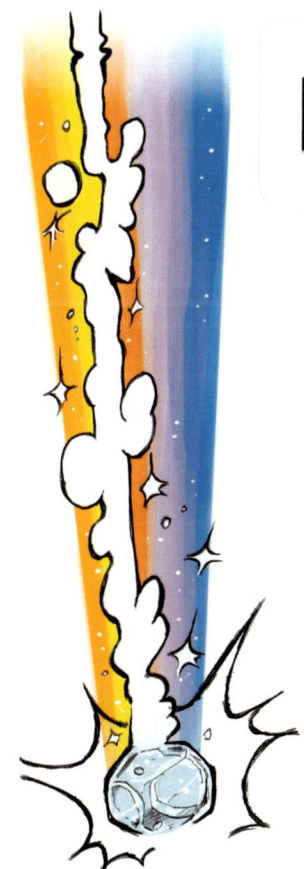

By **Russ Daff**
and
Dr Susannah Redhead

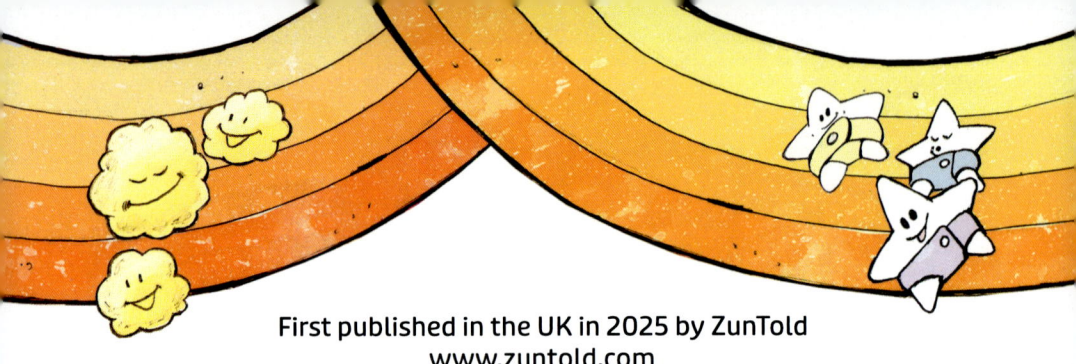

First published in the UK in 2025 by ZunTold
www.zuntold.com

Text and illustrations copyright © AstroVista Ltd 2025
Russ Daff (author and illustrator) and Dr Susannah Redhead (author)
Cover design by Russ Daff & Isla Bousfield-Donohoe

The moral right of the authors has been asserted.

All rights reserved.
Unauthorised duplication contravenes existing laws.

A catalogue record for this book is available from the British Library

ISBN 978-1-915758-29-3
1 2 3 4 5 6 7 8 9 10

Printed and bound by Interak, Poland.

Without in any way limiting the exclusive rights of AstroVista Ltd under copyright, any use of this publication to train generative artificial intelligence (AI) technologies to generate text or images is expressly prohibited. AstroVista Ltd reserve all rights to license uses of this work for generative AI training and development of machine learning language models.

> *Disclaimer. For carers: Tales of the Emotosphere includes general information on resilience and wellbeing. This is not intended as medical advice, diagnosis or treatment. Please discuss with a medical professional if specific help is needed.*

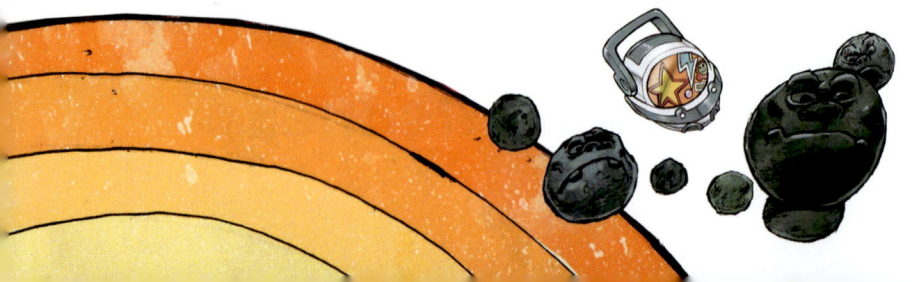

"For Emmeline, Johnny and especially Kerry, the third amigo!"

– Russ Daff

"For Billy and Max, my heart and soul, and to Kerry Daff, for your vision, belief and drive to bring the Emotosphere to life!"

– Dr Susannah Redhead

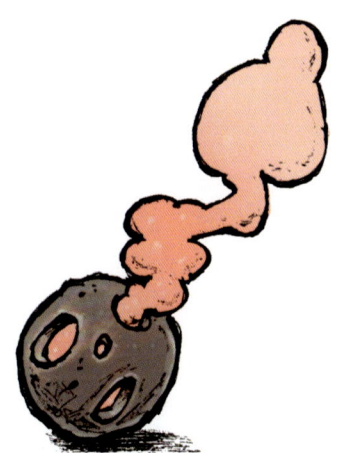

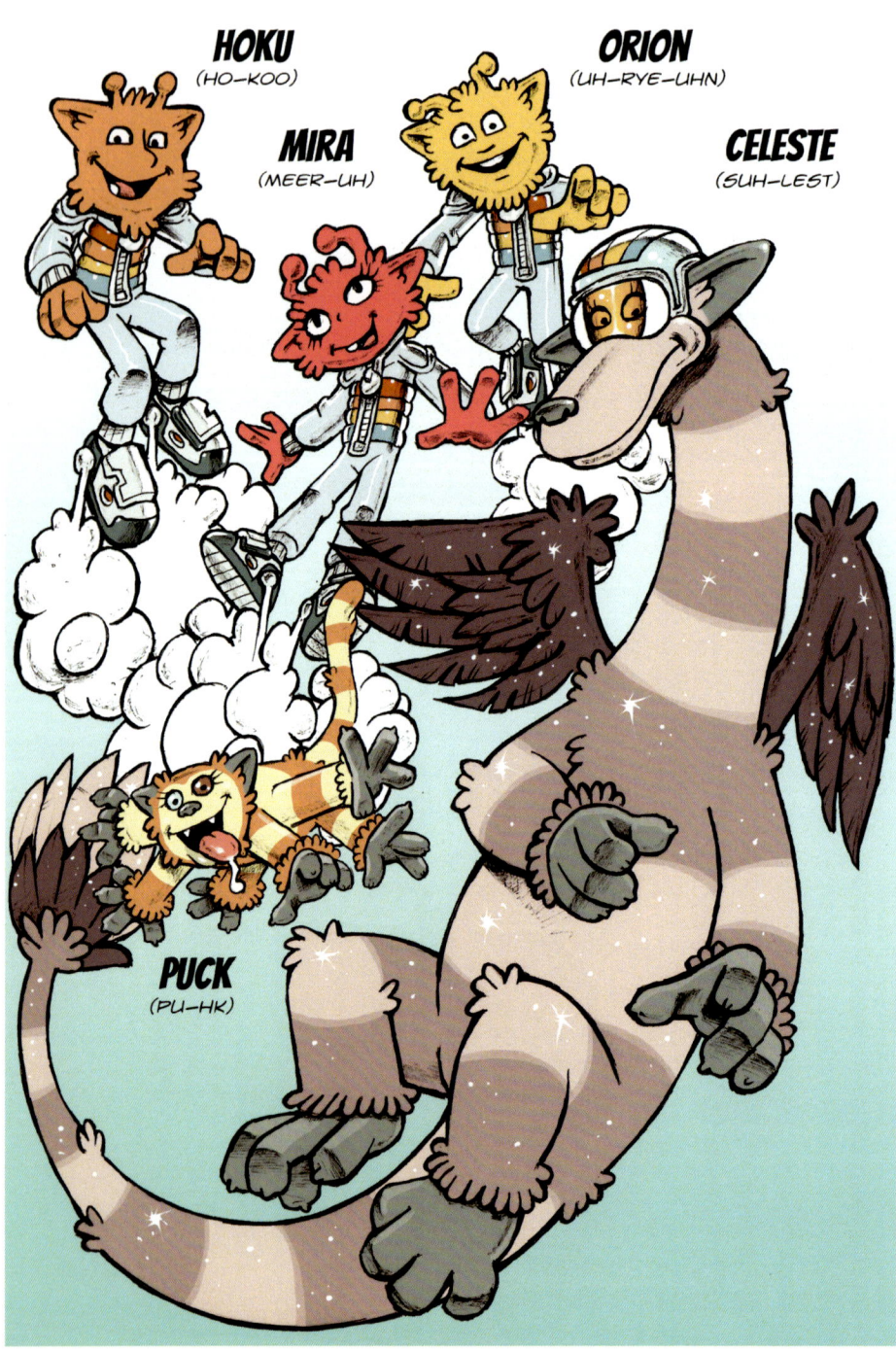

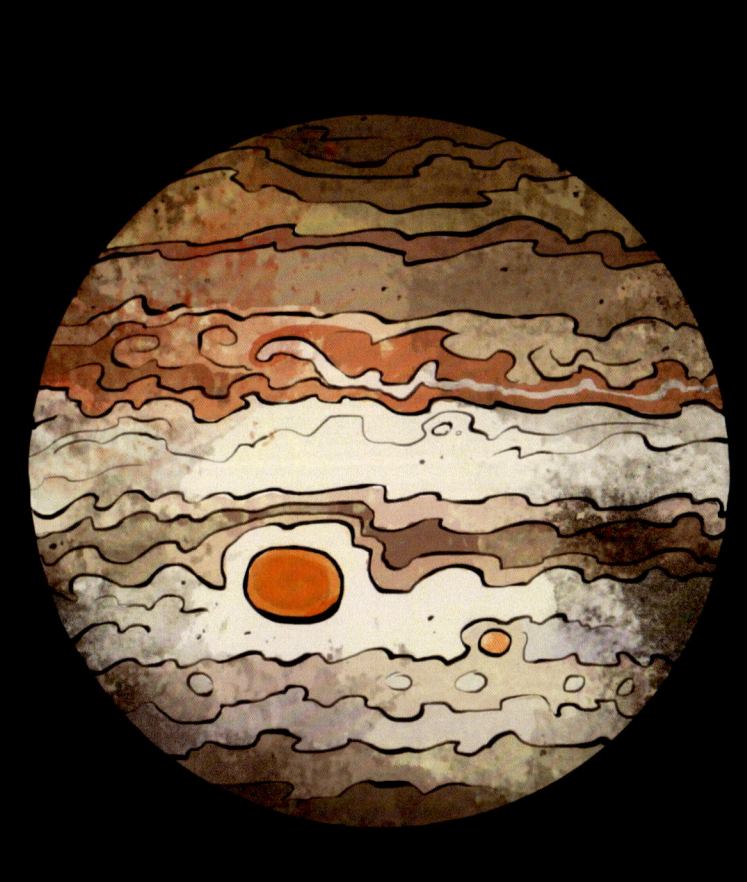

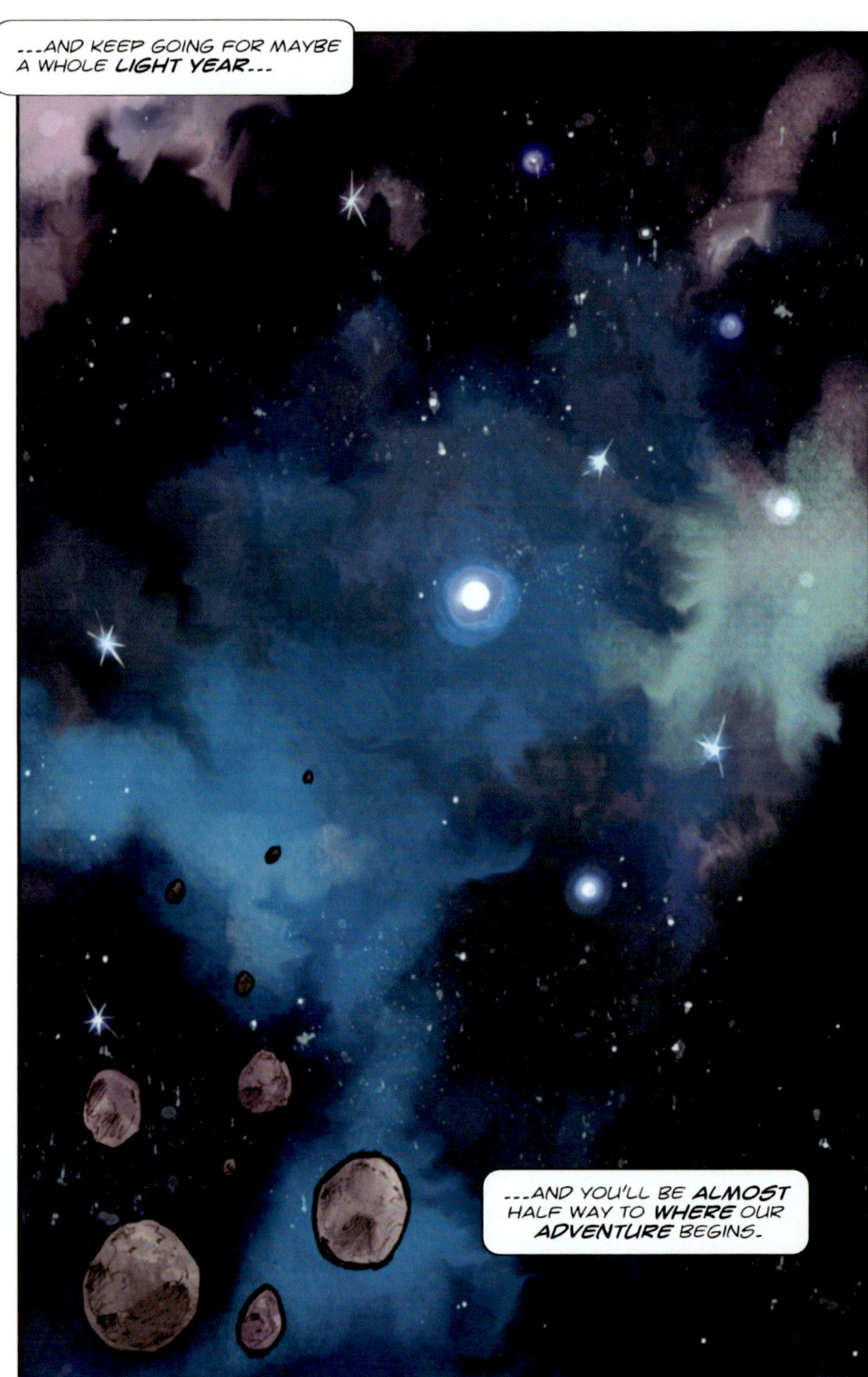

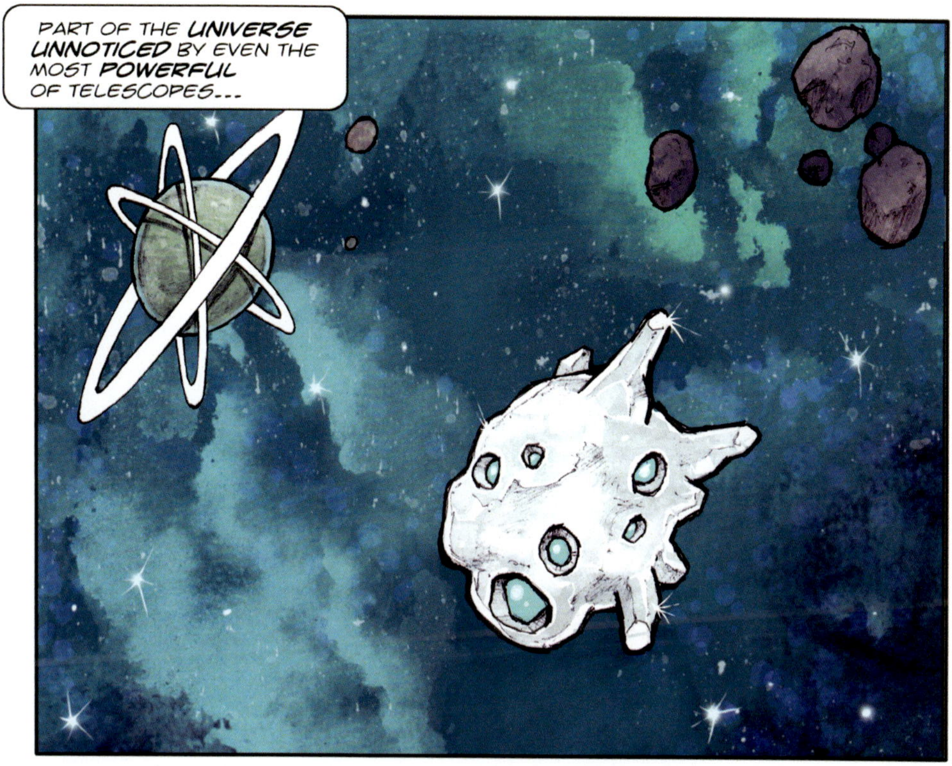

PART OF THE **UNIVERSE UNNOTICED** BY EVEN THE MOST **POWERFUL** OF TELESCOPES...

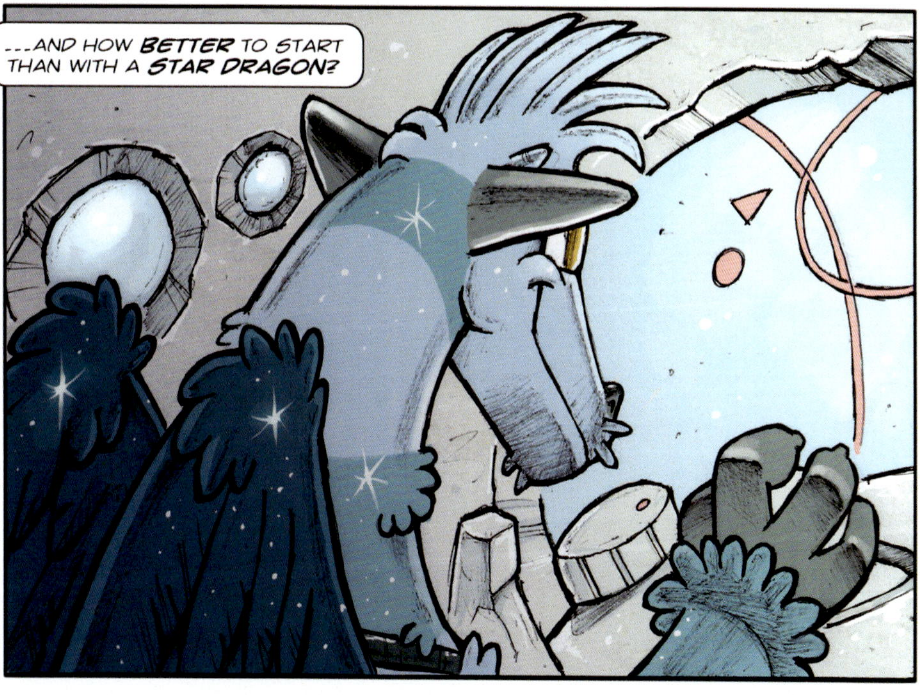

...AND HOW **BETTER** TO START THAN WITH A **STAR DRAGON?**

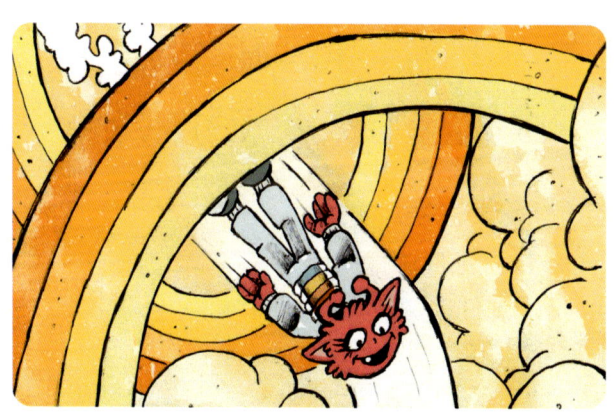

PART ONE

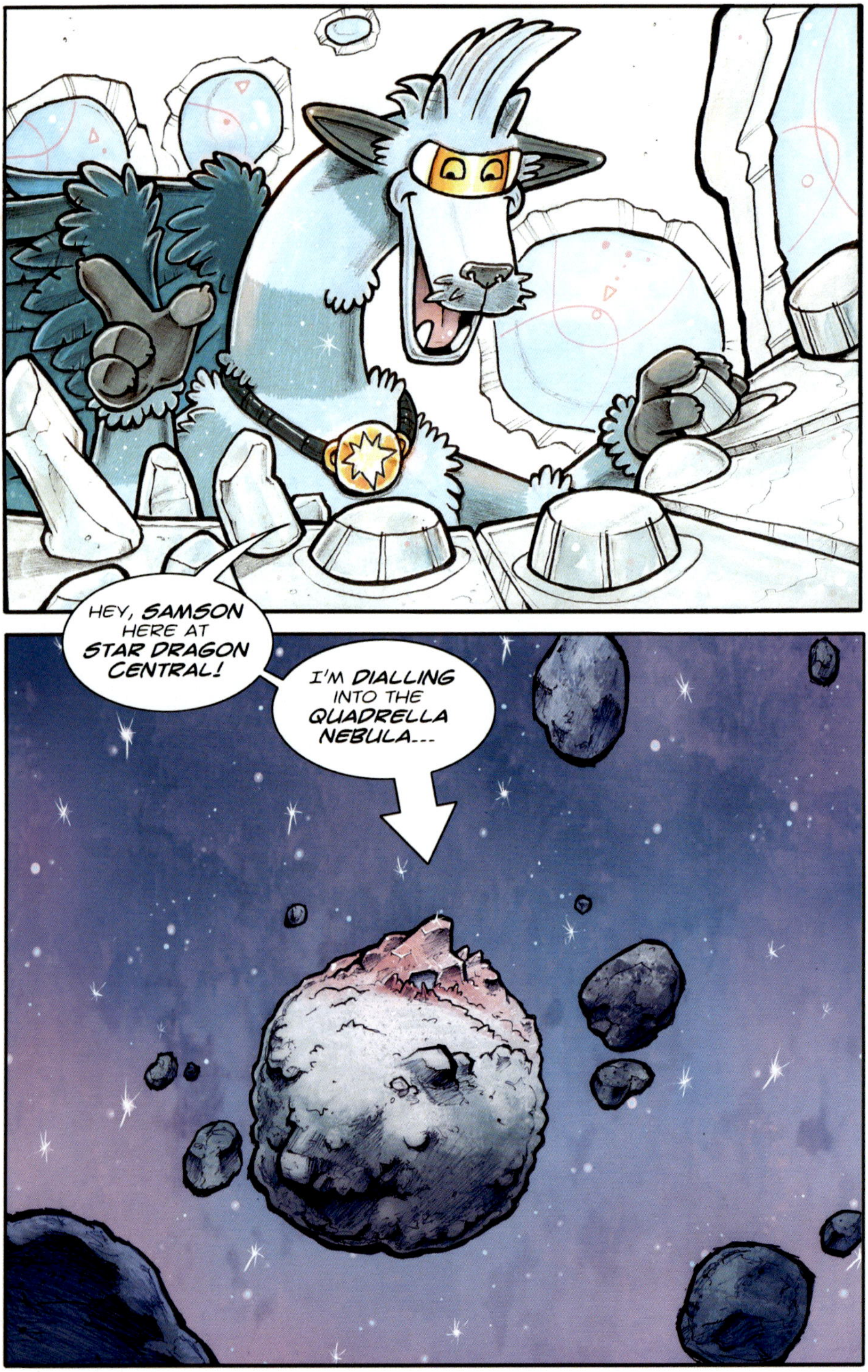

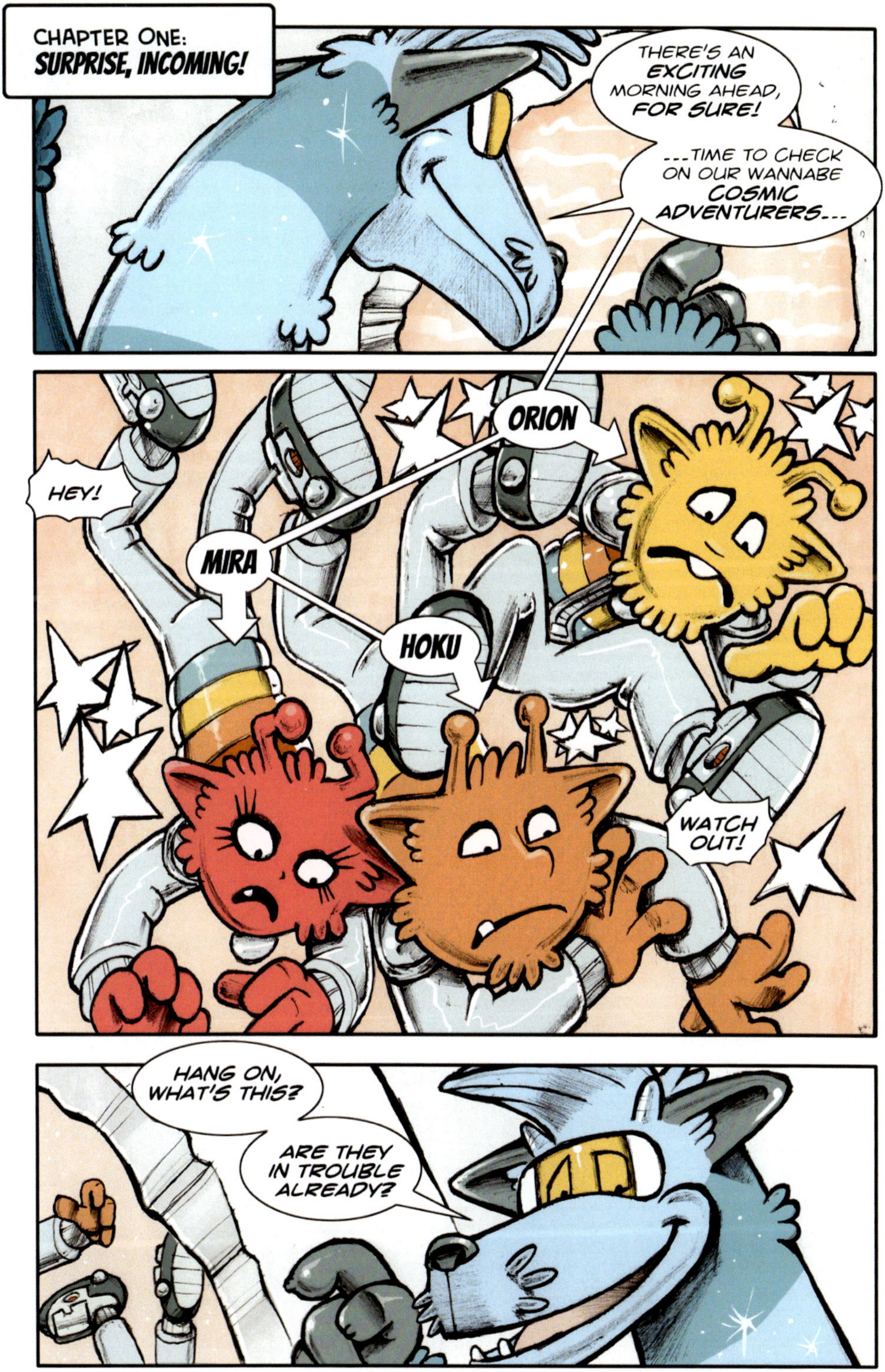

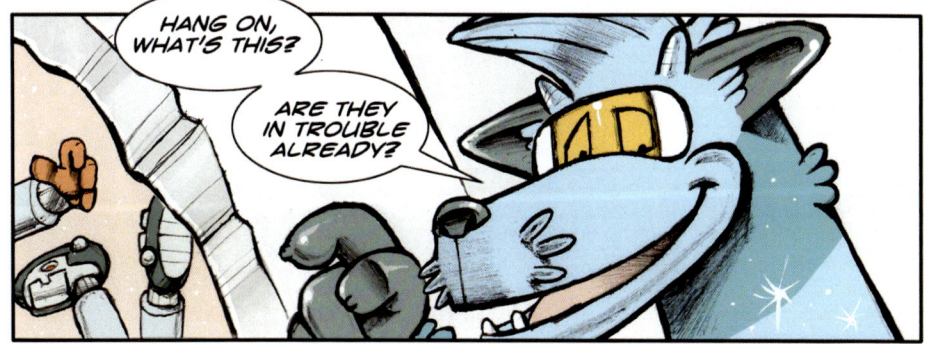

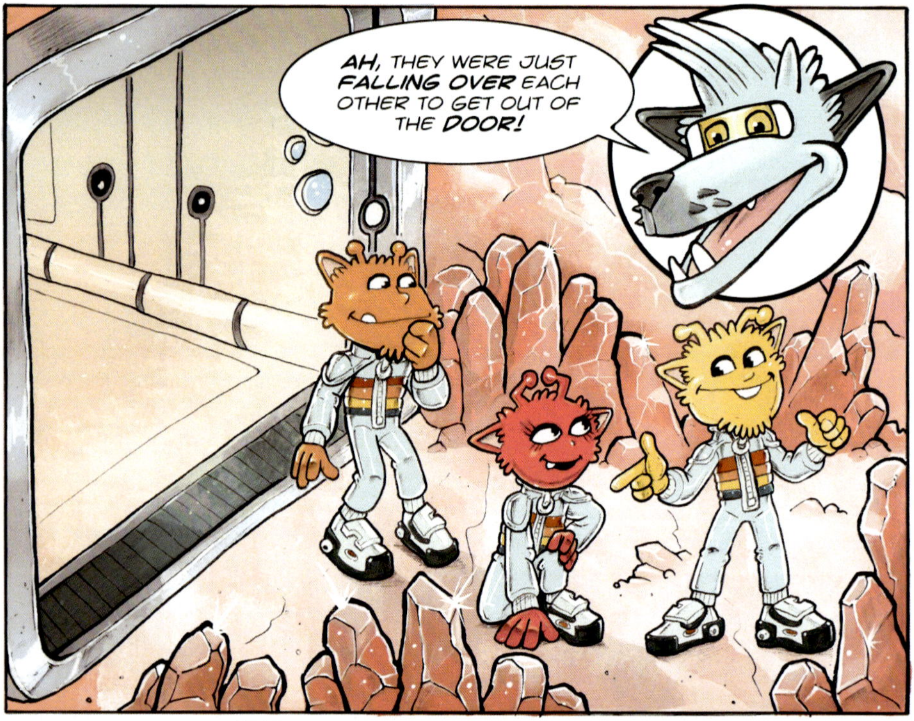

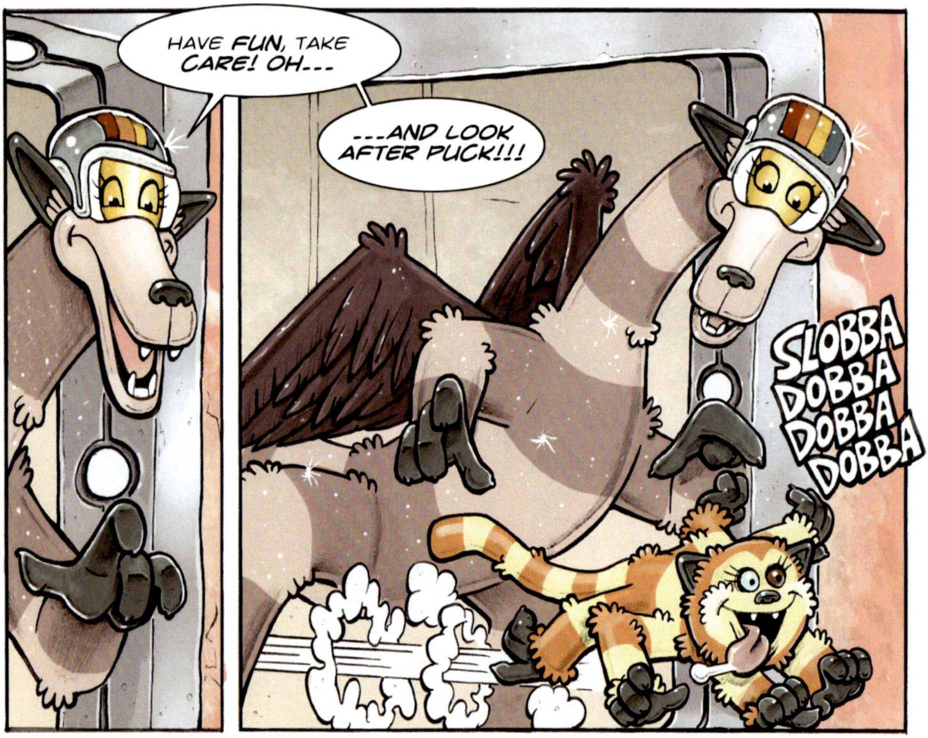

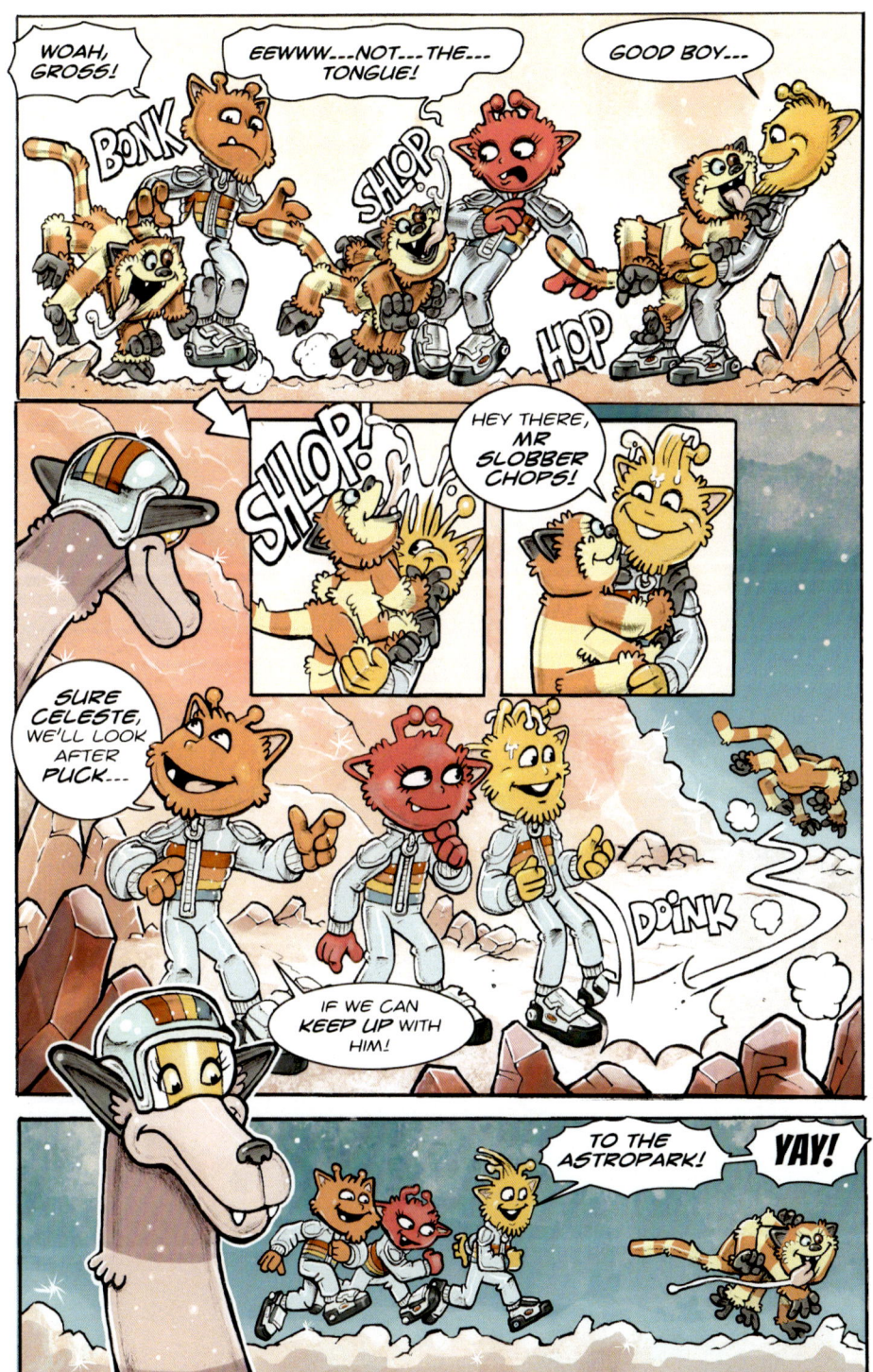

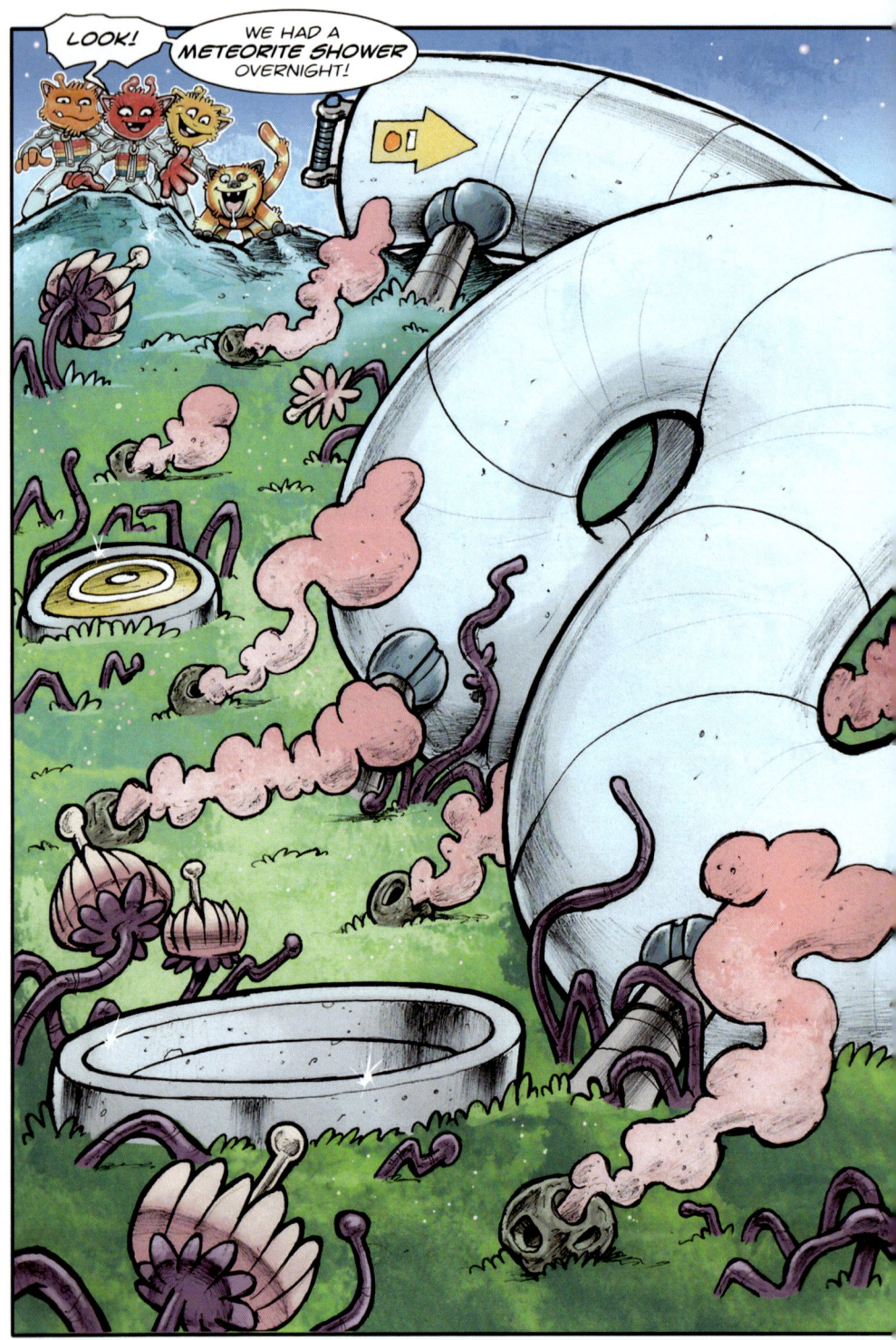

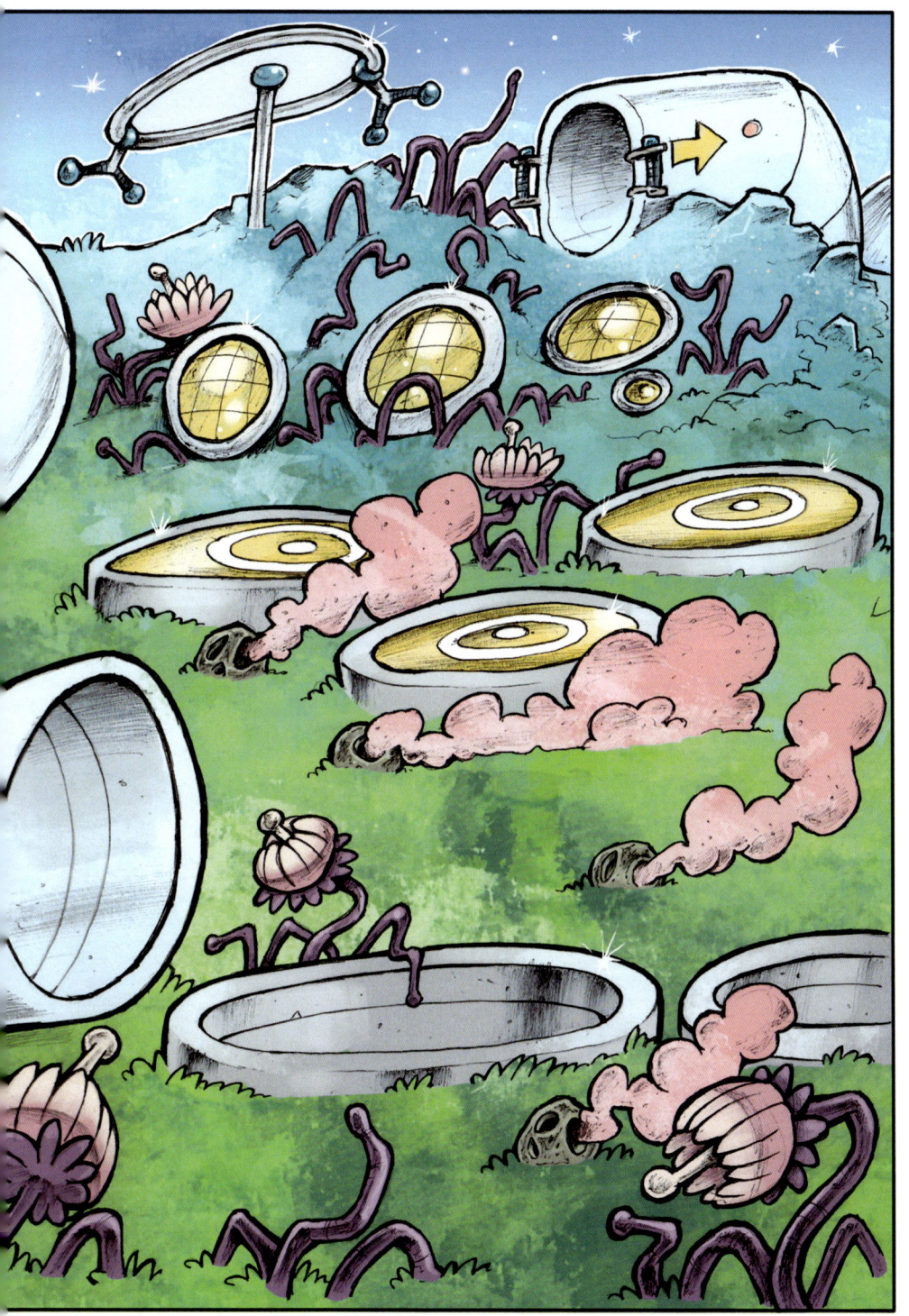

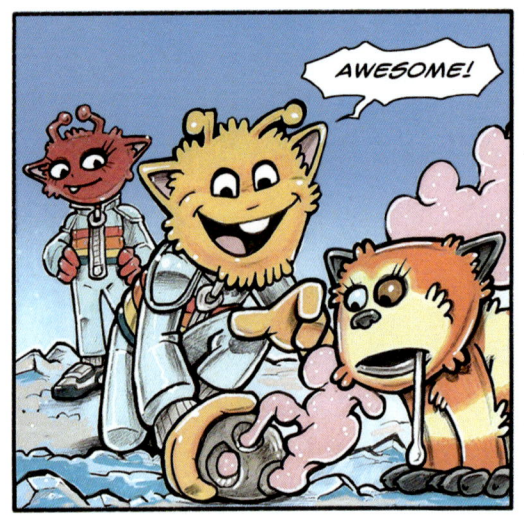
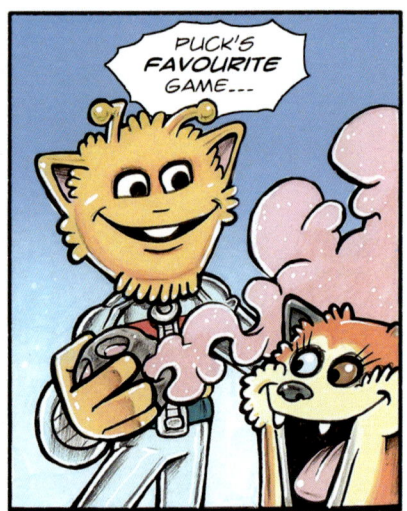
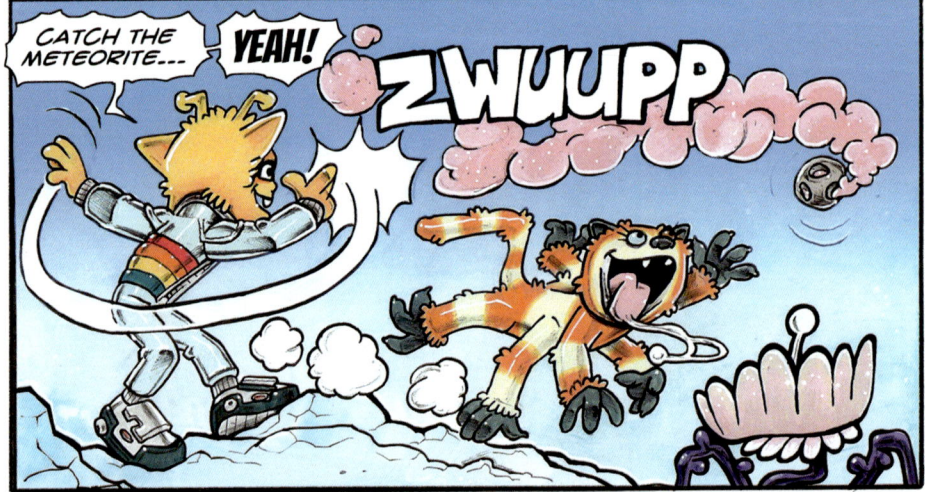
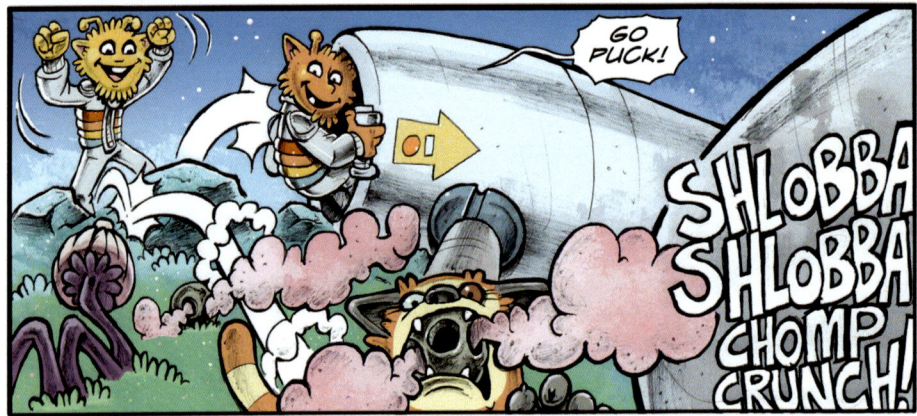

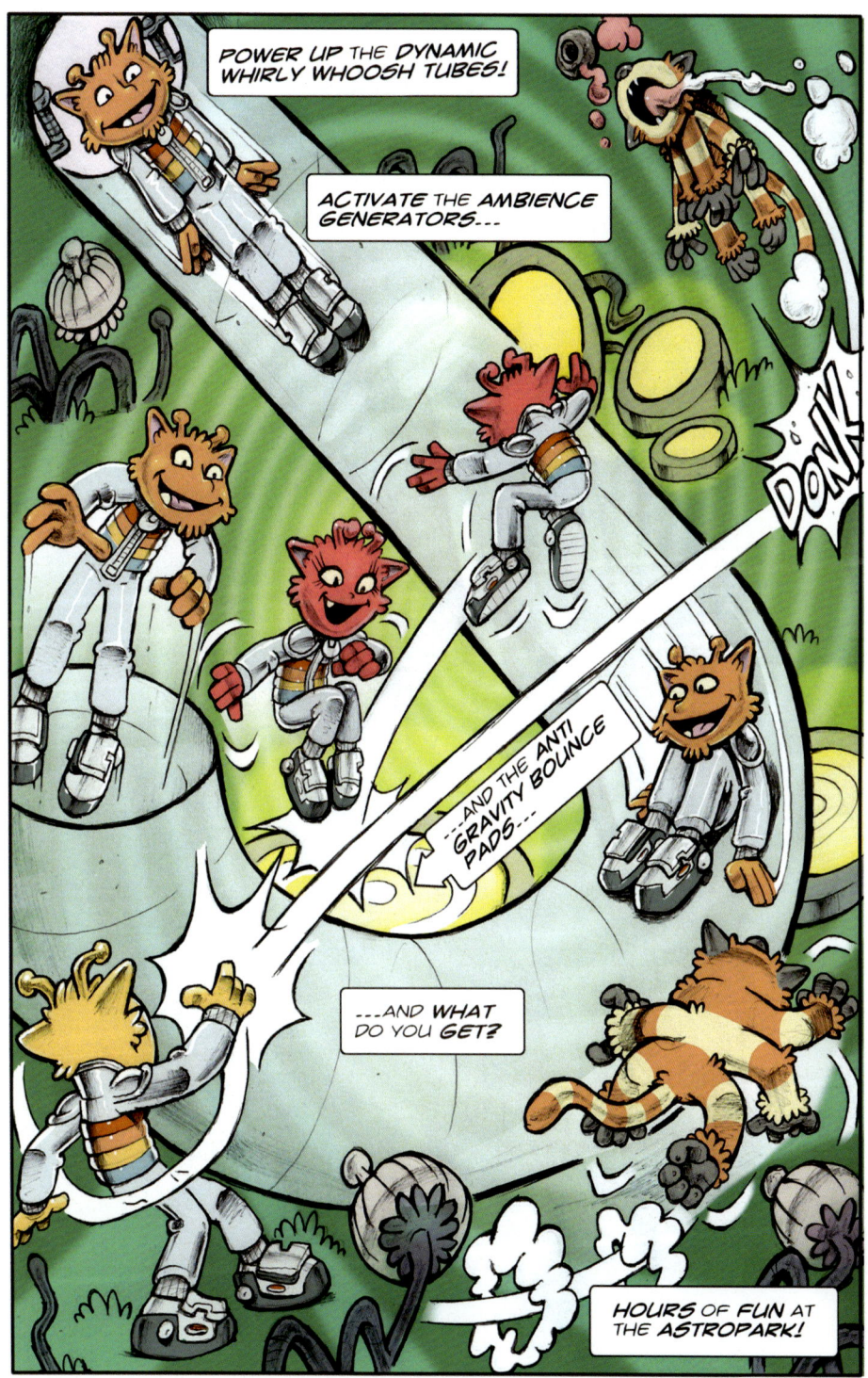

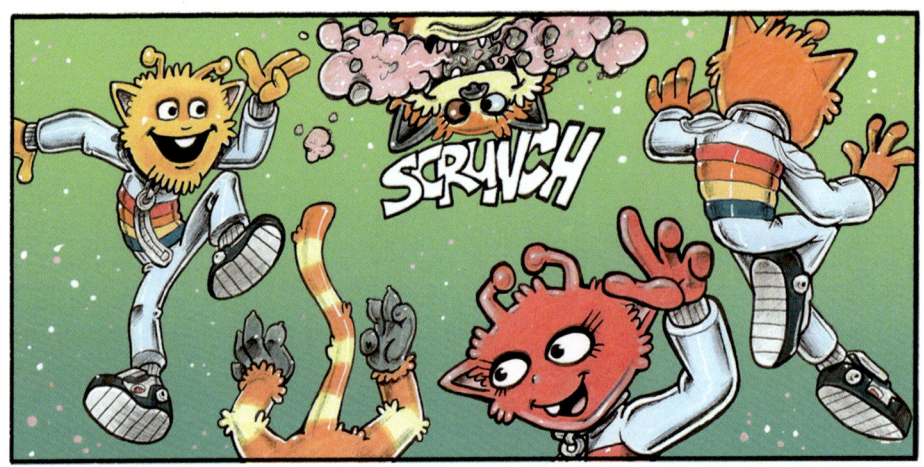
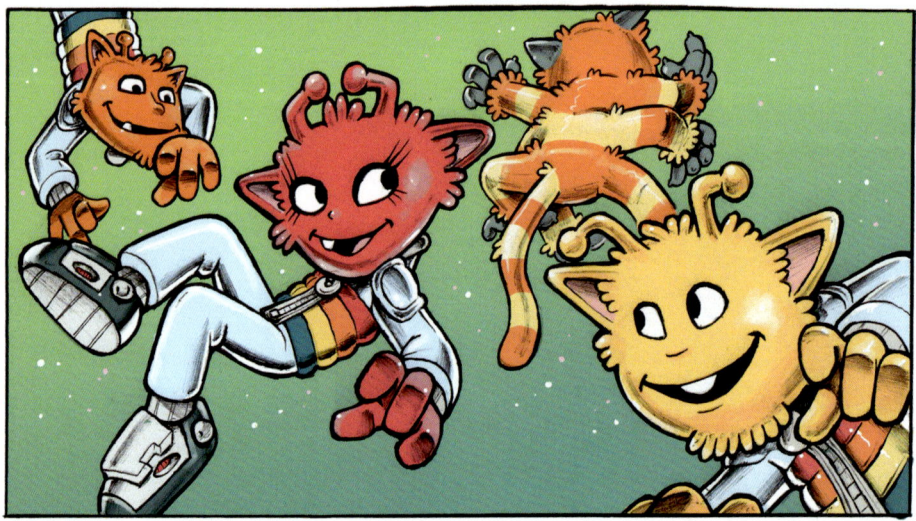
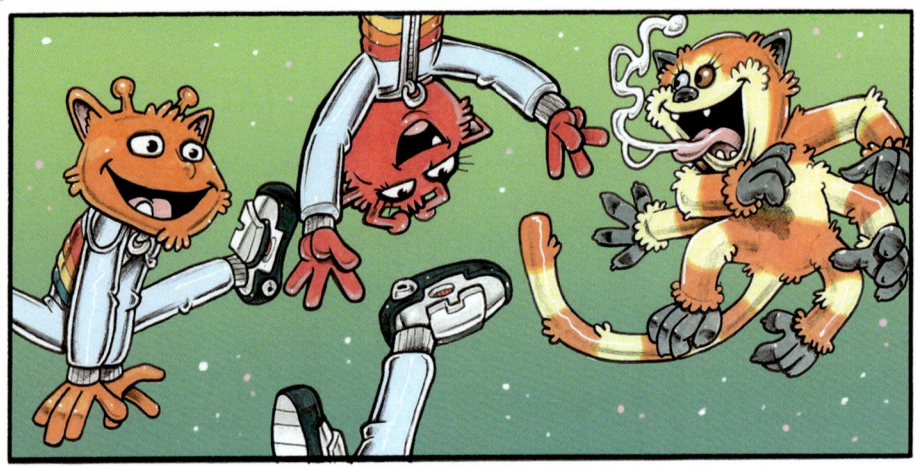

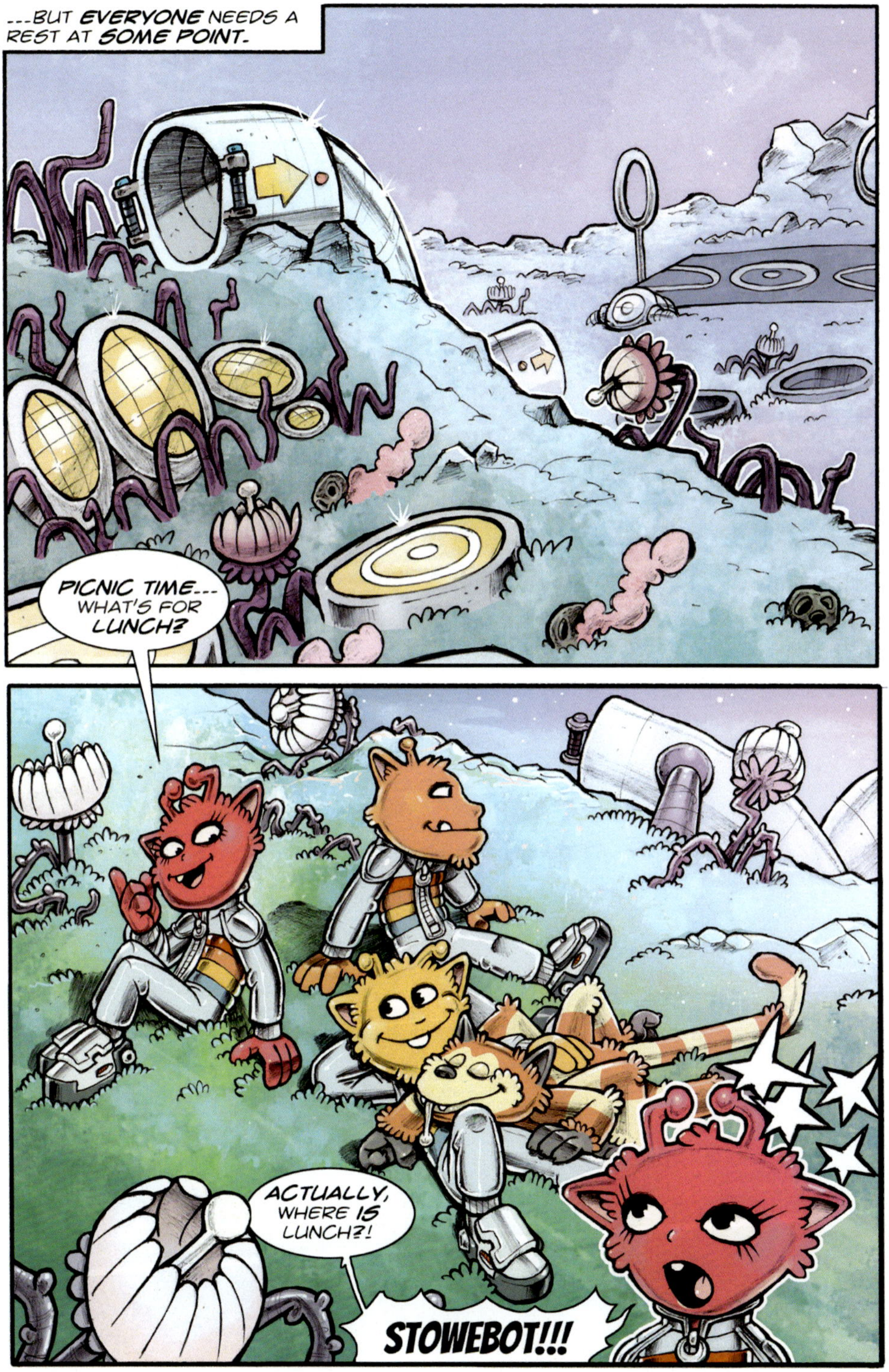

...BUT *EVERYONE* NEEDS A REST AT *SOME POINT*.

PICNIC TIME... WHAT'S FOR *LUNCH*?

ACTUALLY, WHERE *IS* LUNCH?!

STOWEBOT!!!

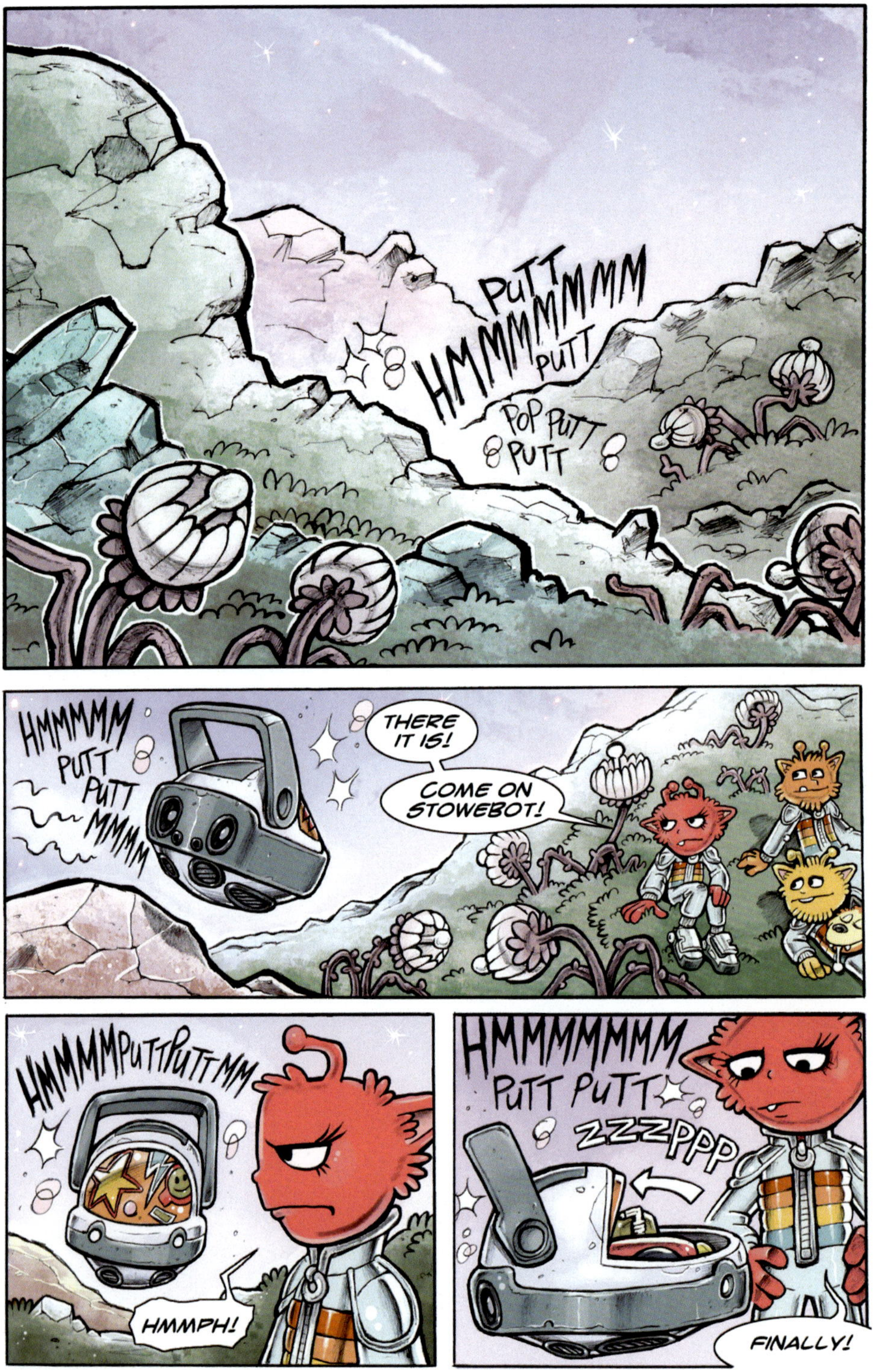

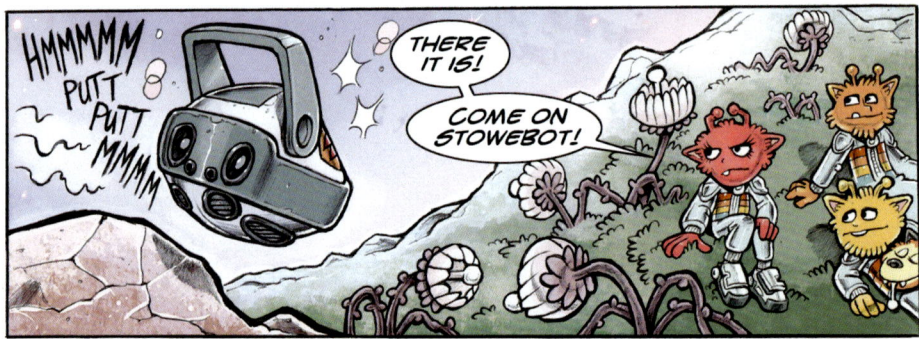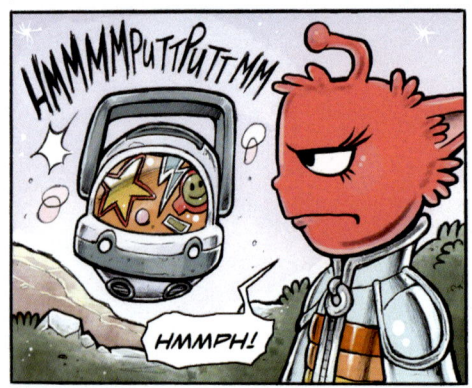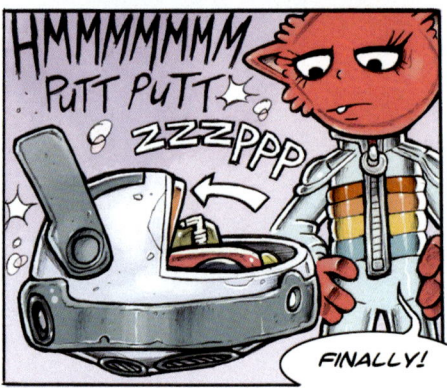

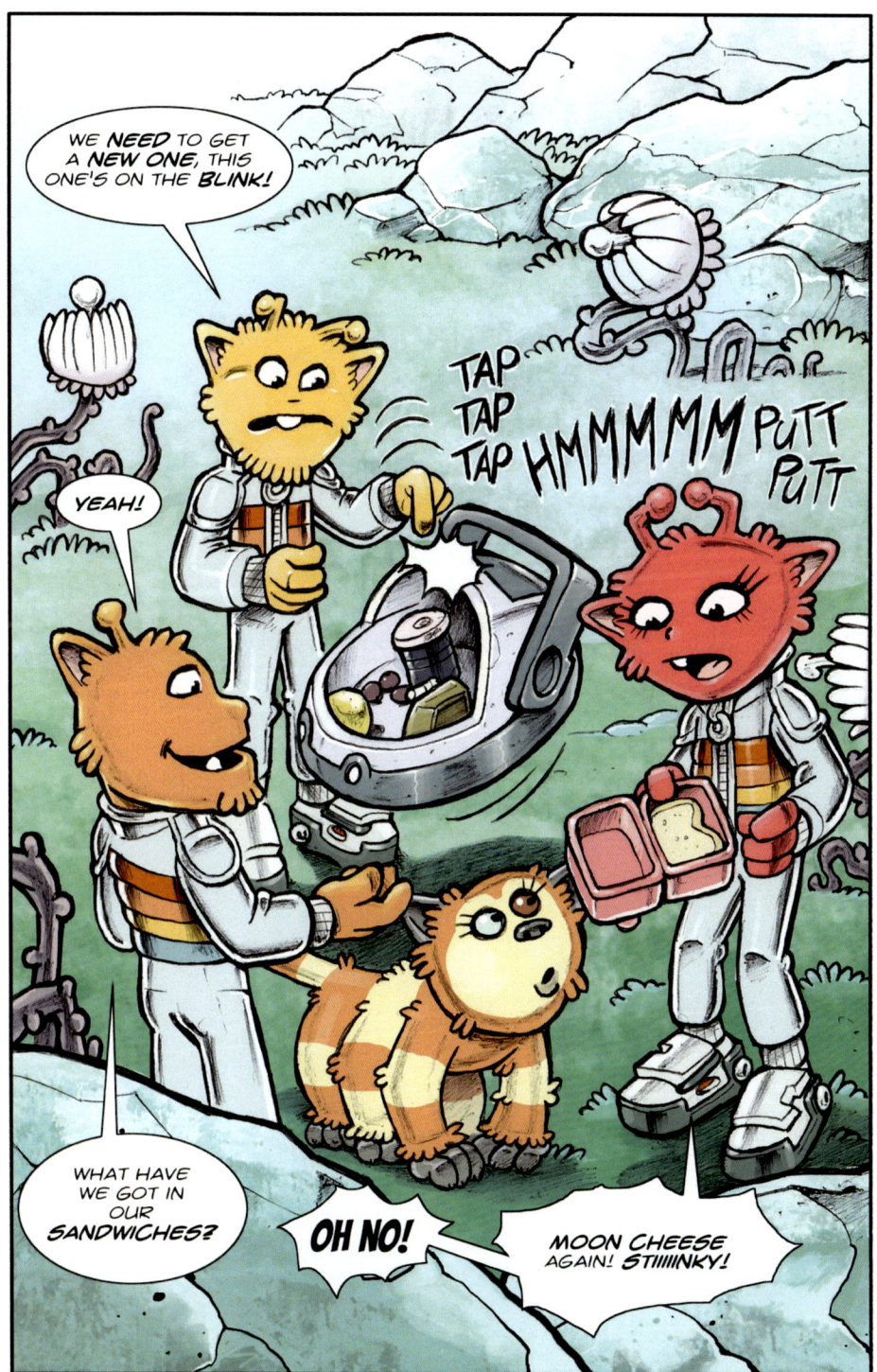

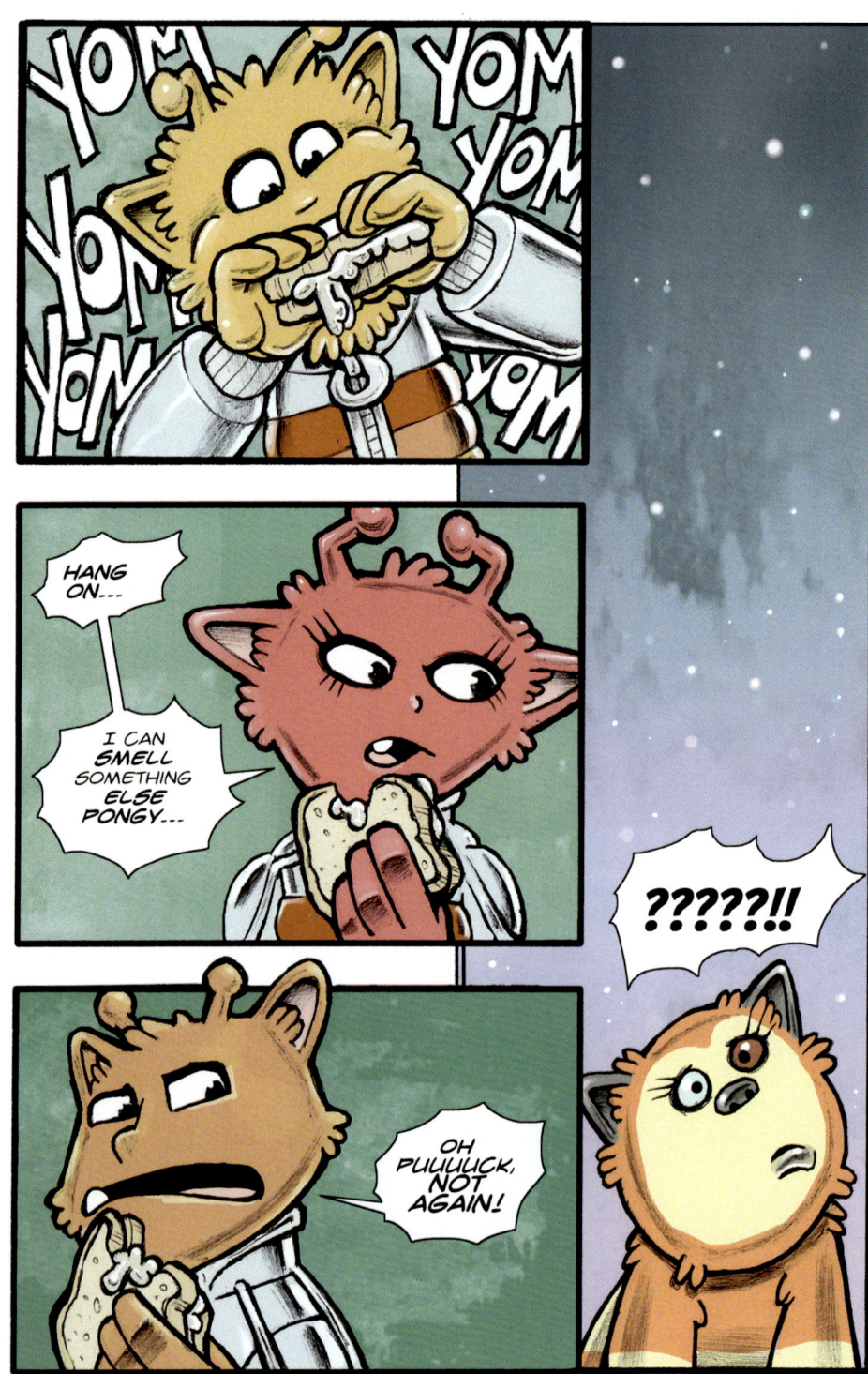

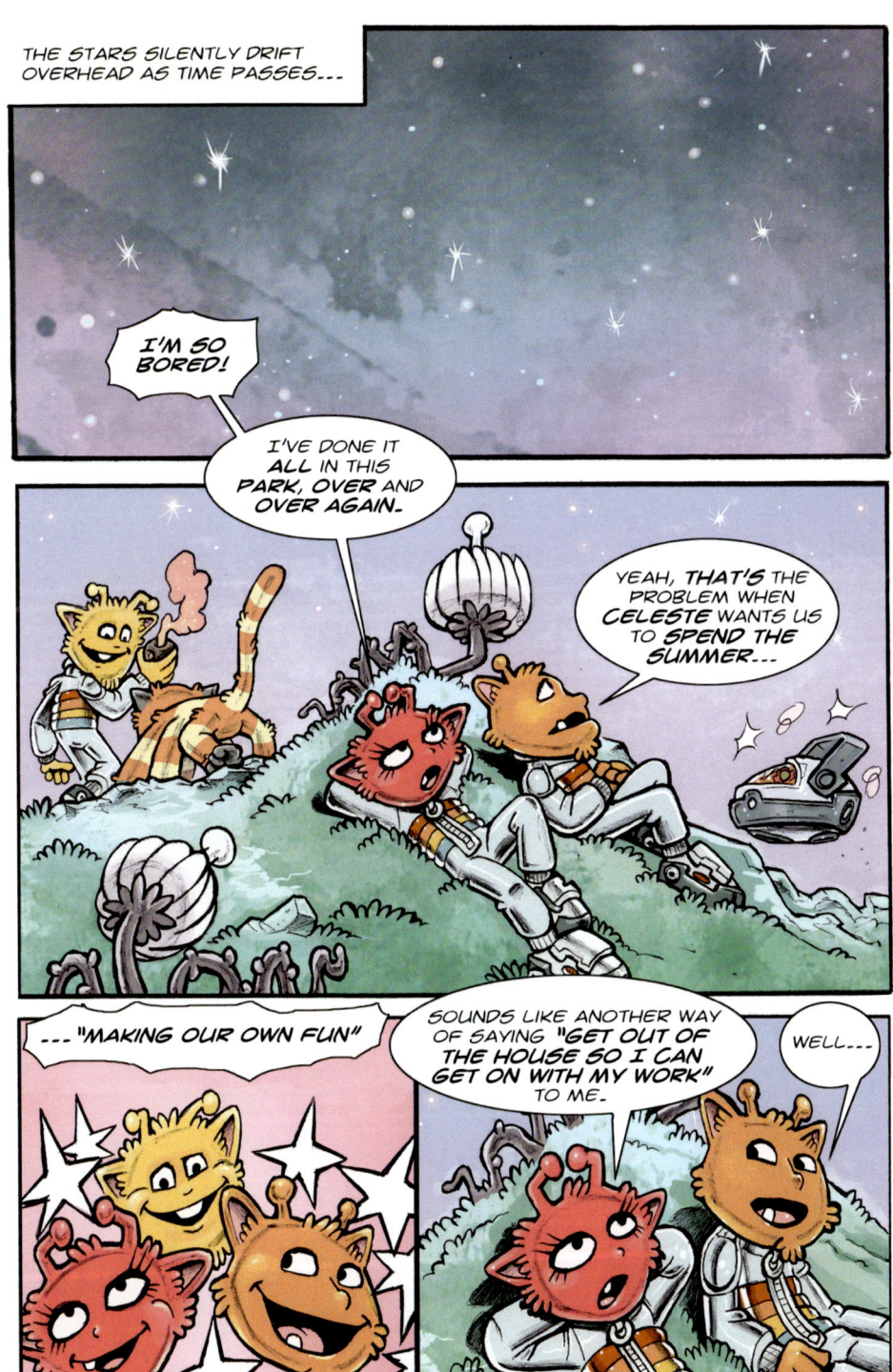

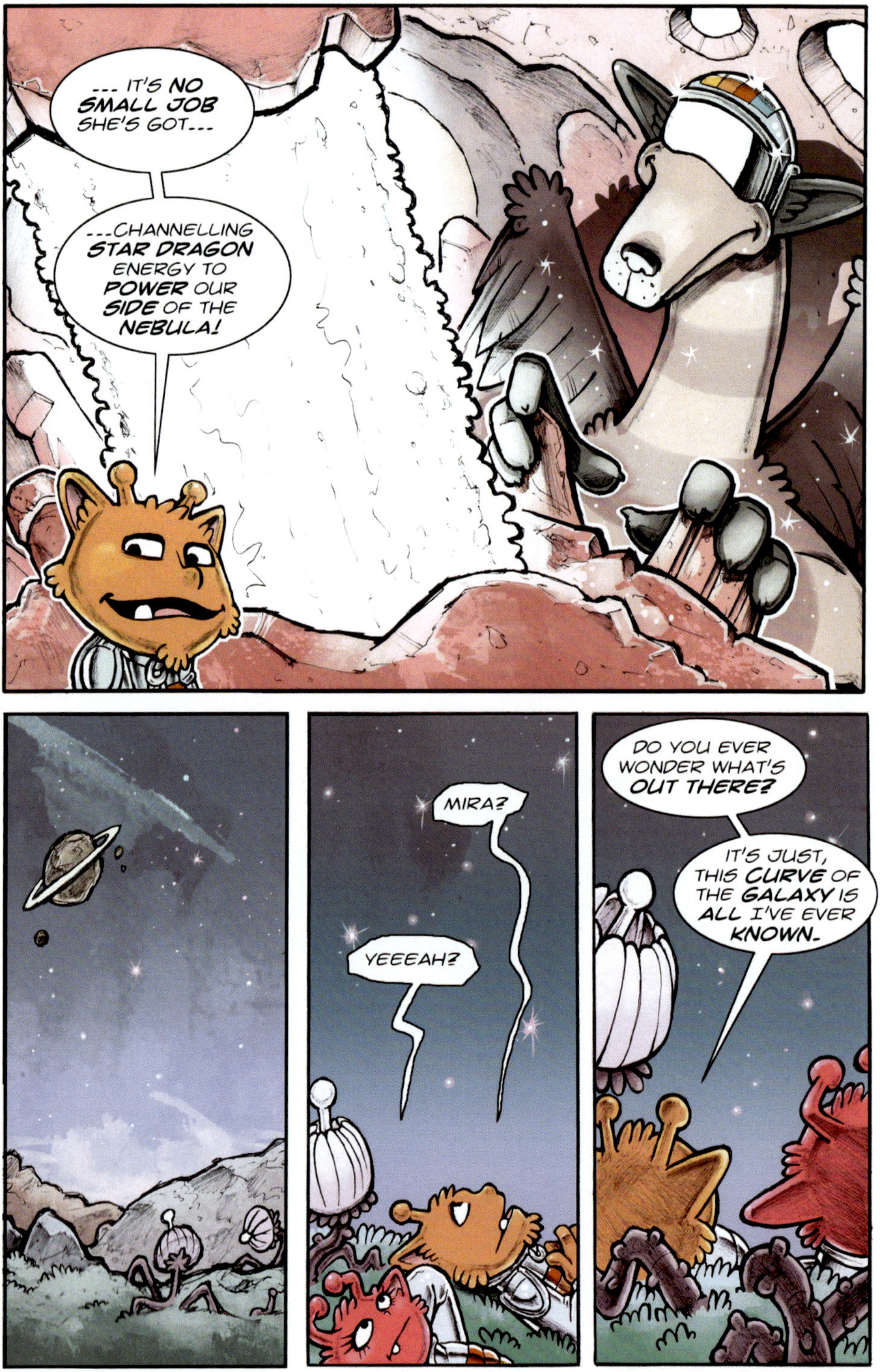

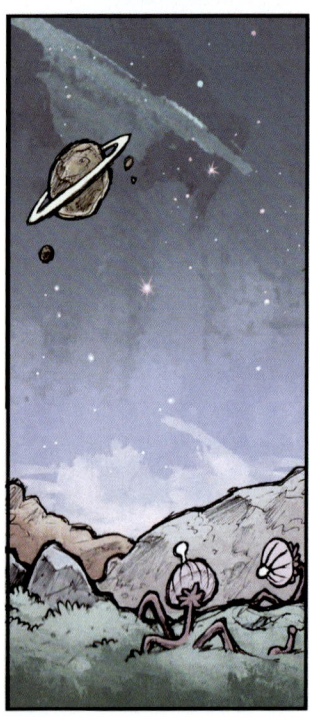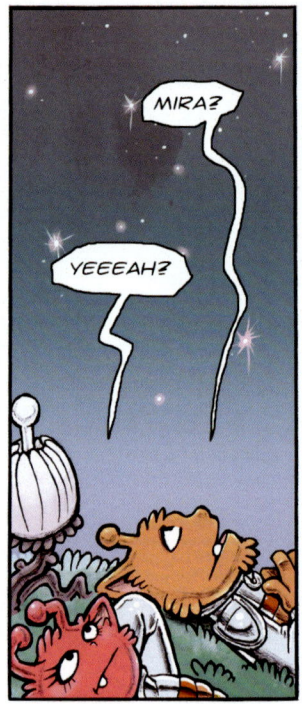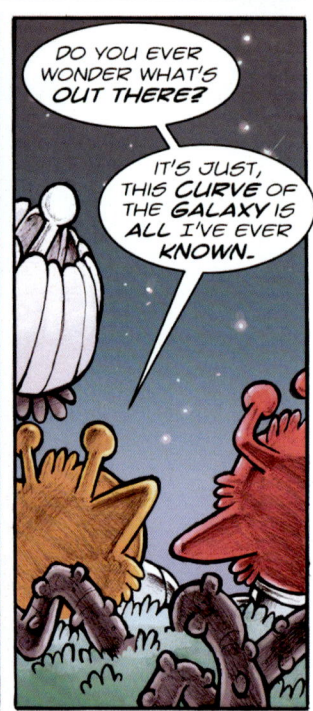

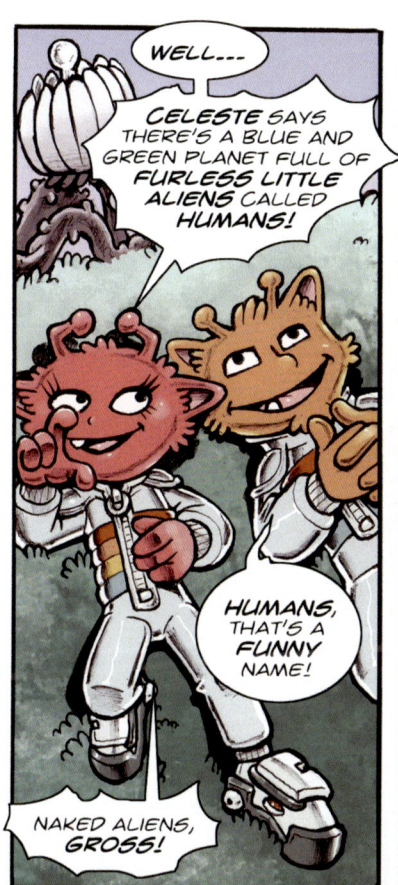
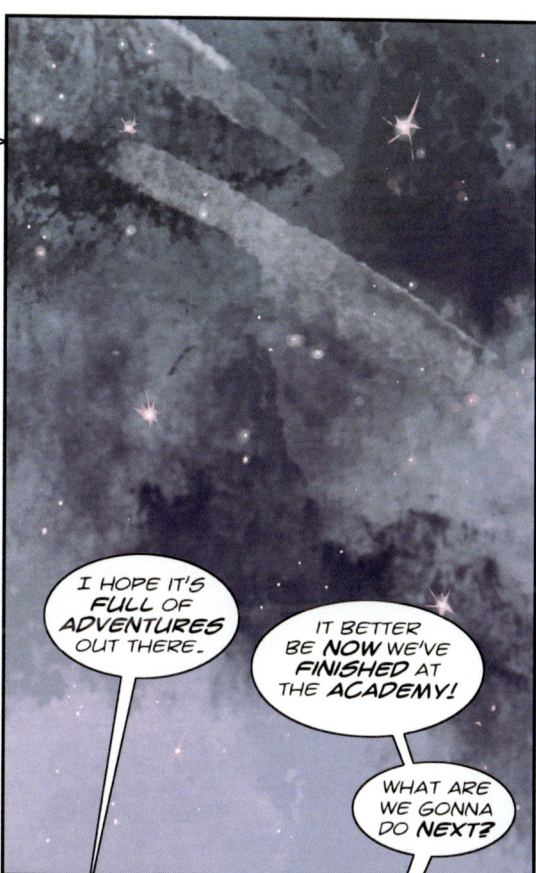
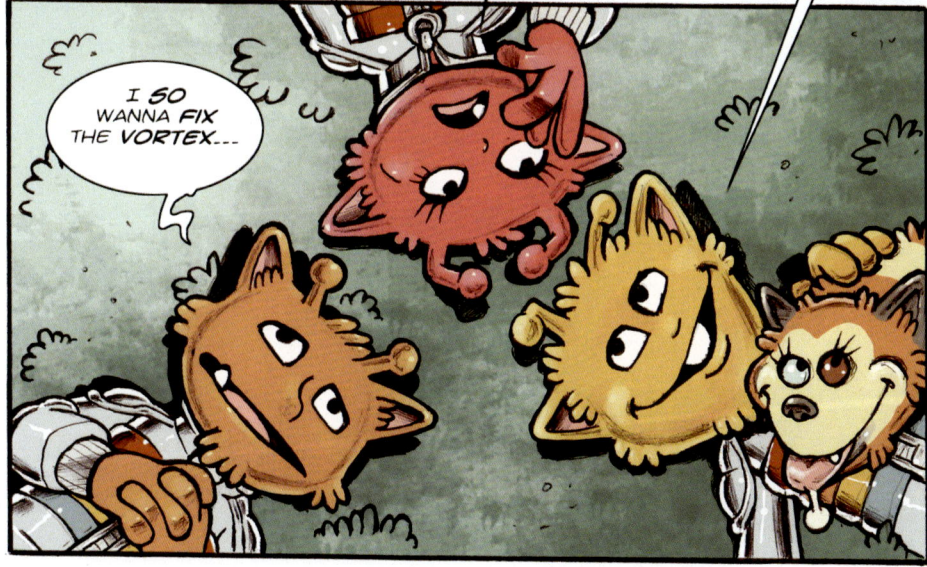

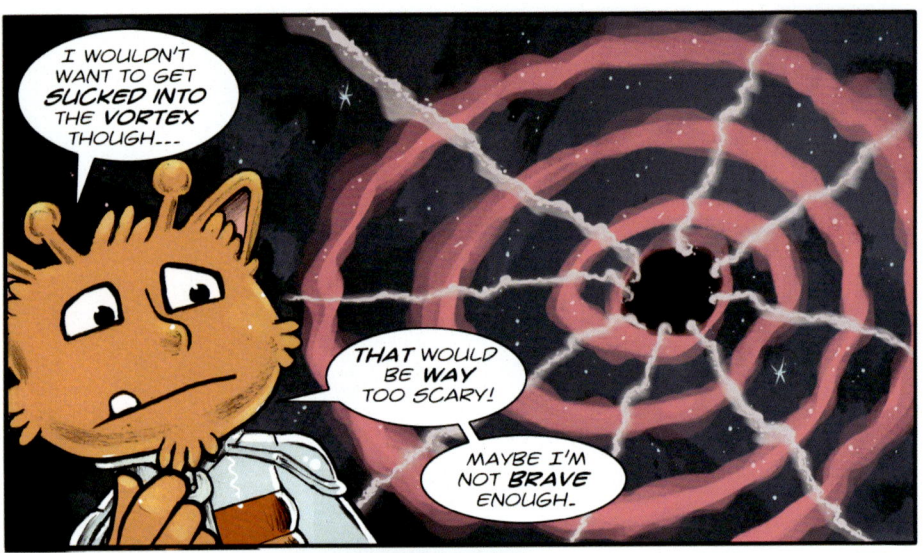
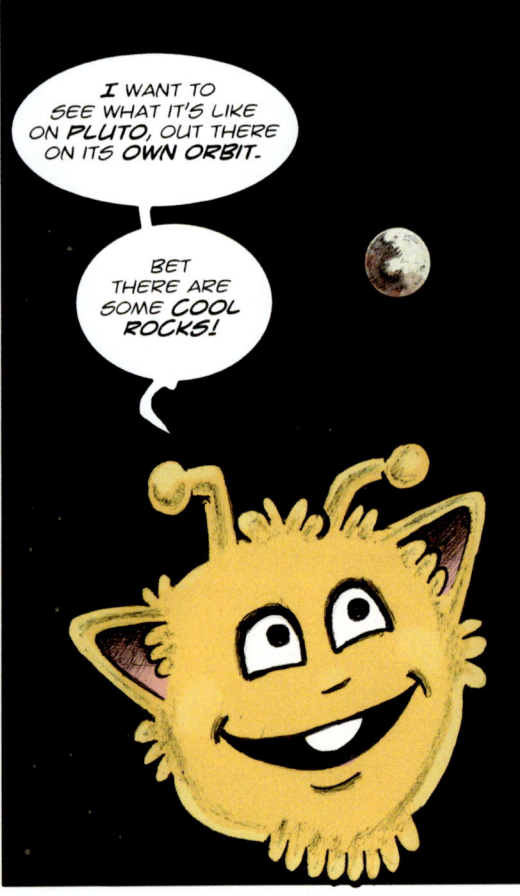
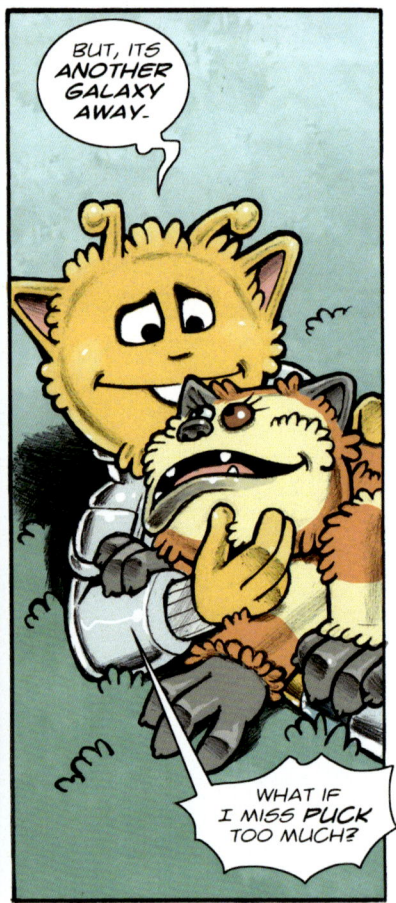

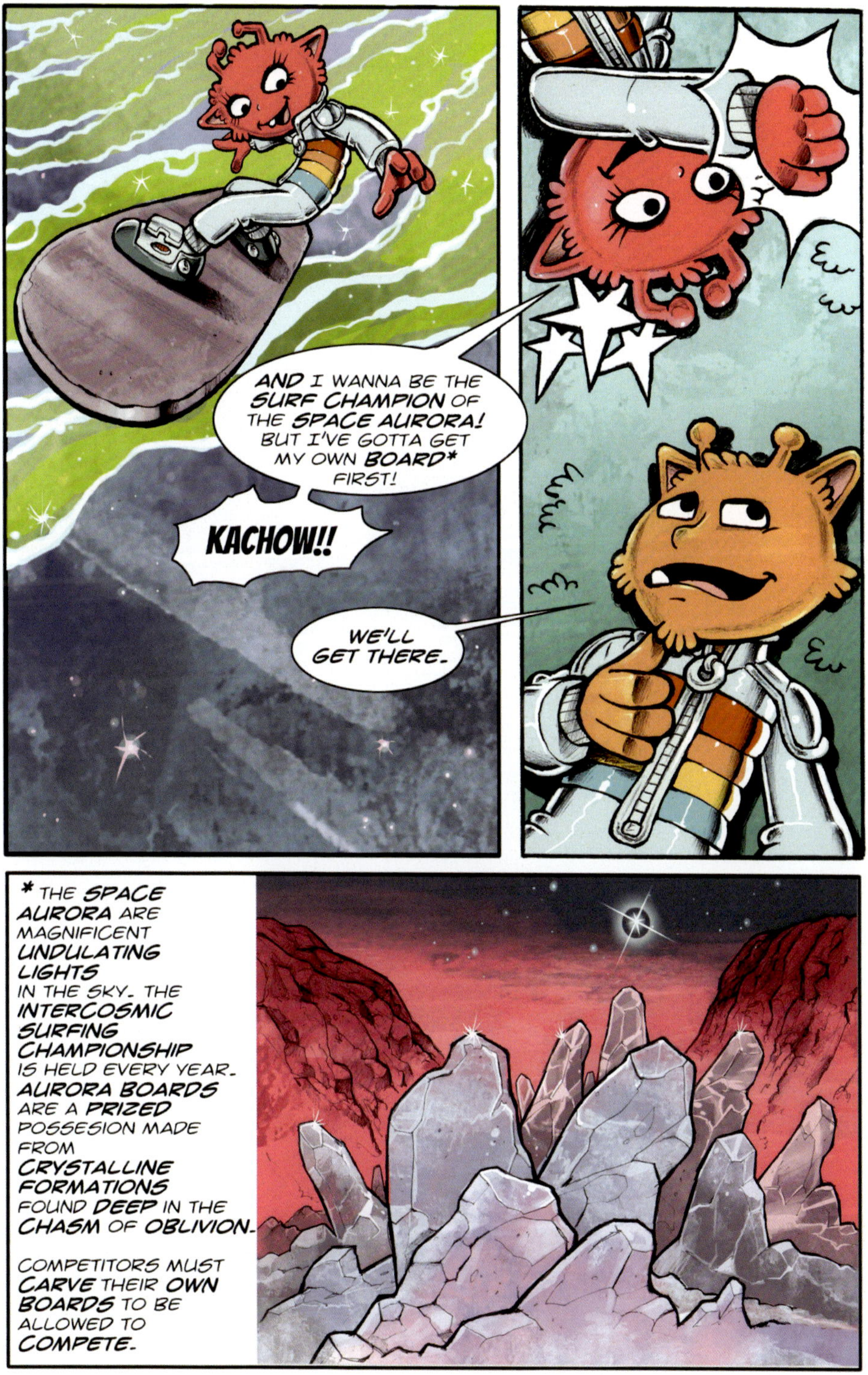

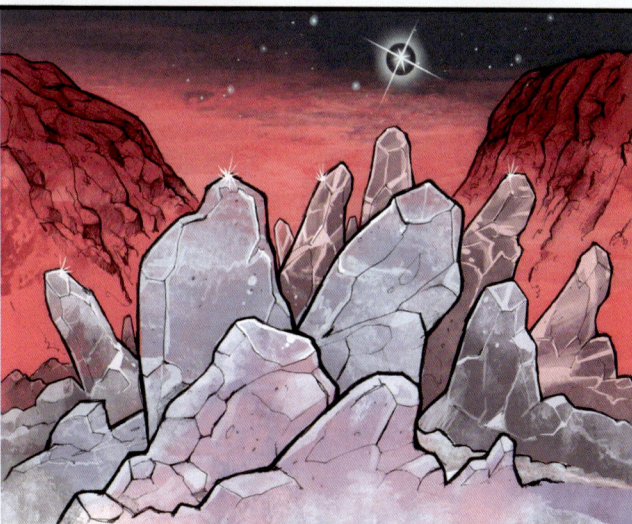

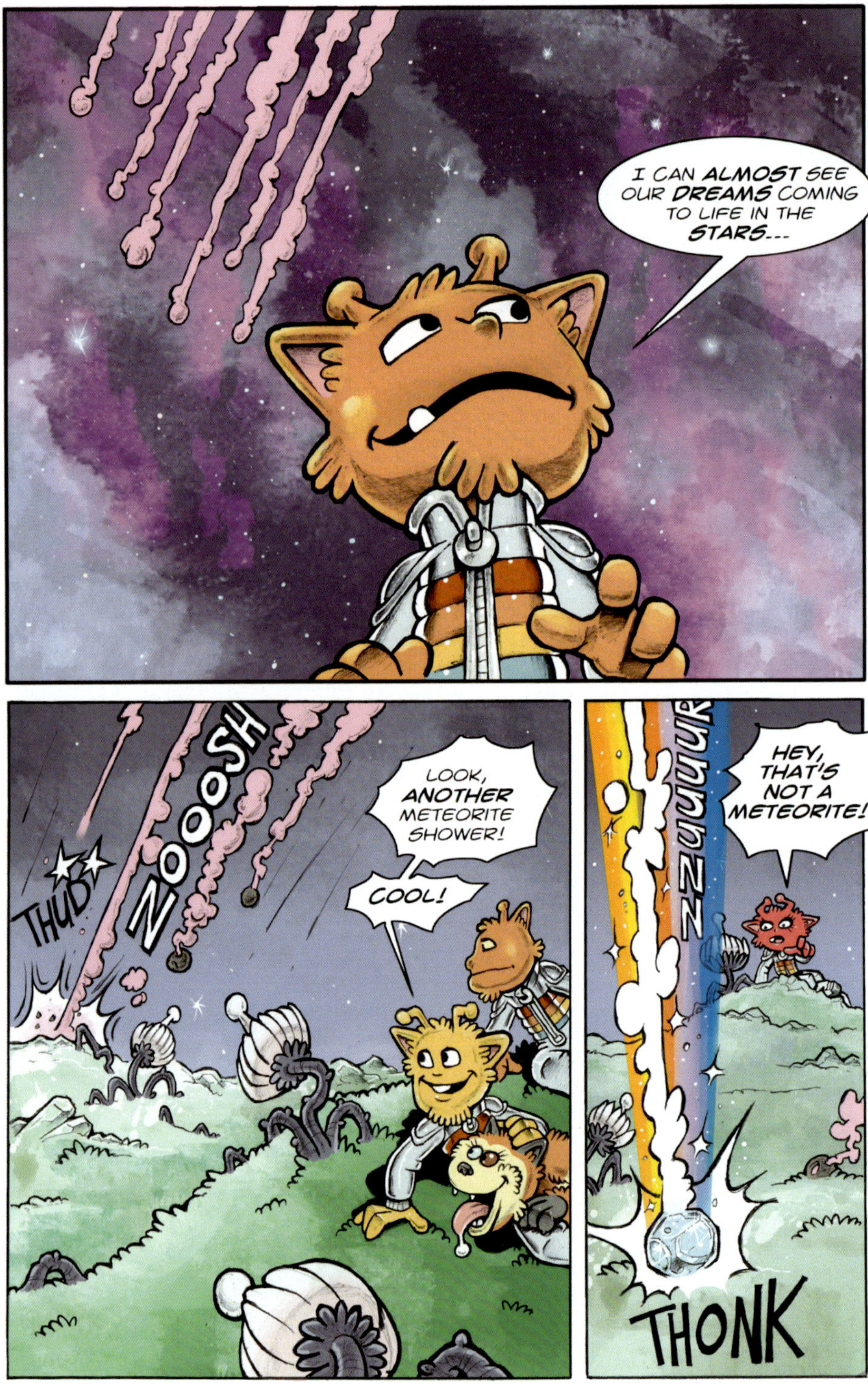

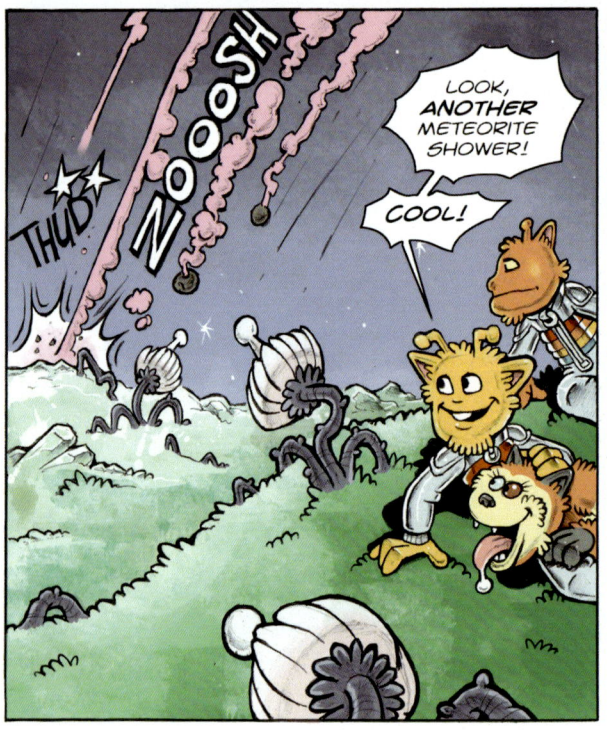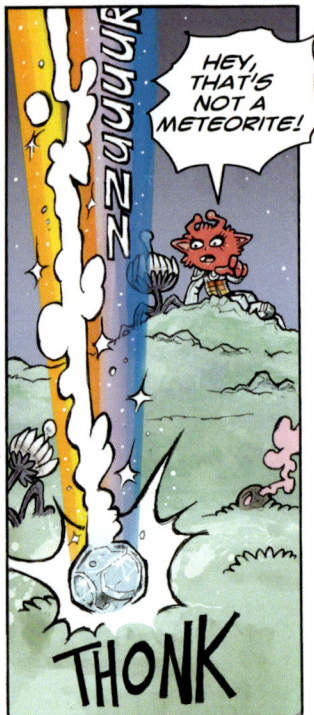

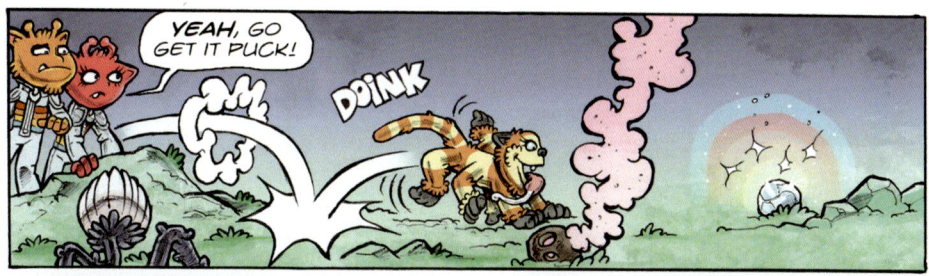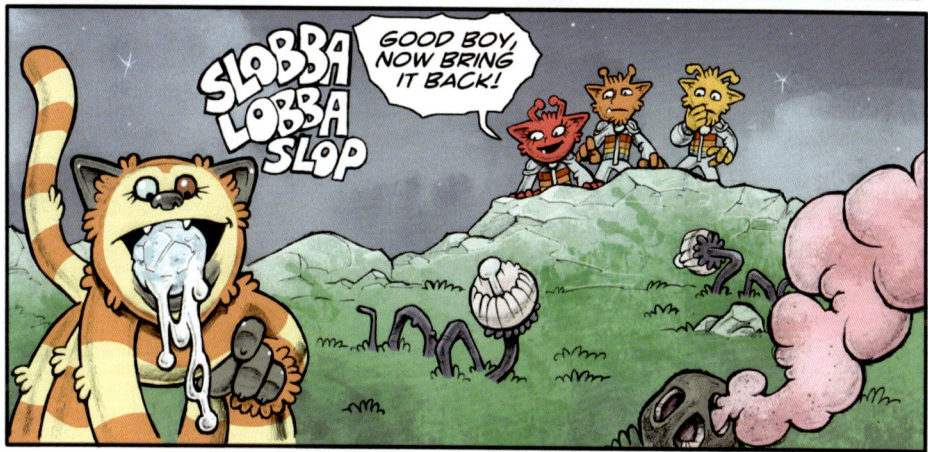

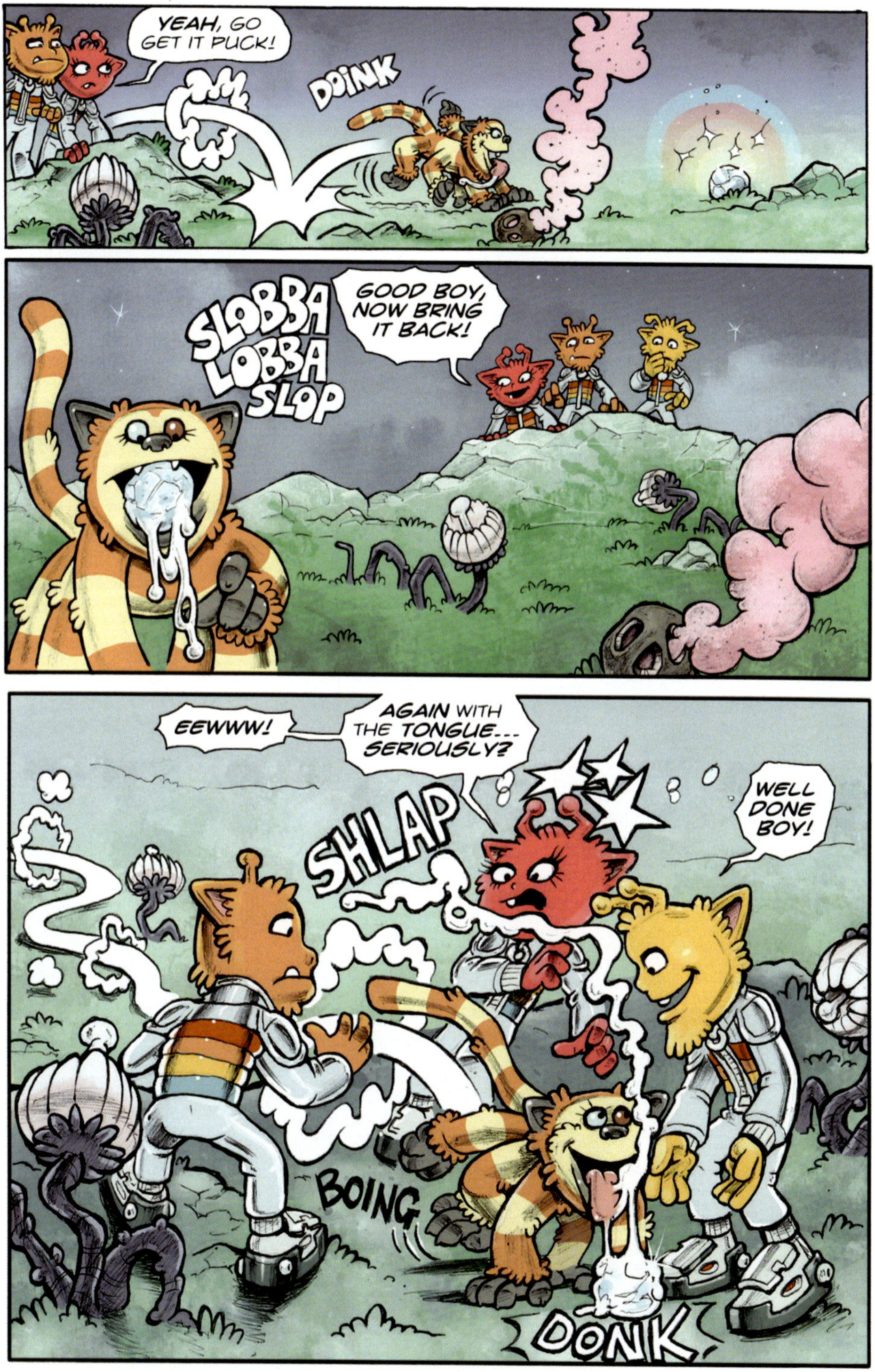

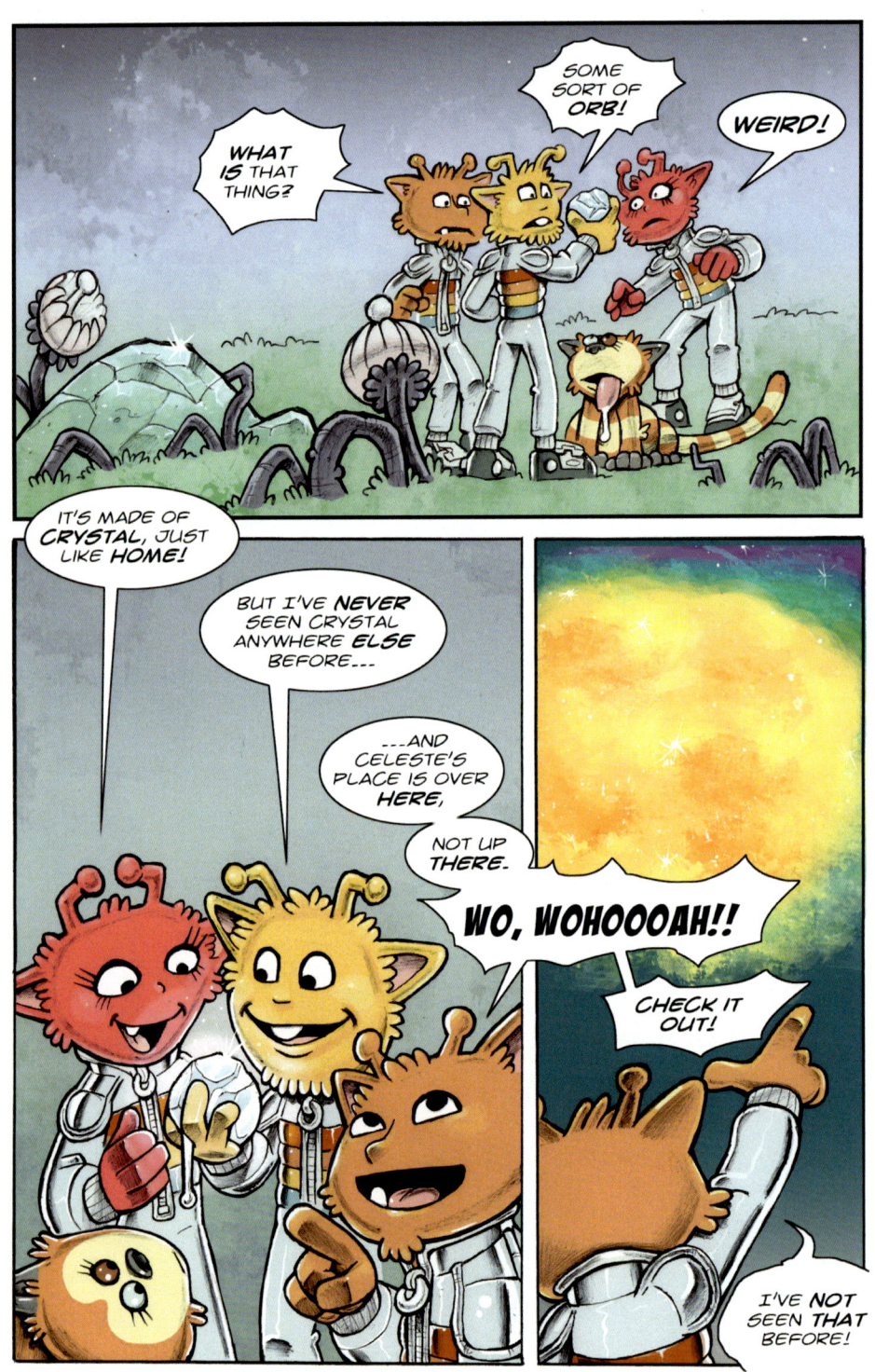

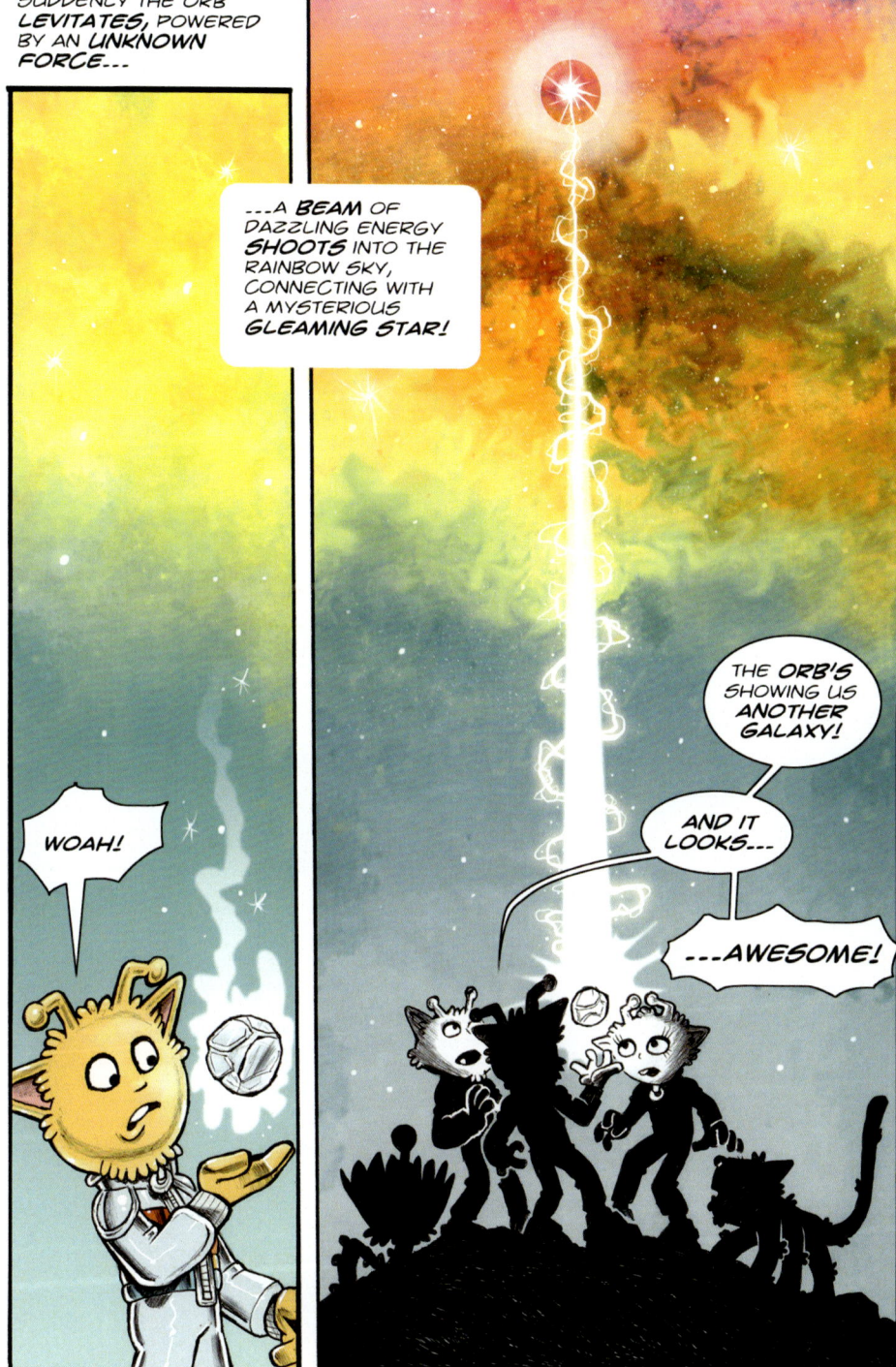

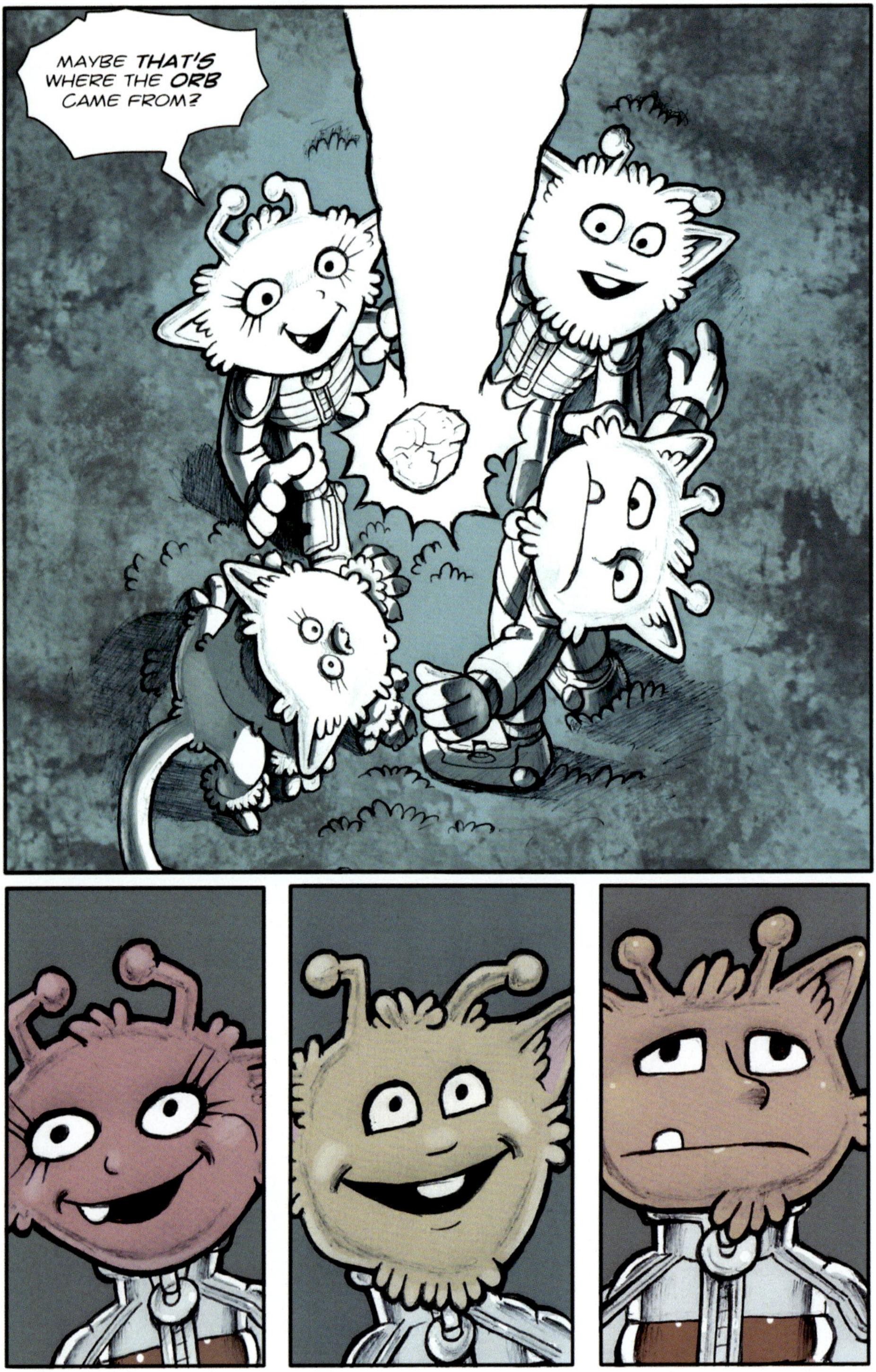

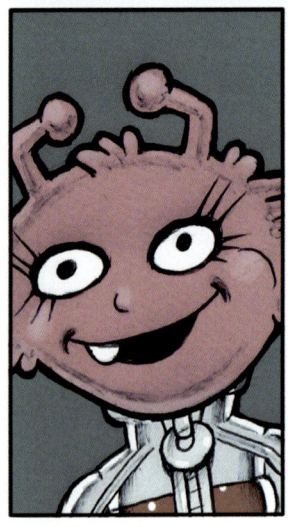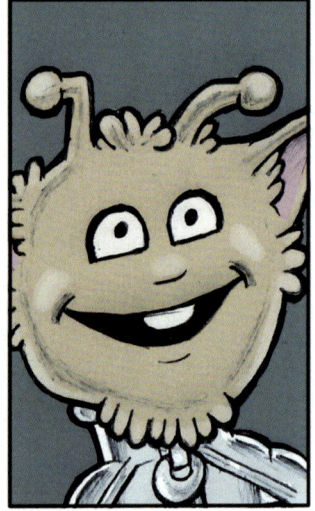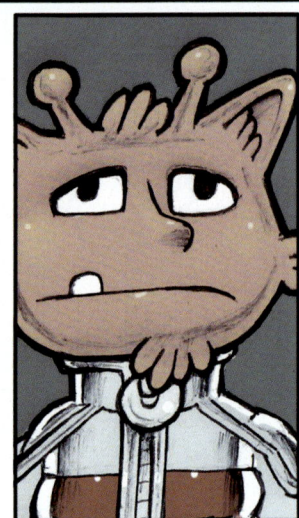

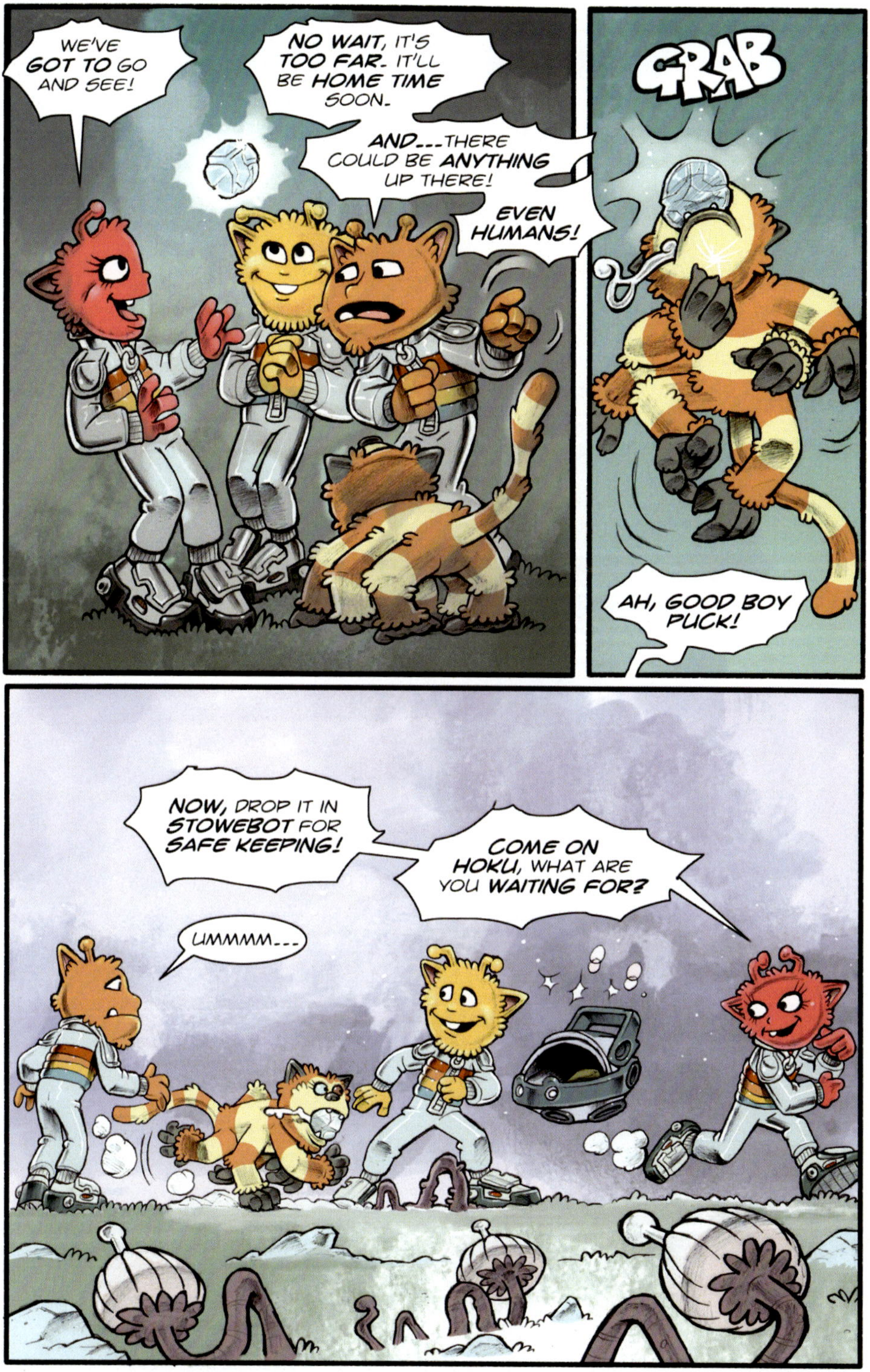

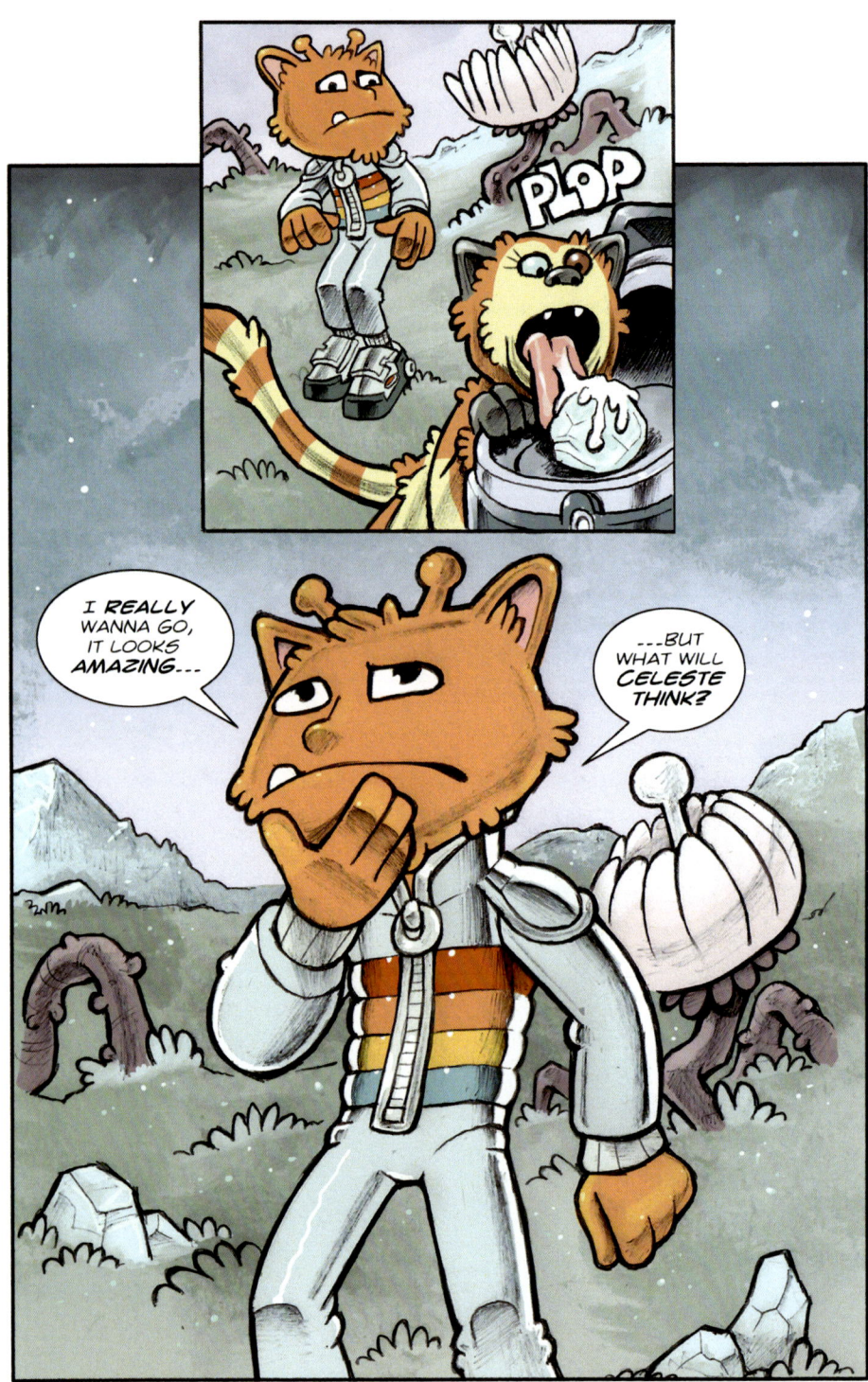

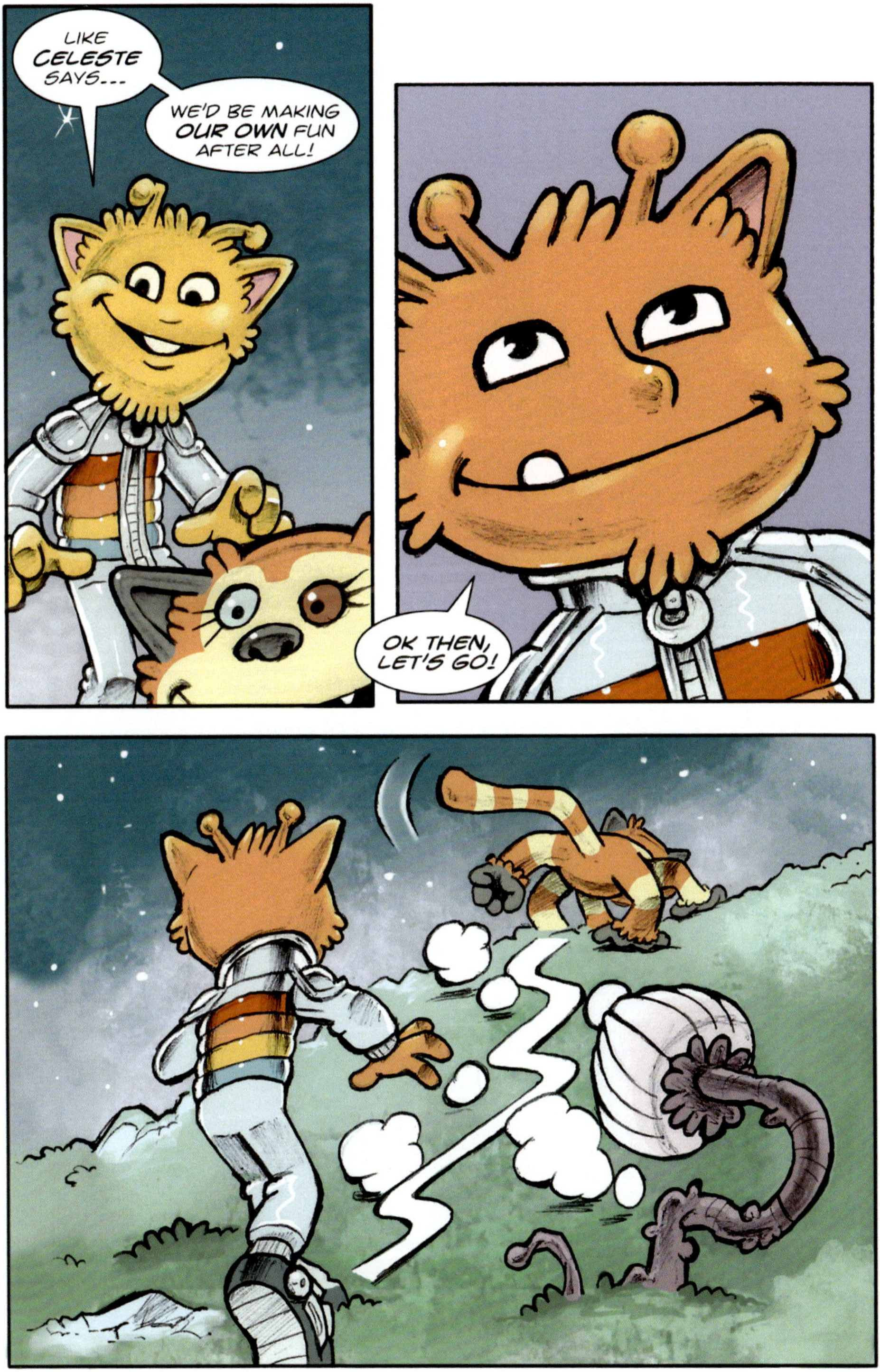

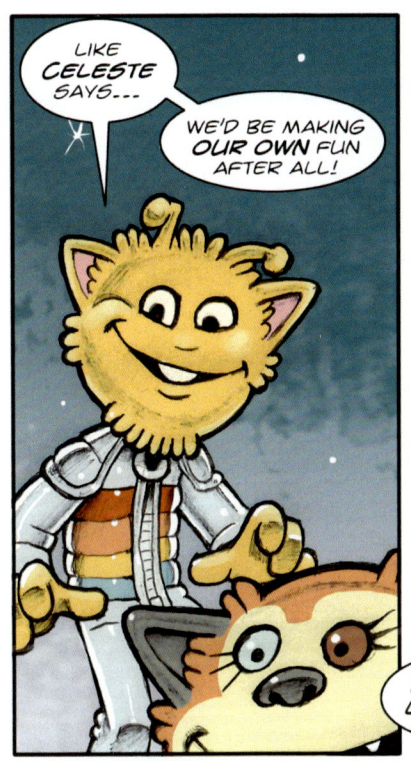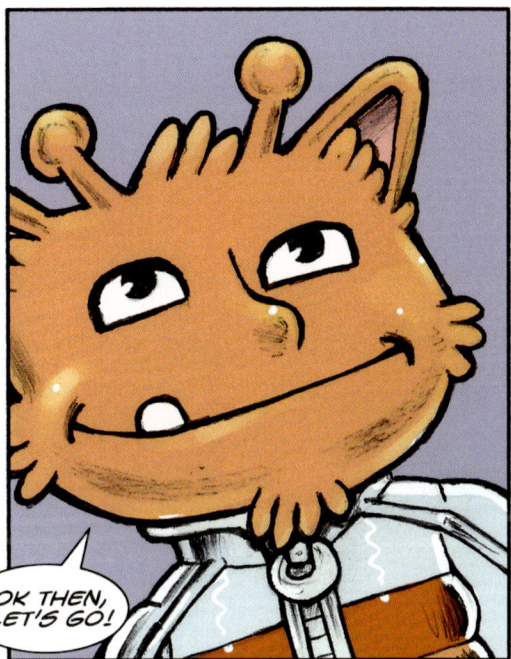

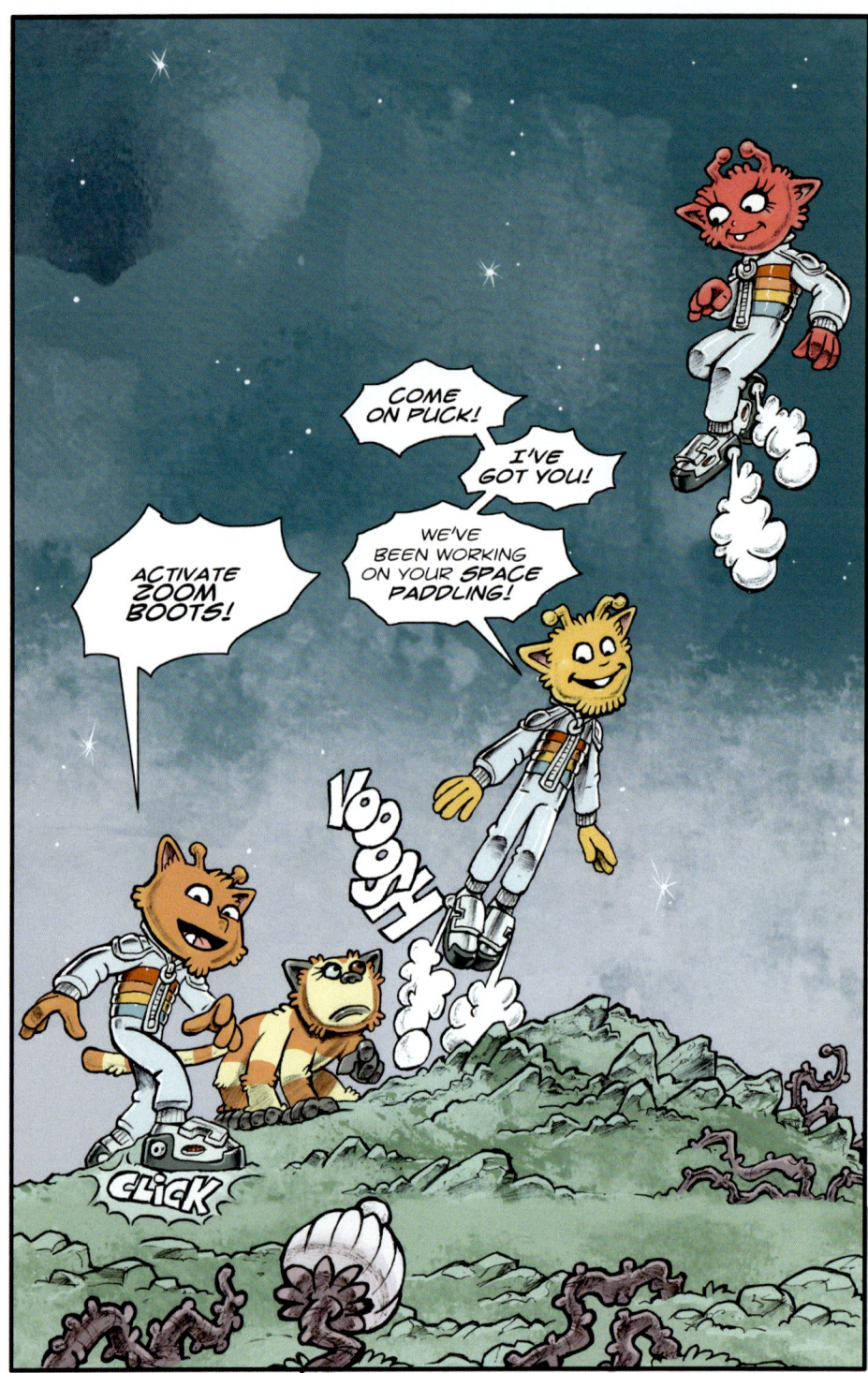

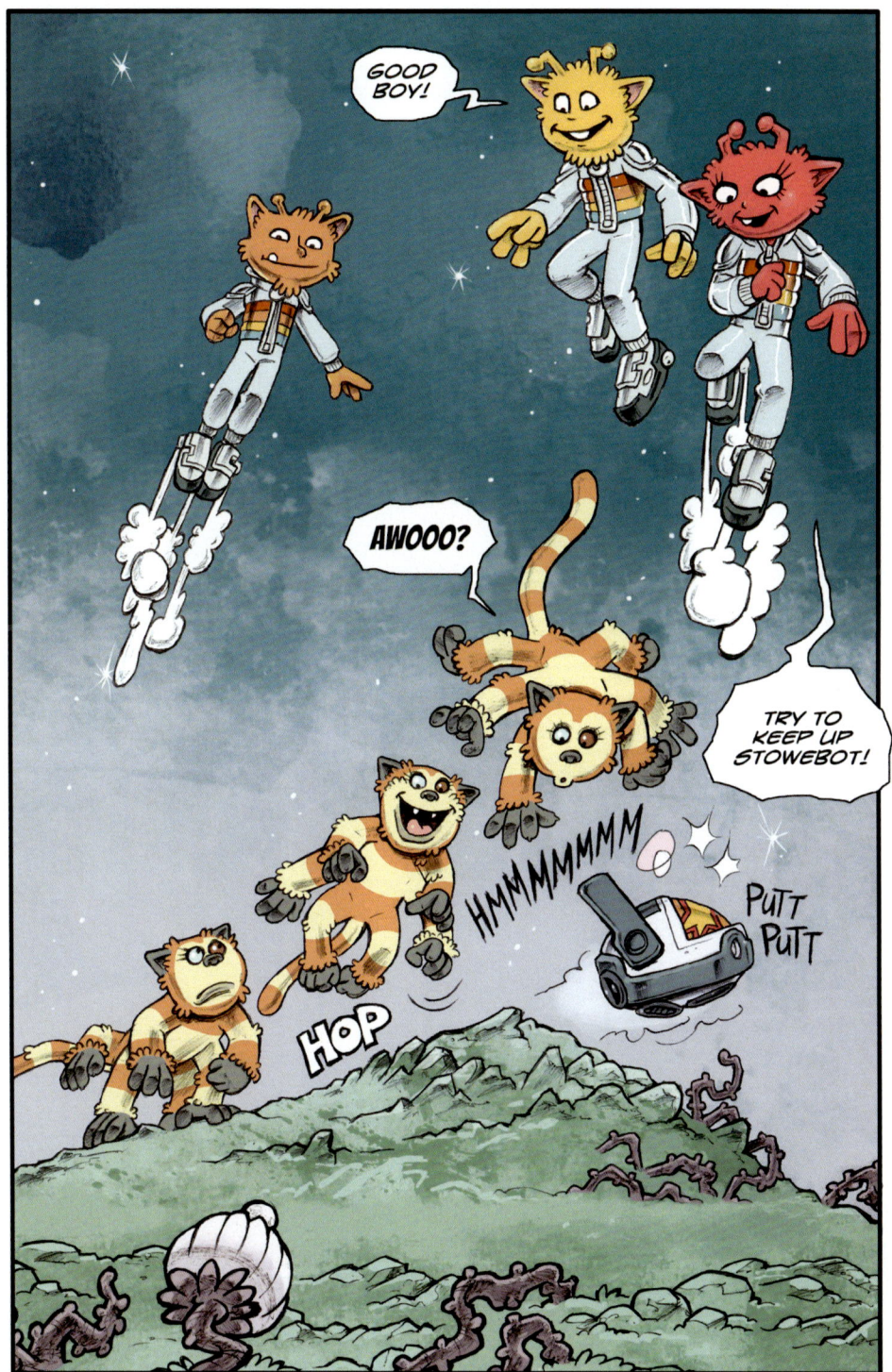

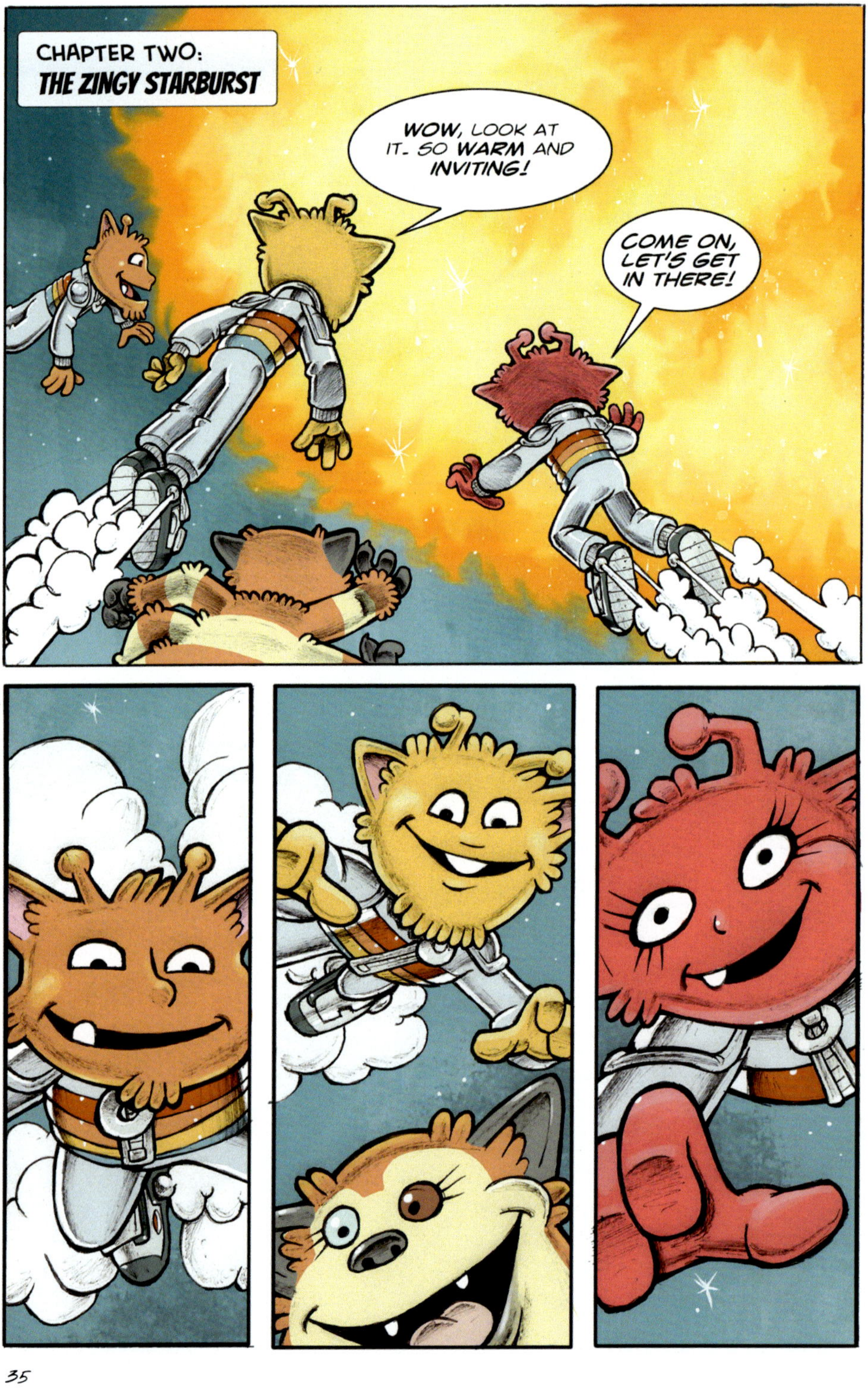

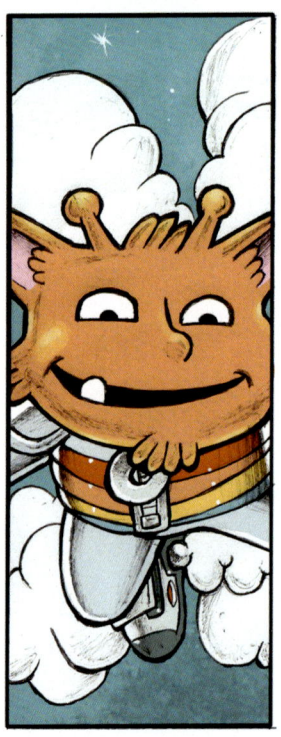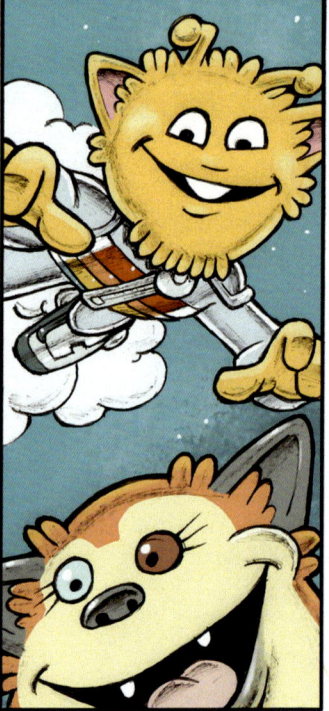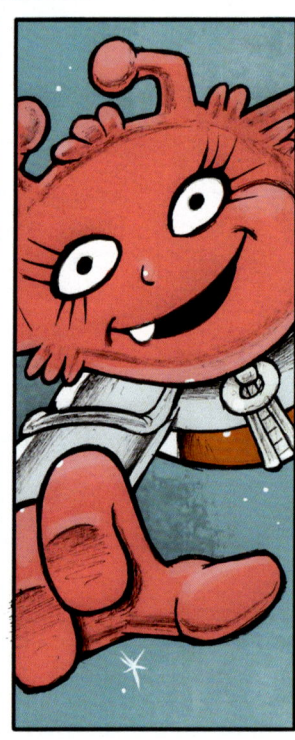

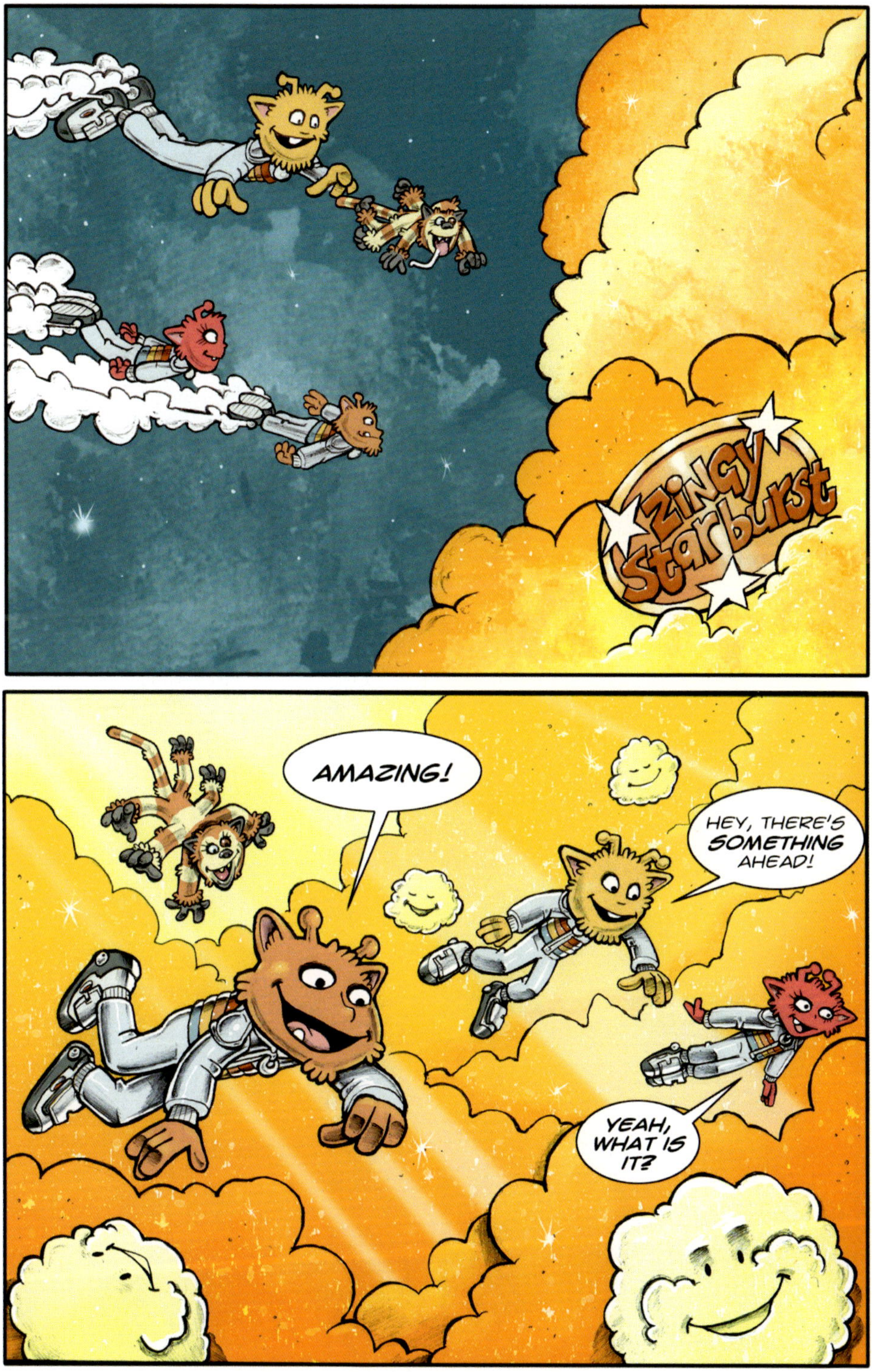

36

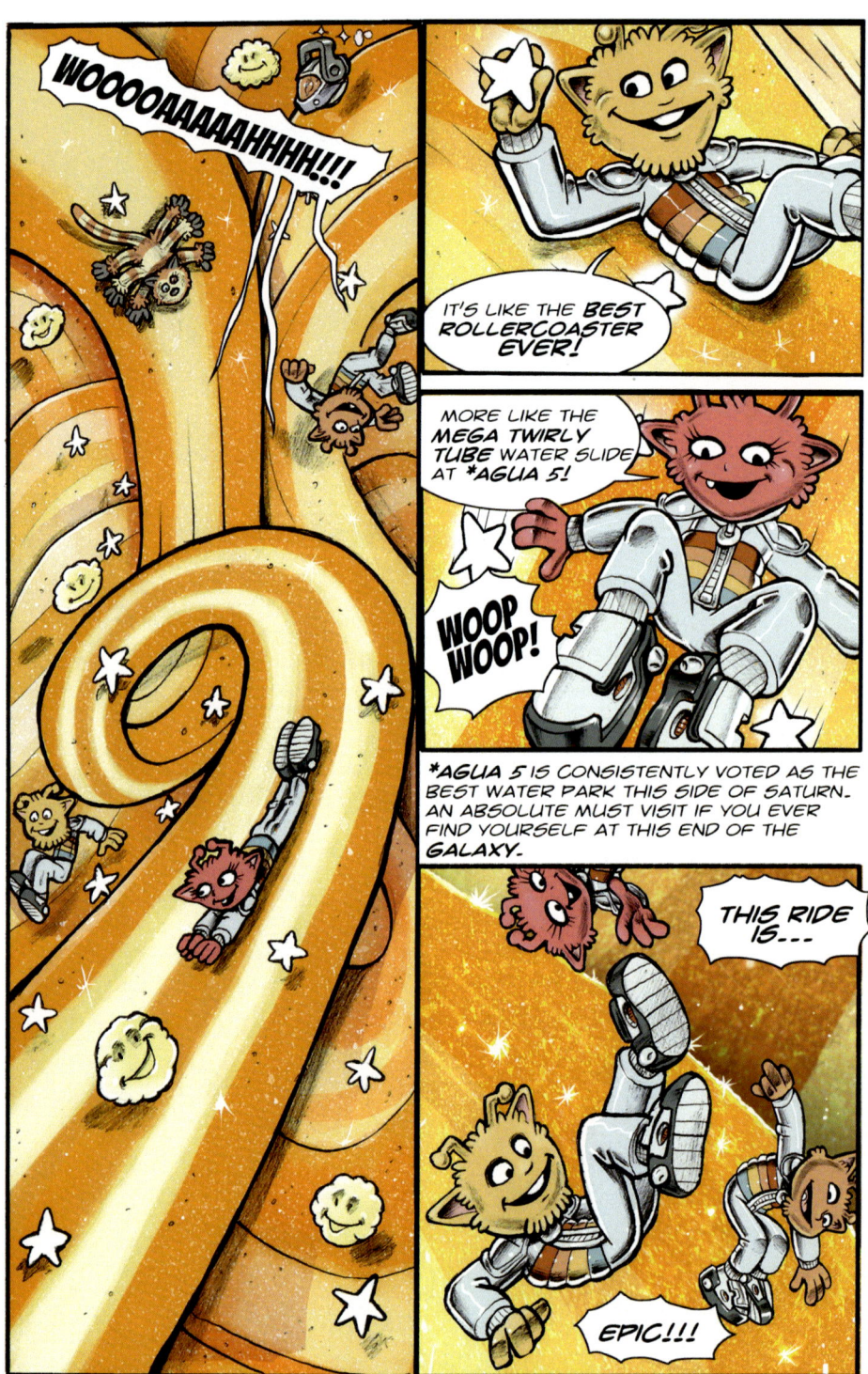

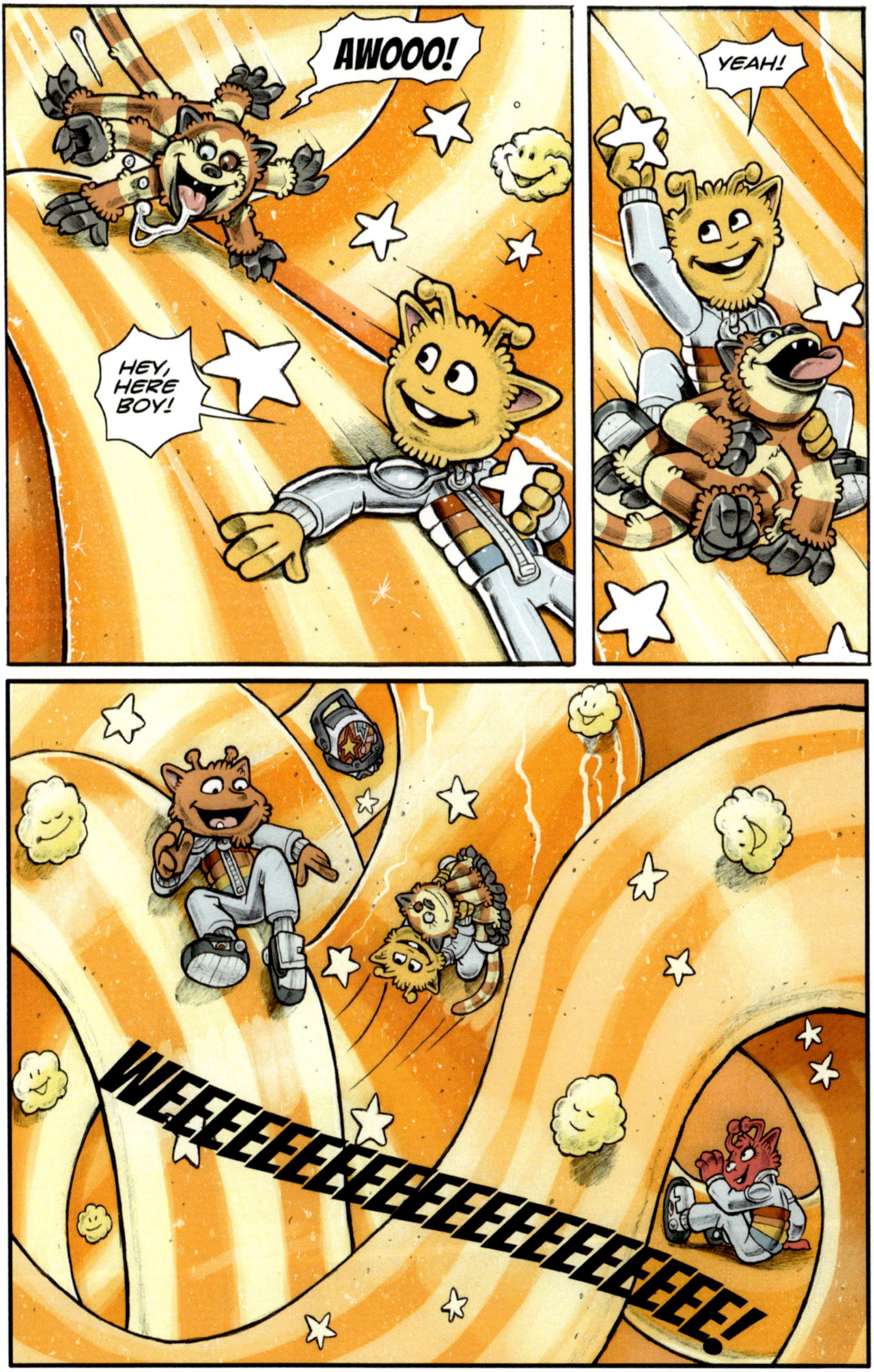

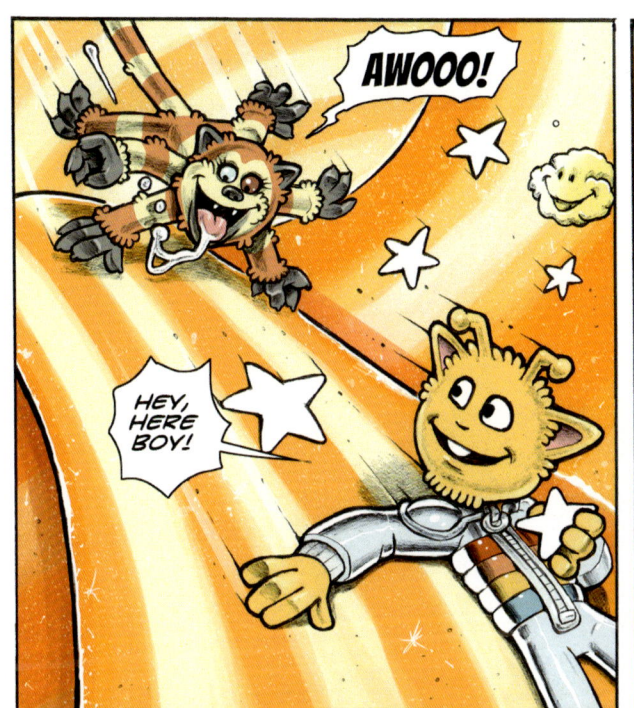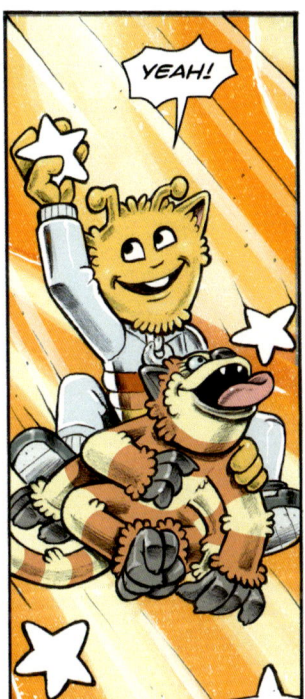

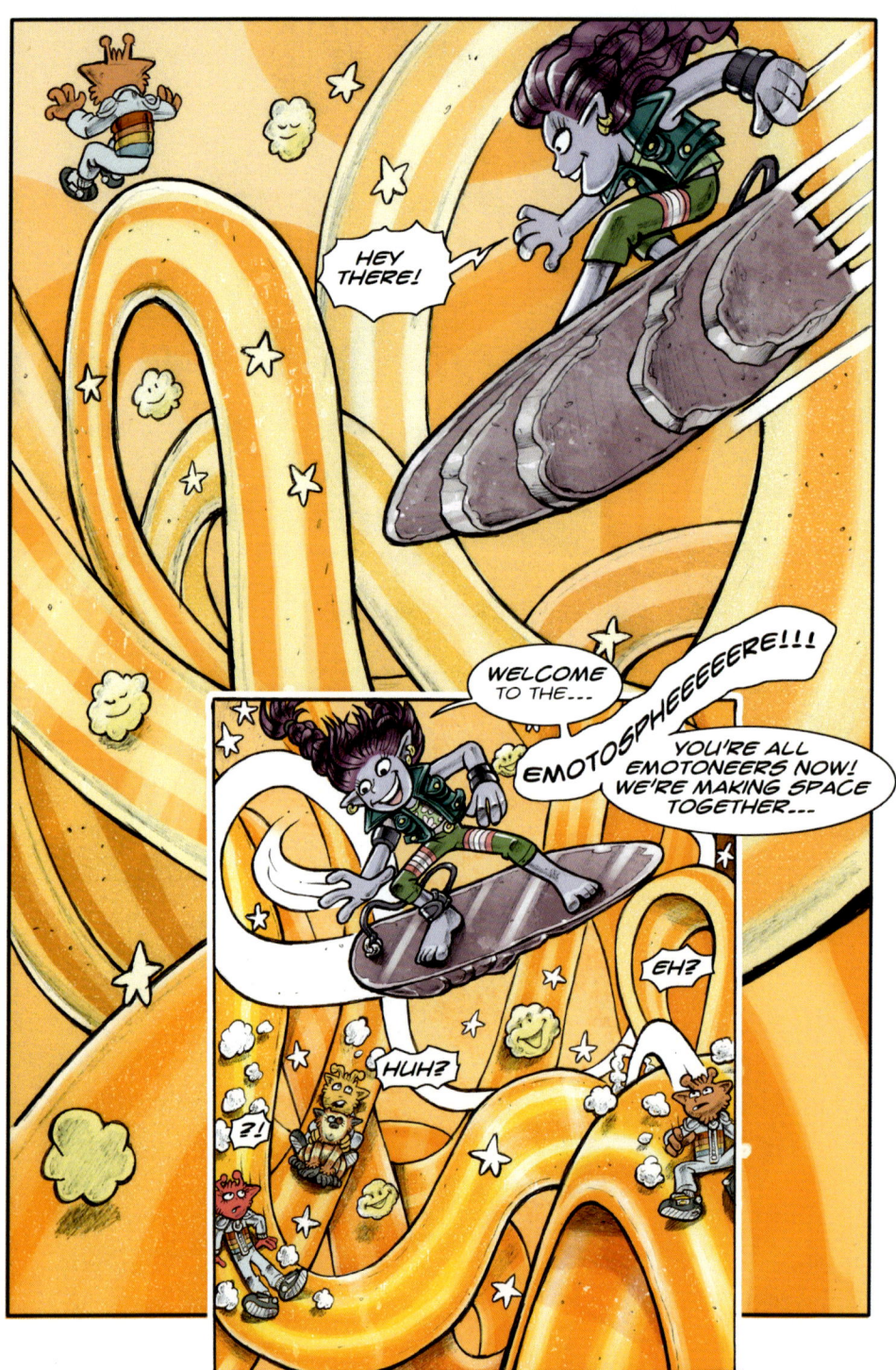

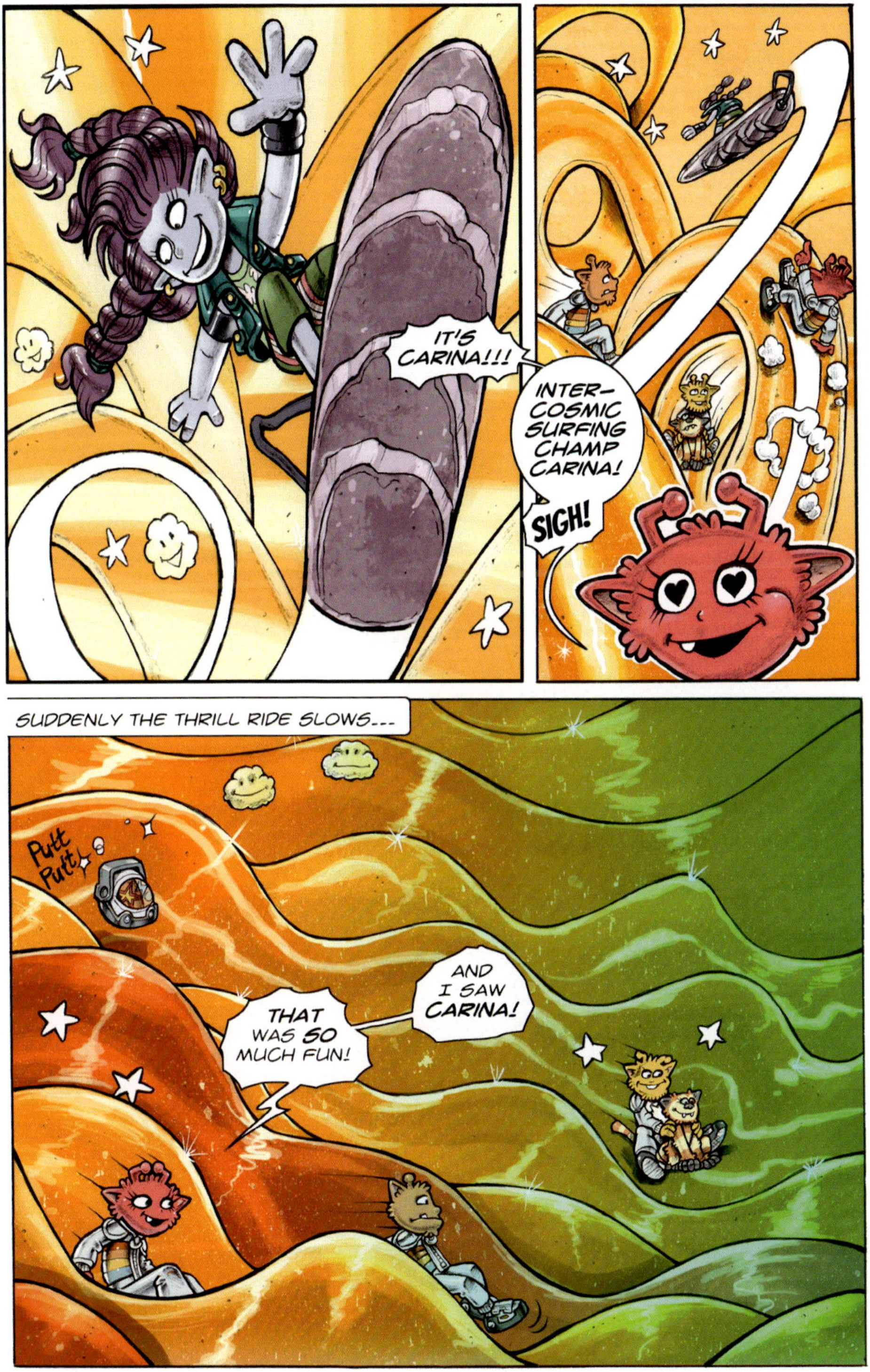

IT'S CARINA!!!

INTER-COSMIC SURFING CHAMP CARINA!

SIGH!

SUDDENLY THE THRILL RIDE SLOWS...

Putt Putt

THAT WAS *SO* MUCH FUN!

AND I SAW *CARINA!*

40

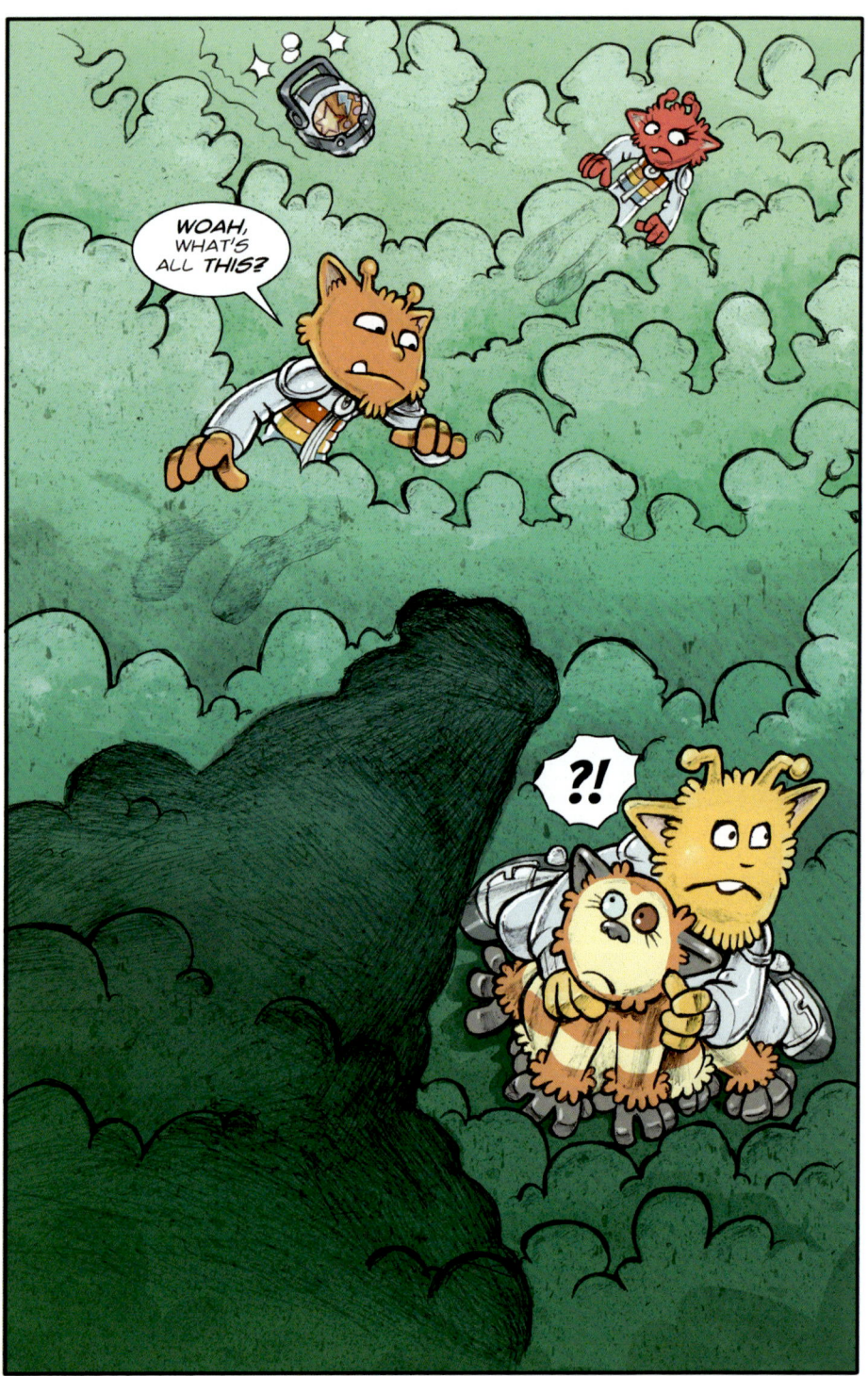

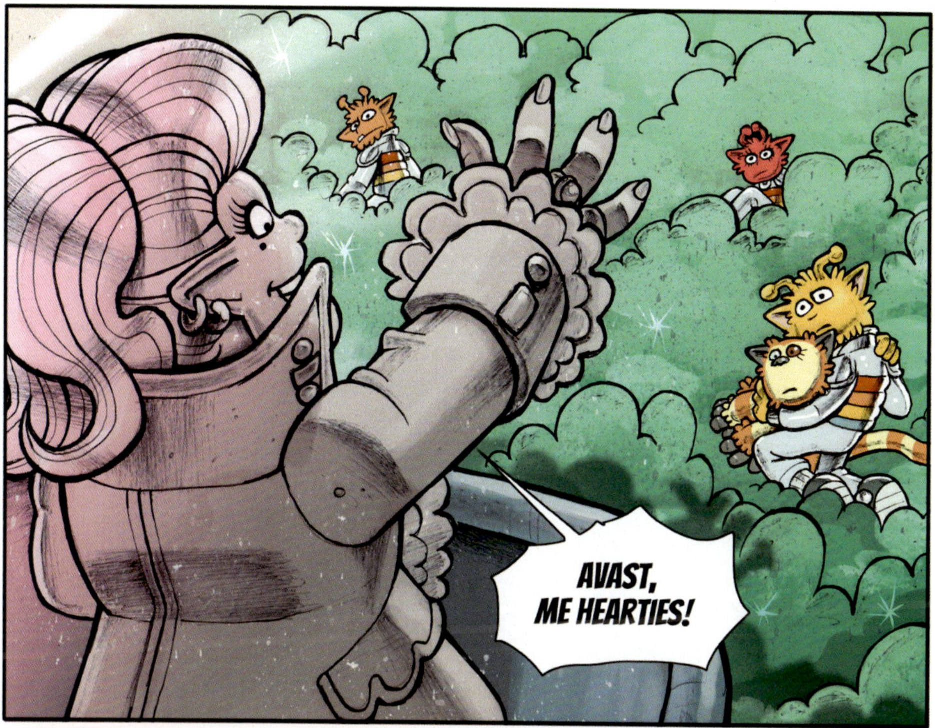

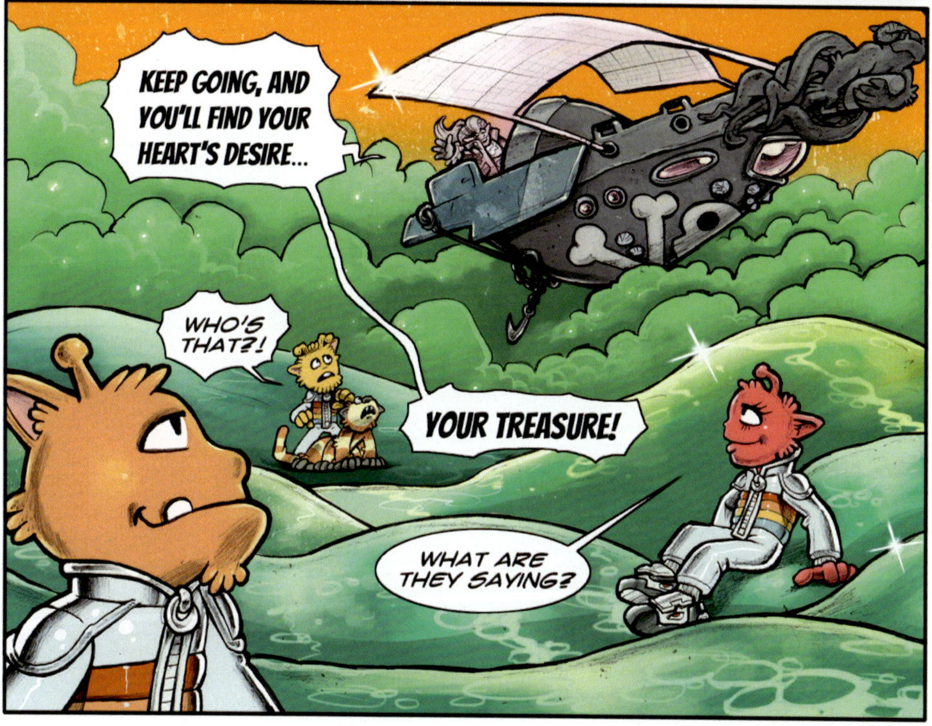

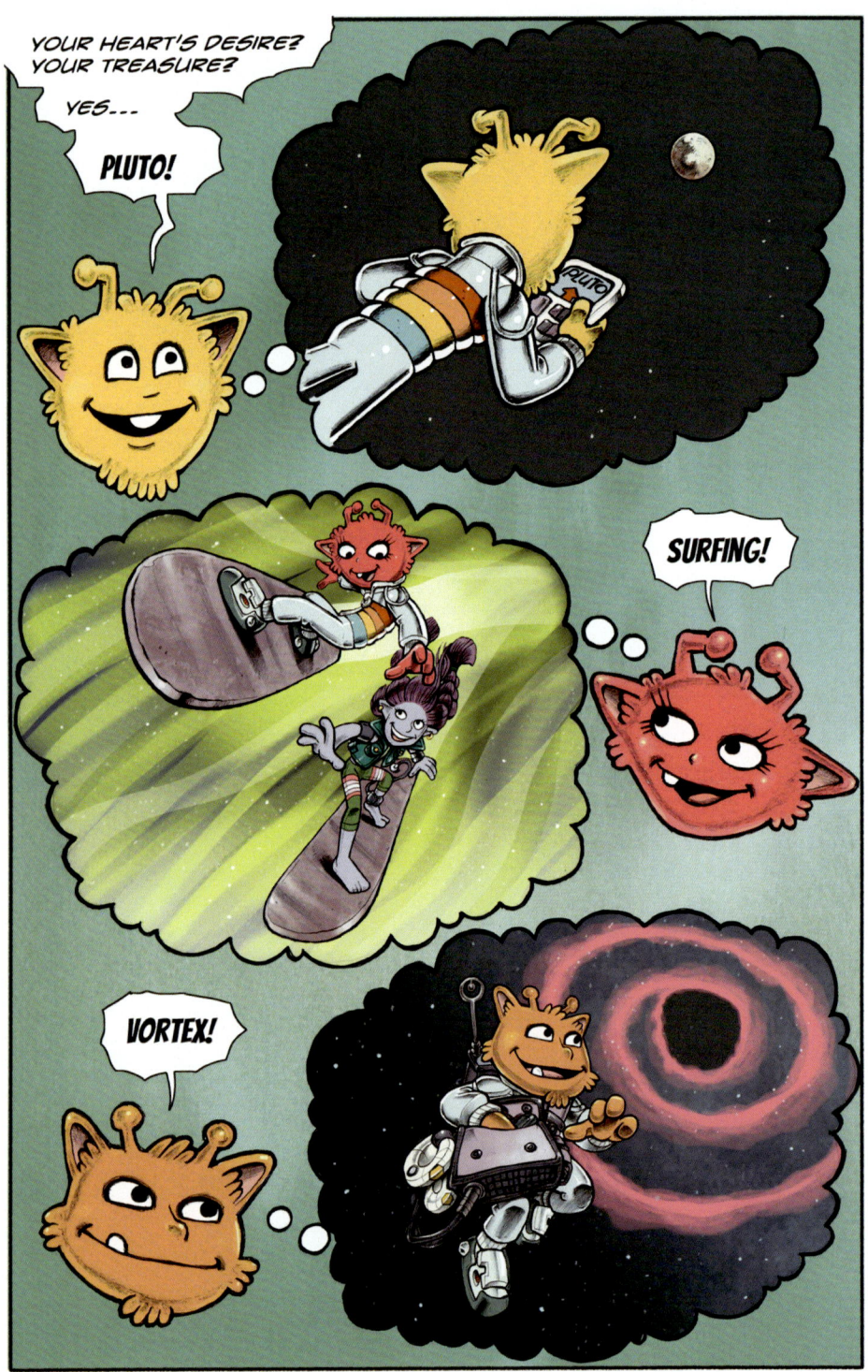

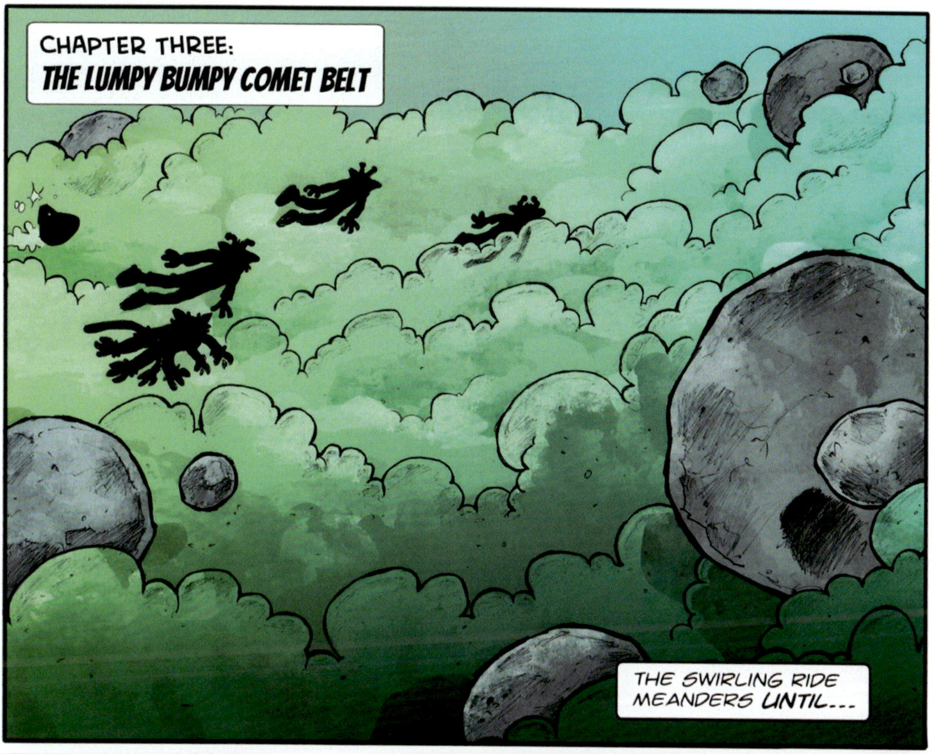

CHAPTER THREE:
THE LUMPY BUMPY COMET BELT

THE SWIRLING RIDE MEANDERS *UNTIL*....

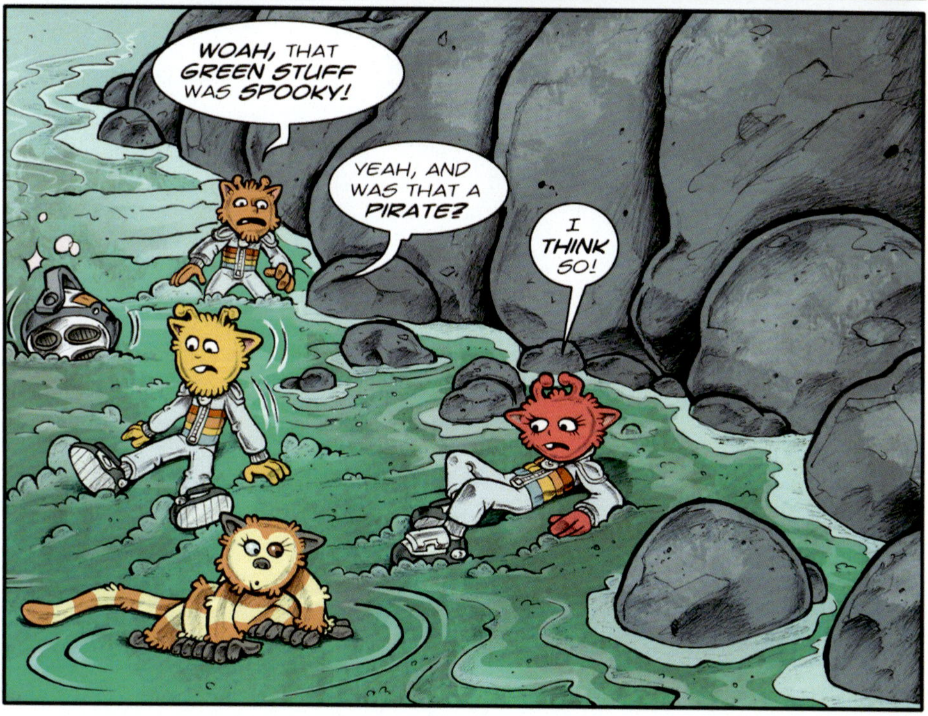

WOAH, THAT *GREEN STUFF* WAS *SPOOKY!*

YEAH, AND WAS THAT A *PIRATE?*

I THINK SO!

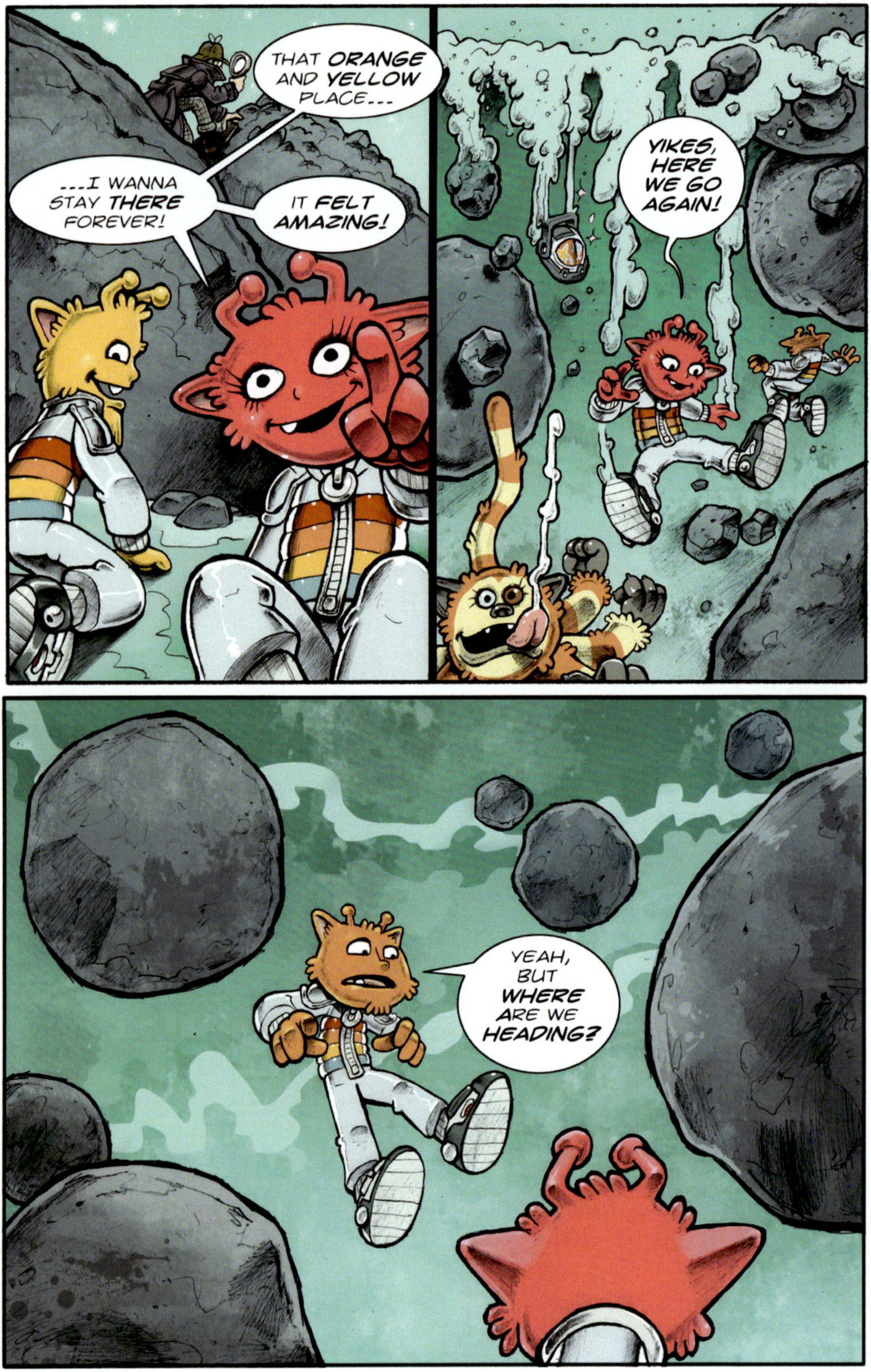

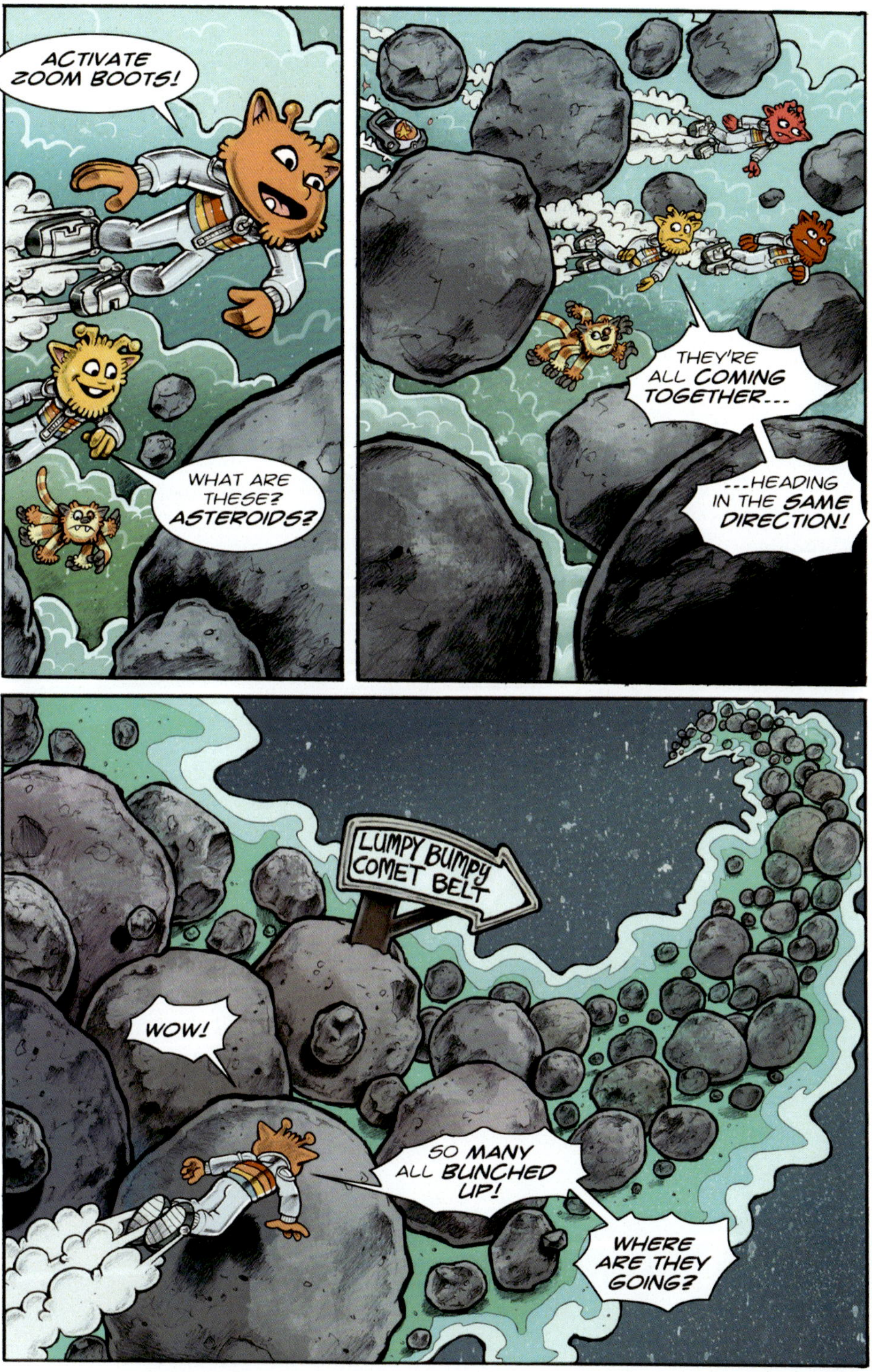

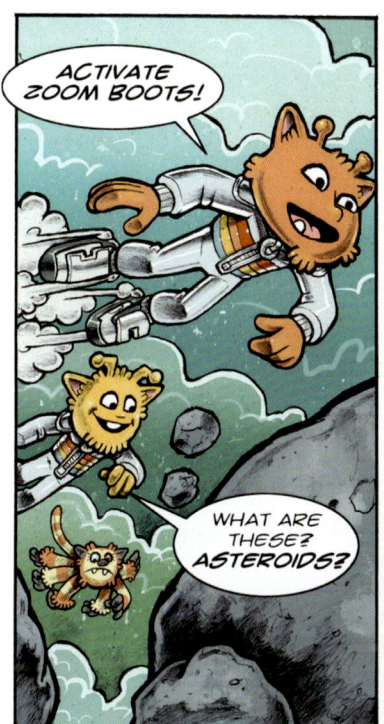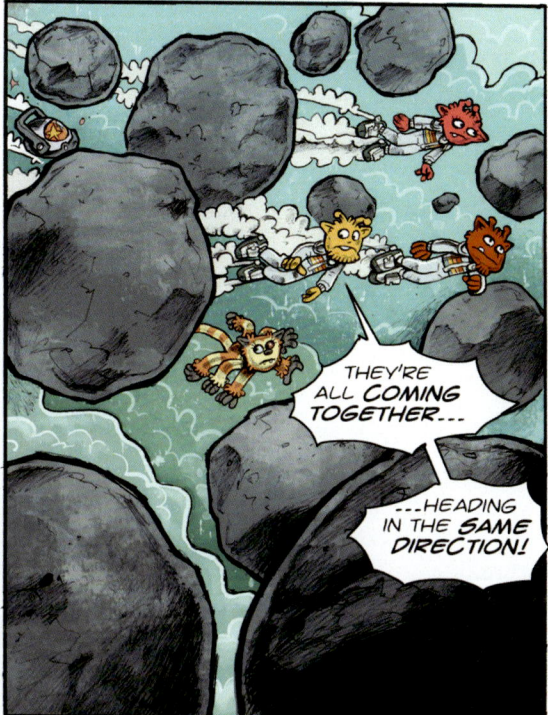

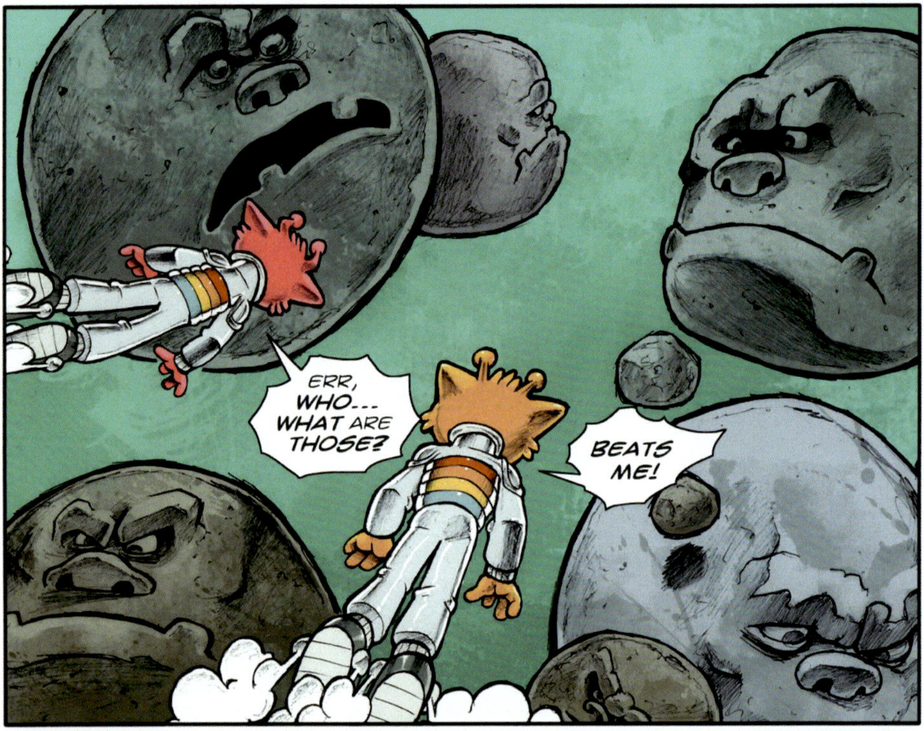

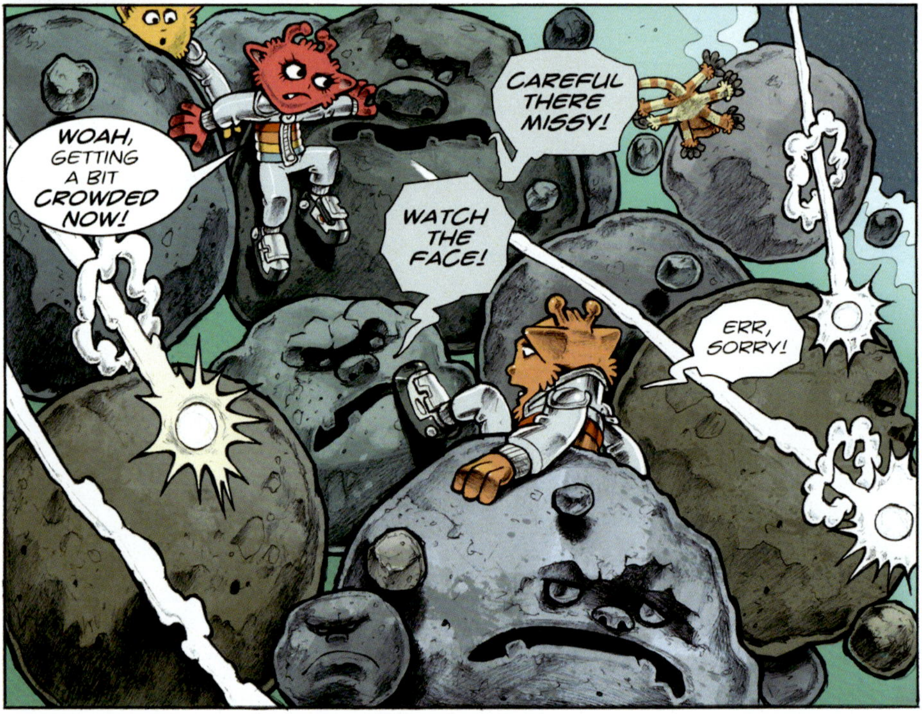

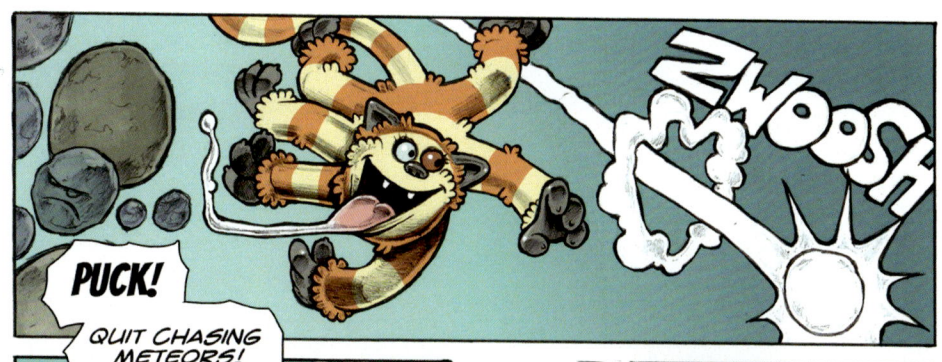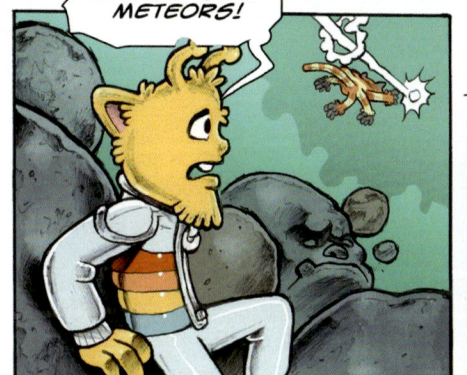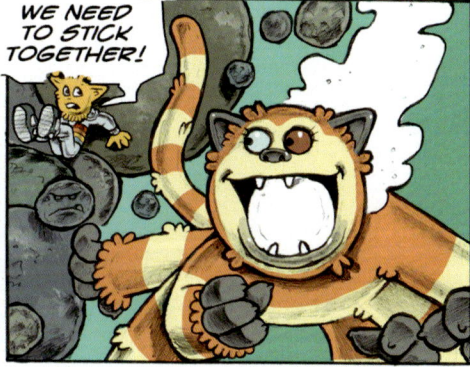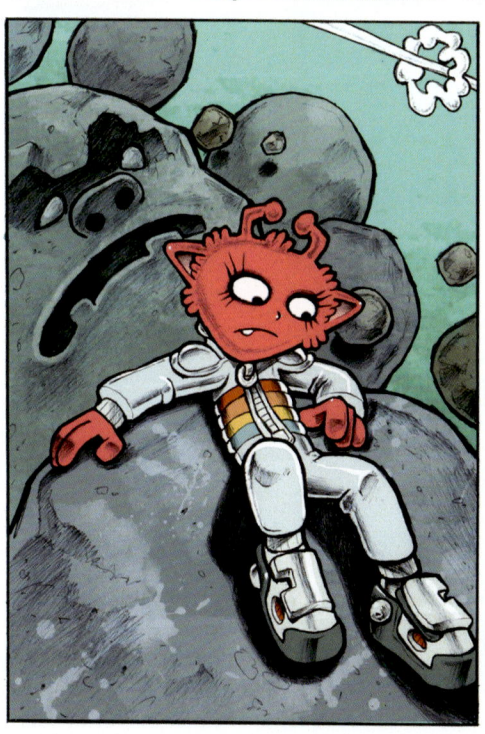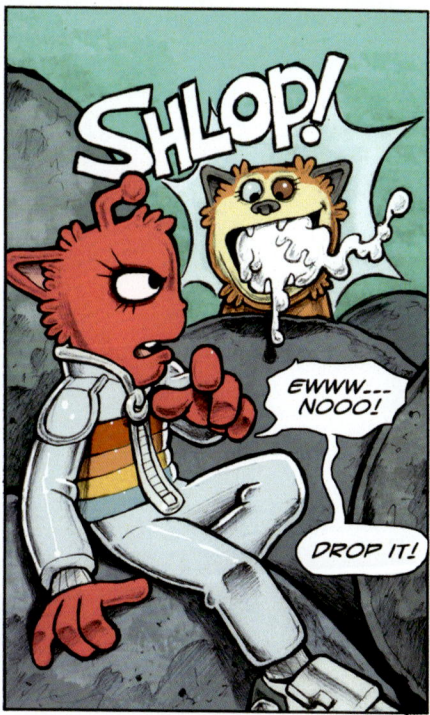

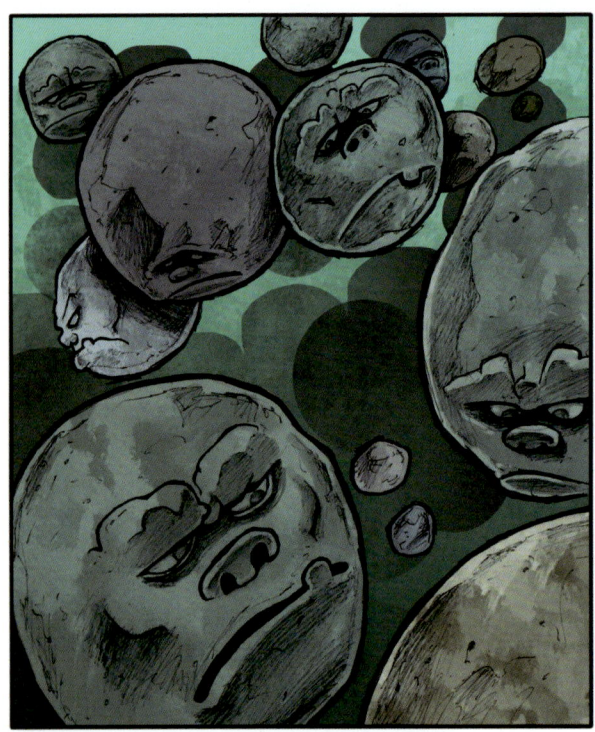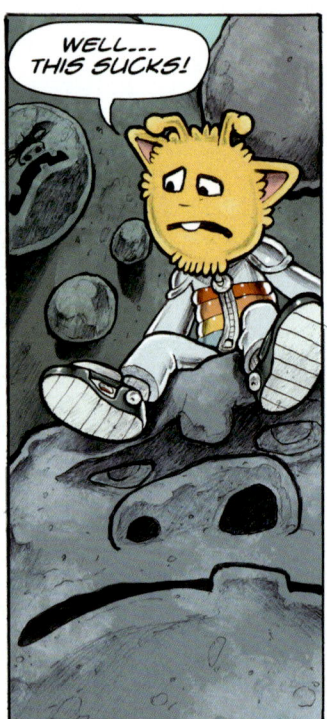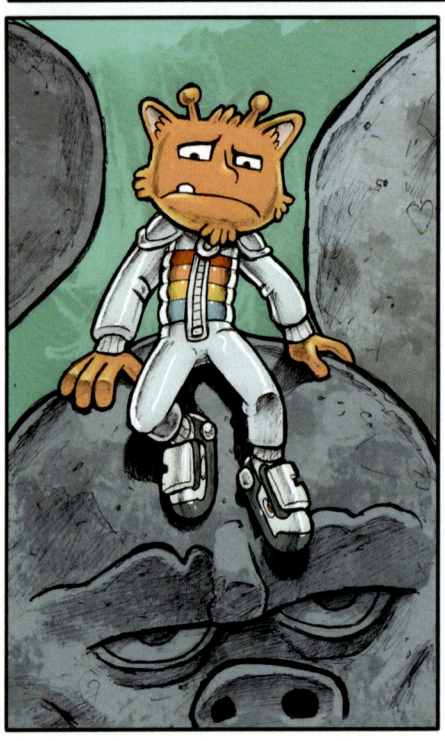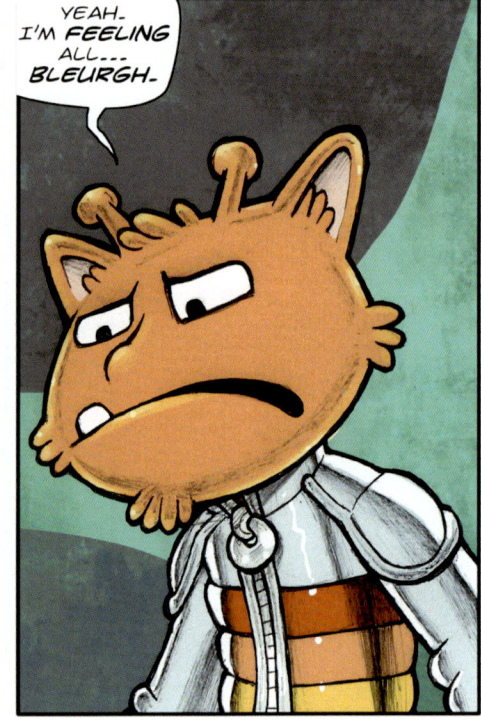

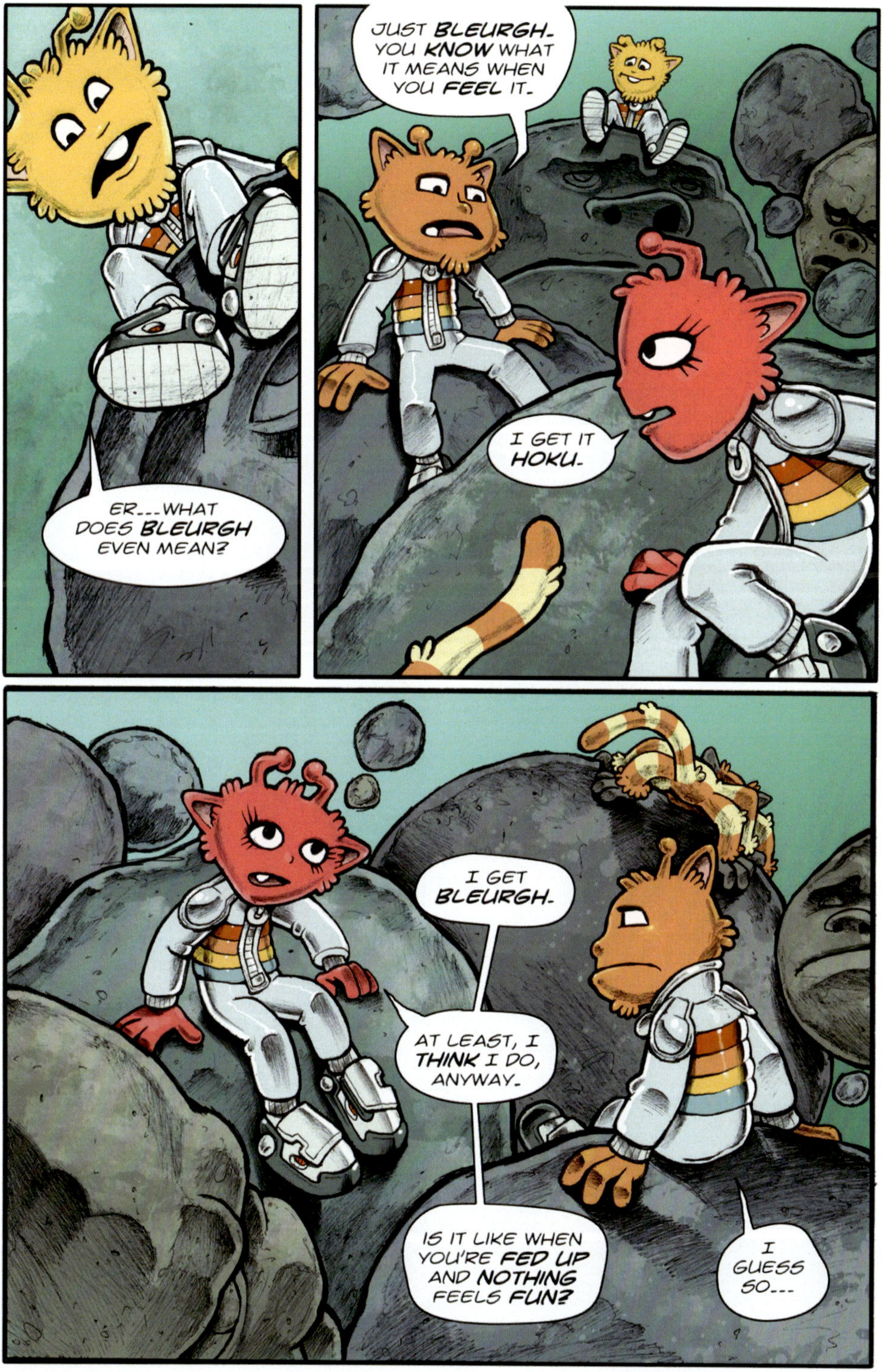

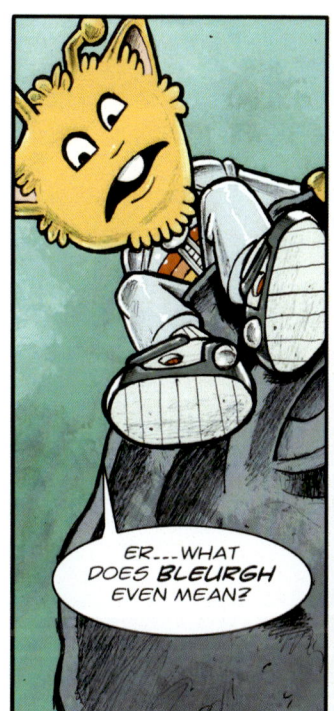
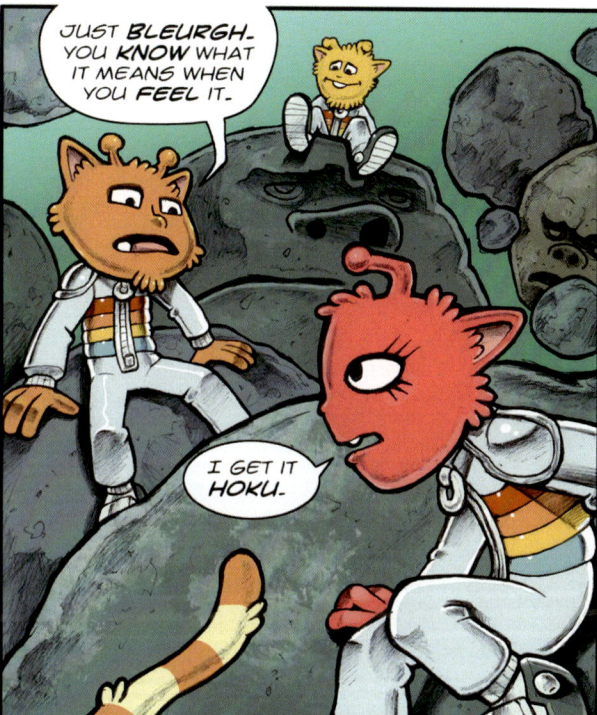

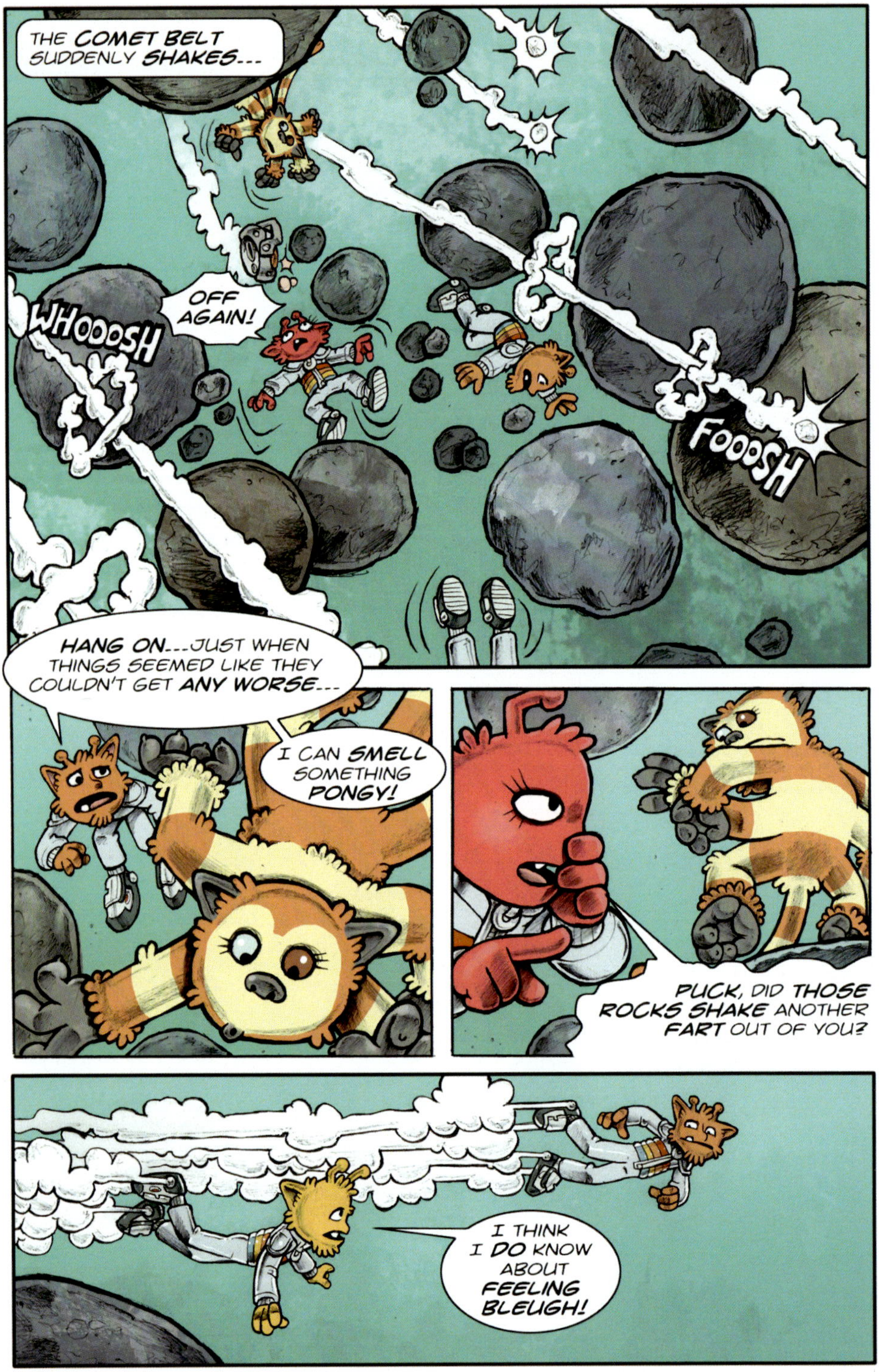

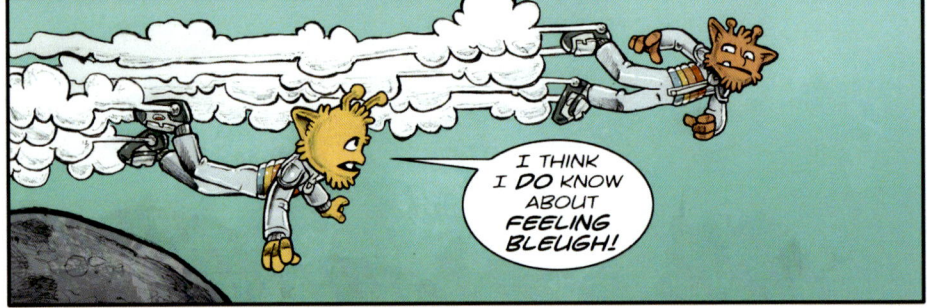

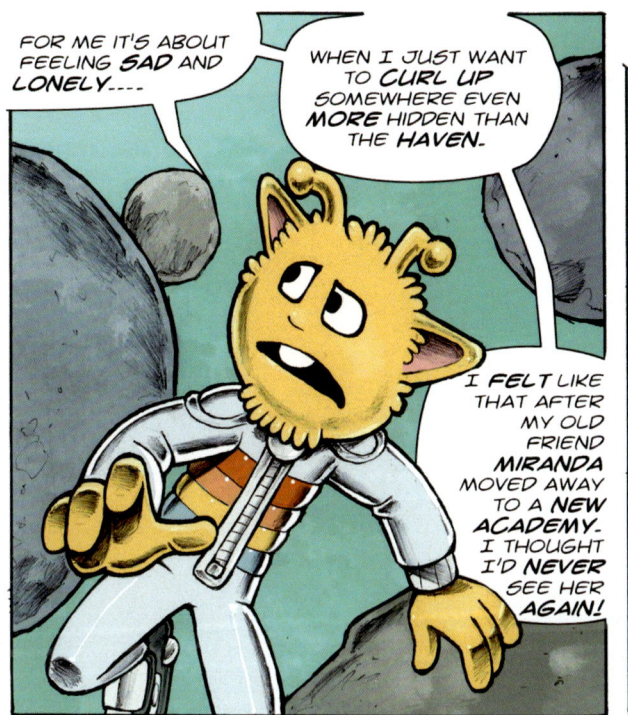
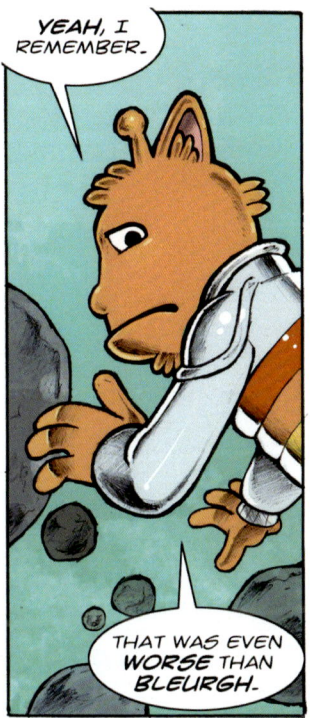
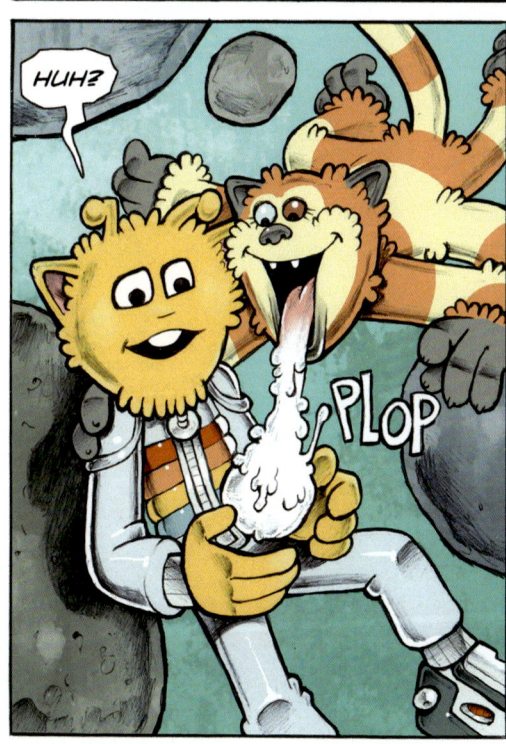
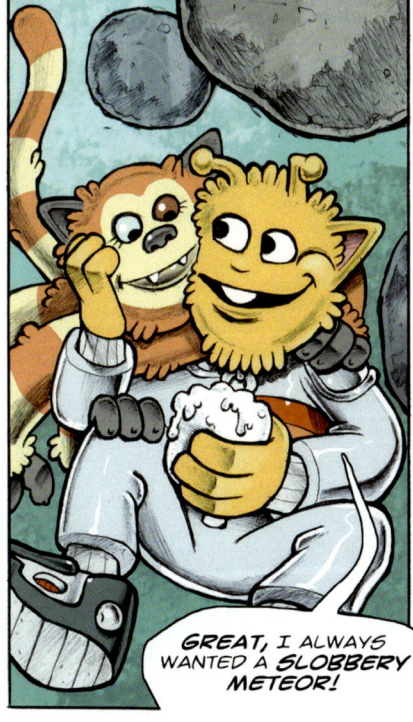

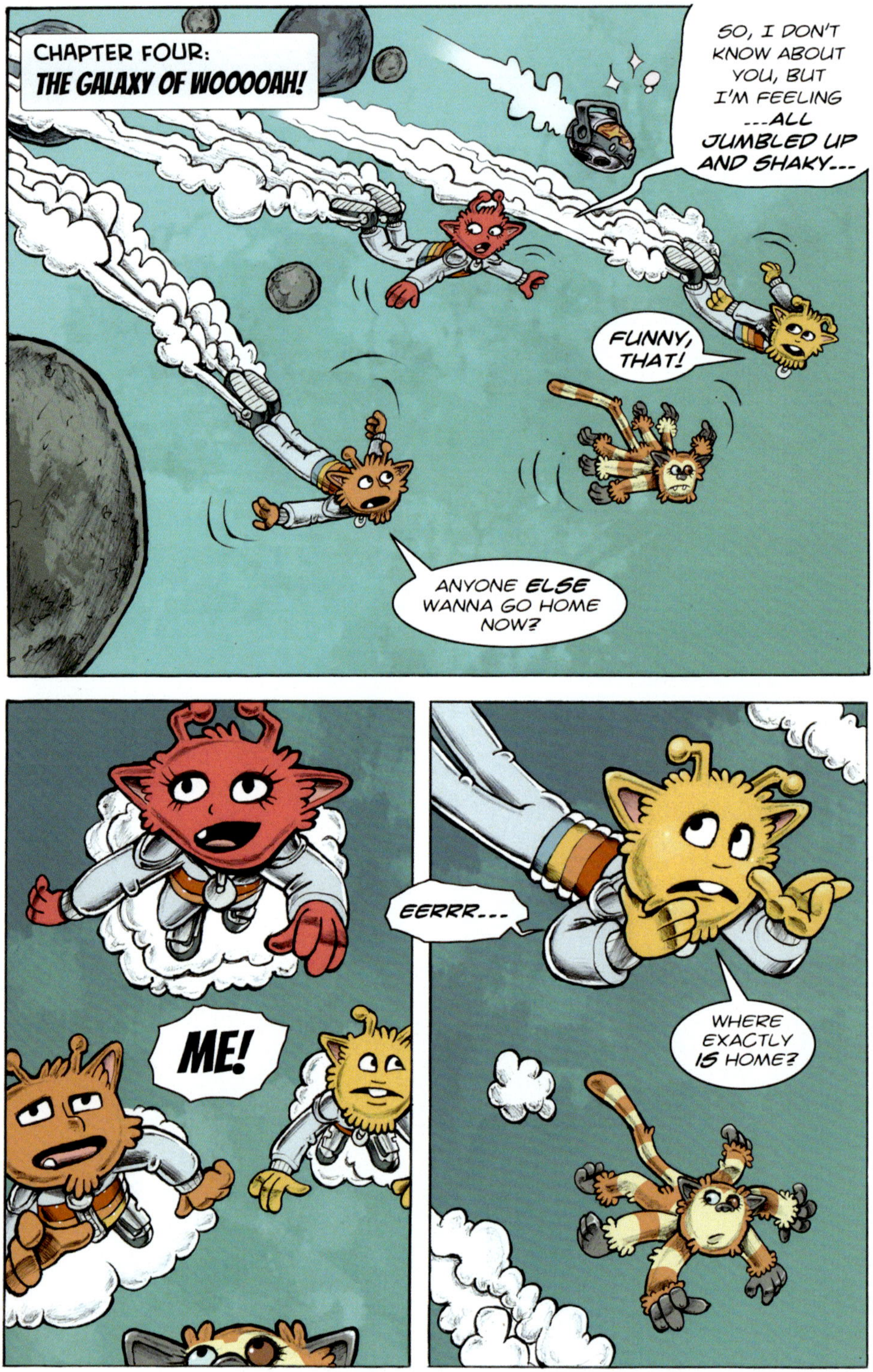

53

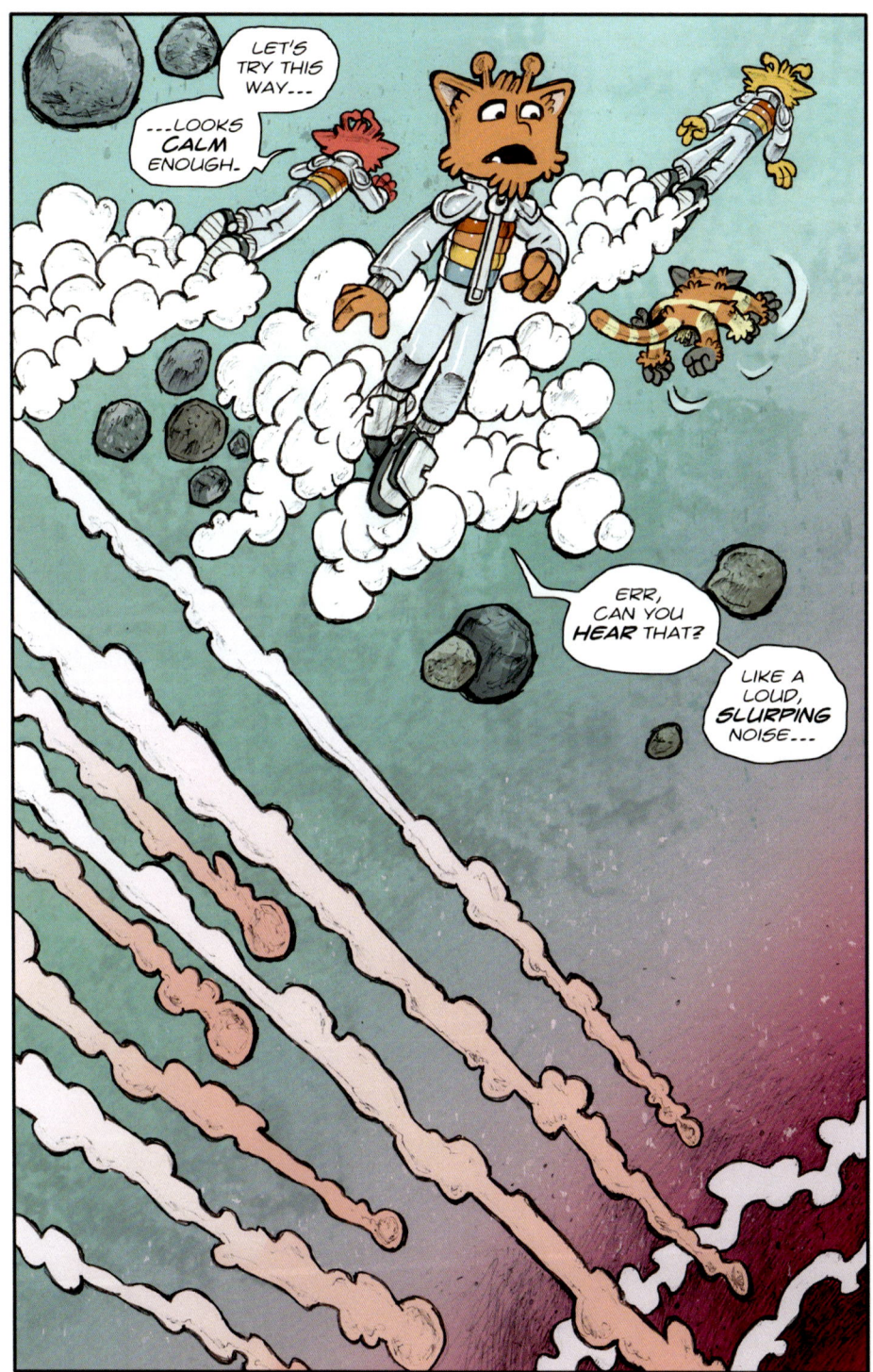

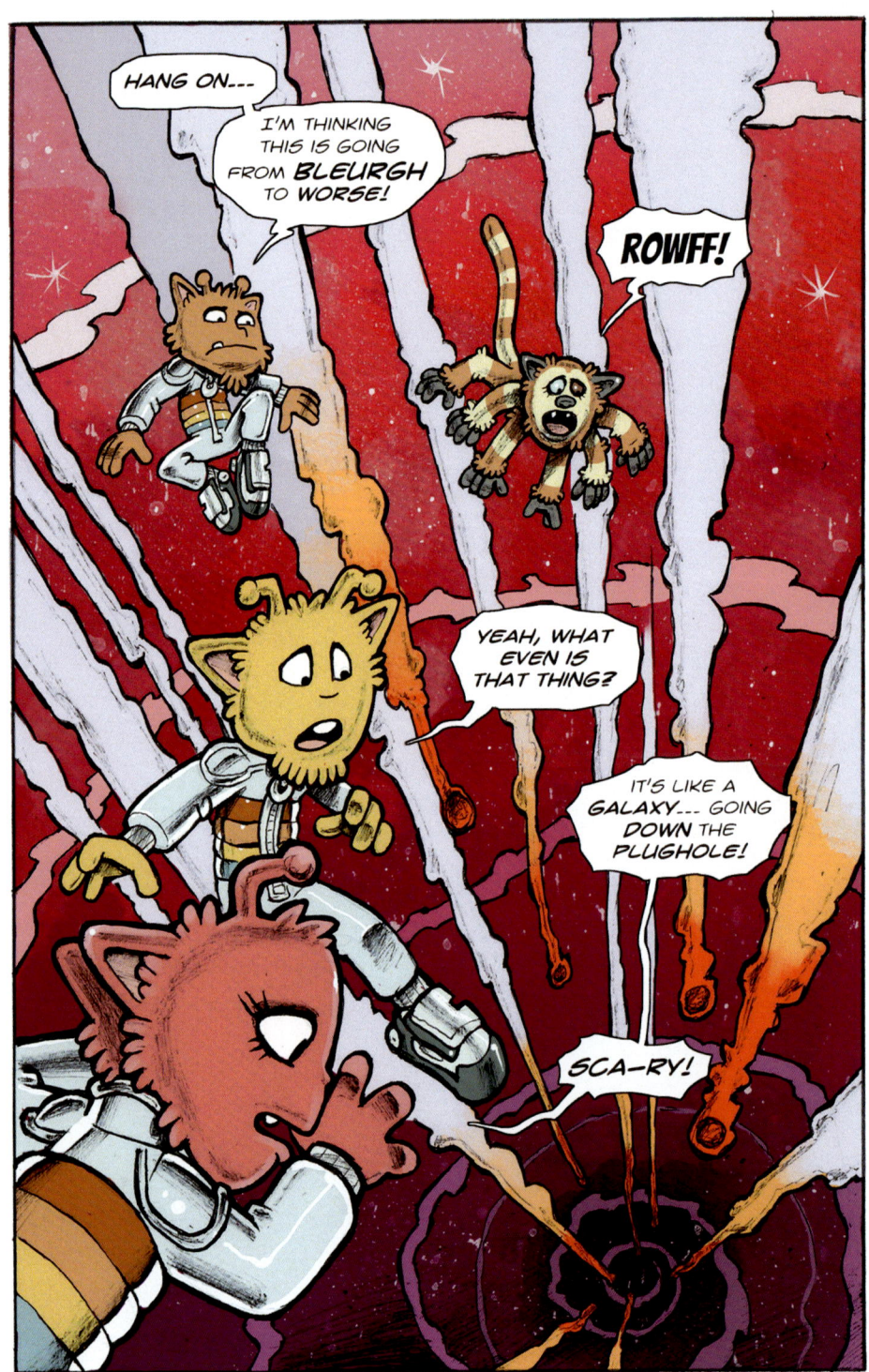

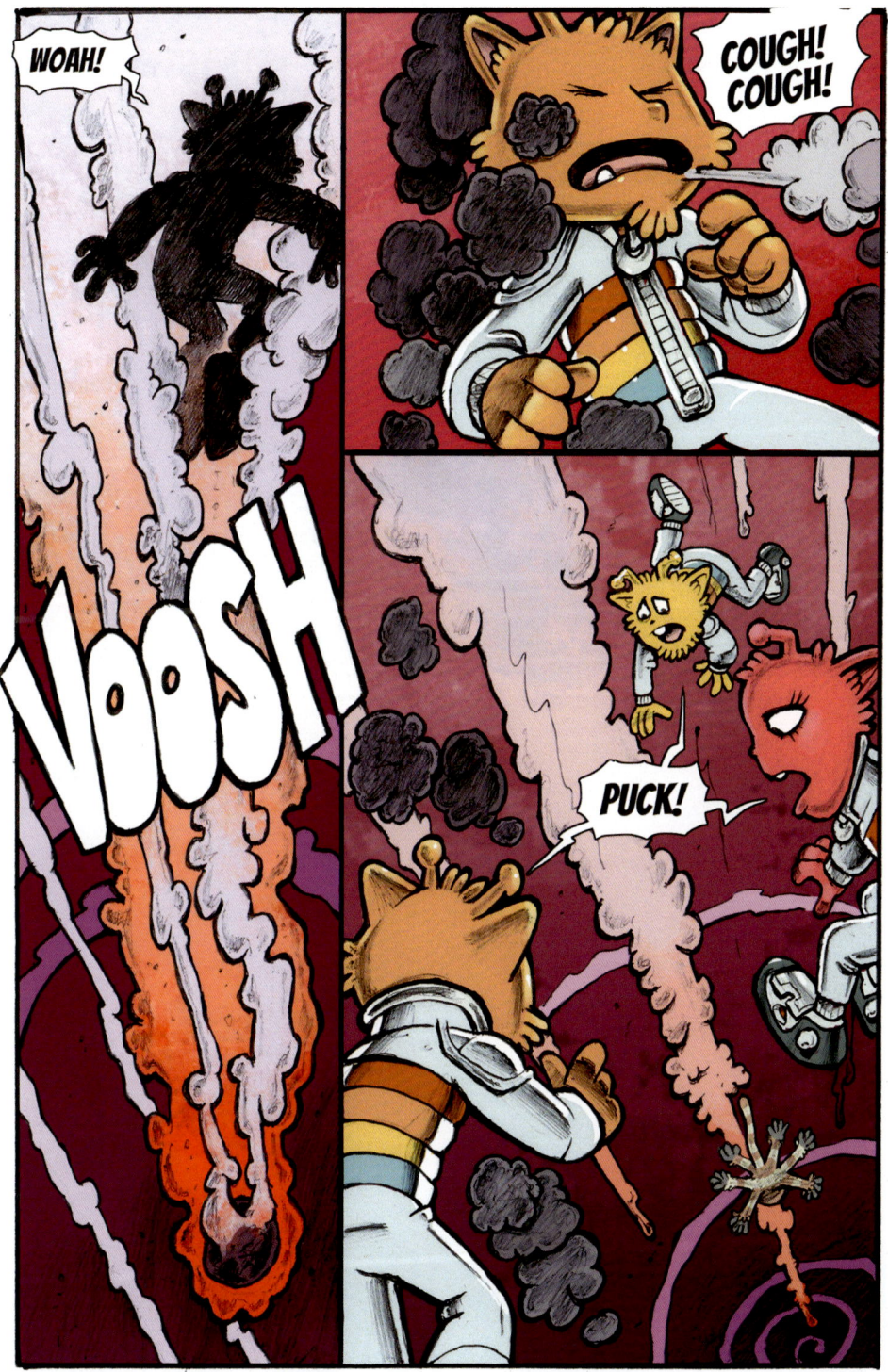

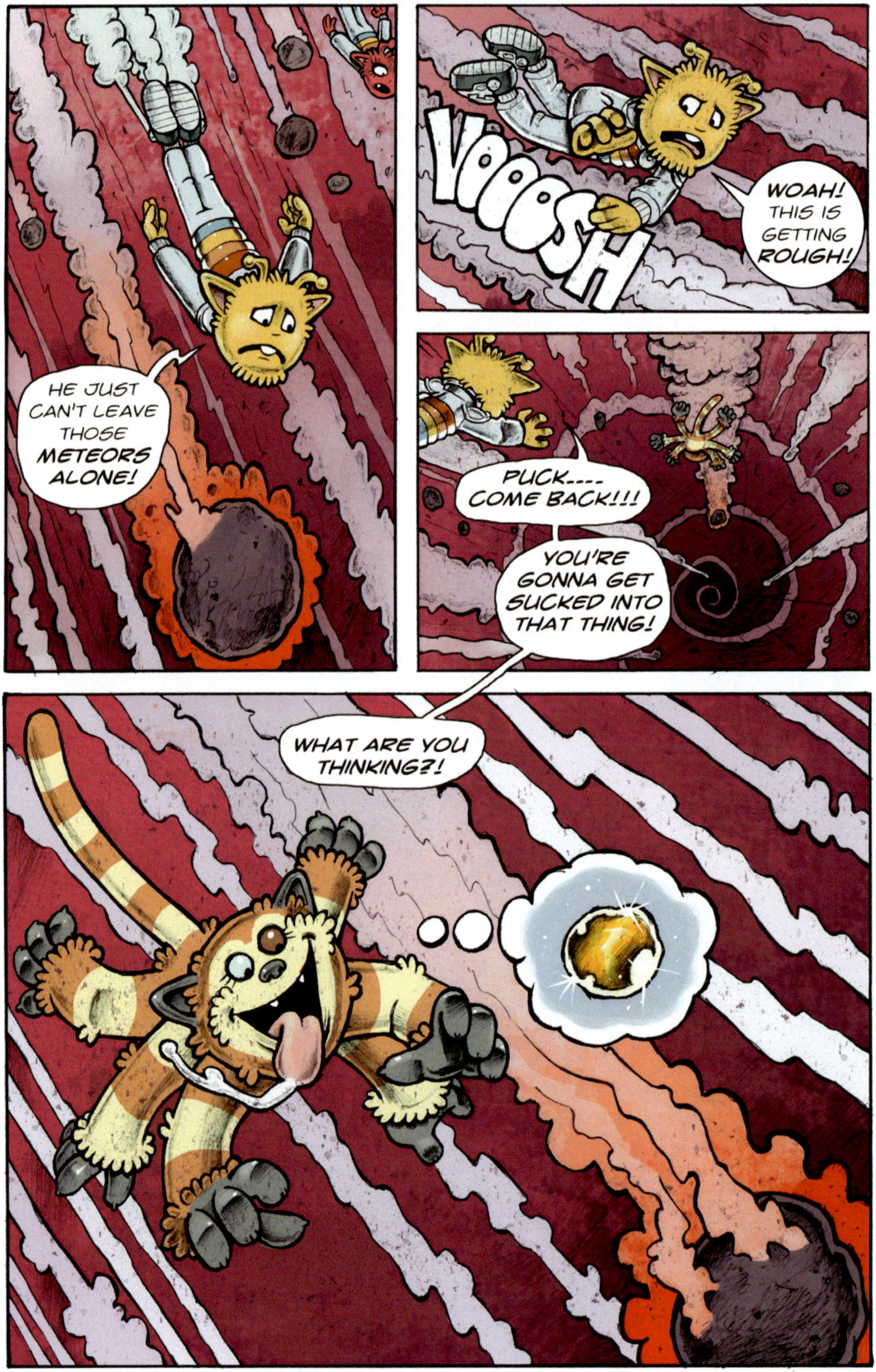

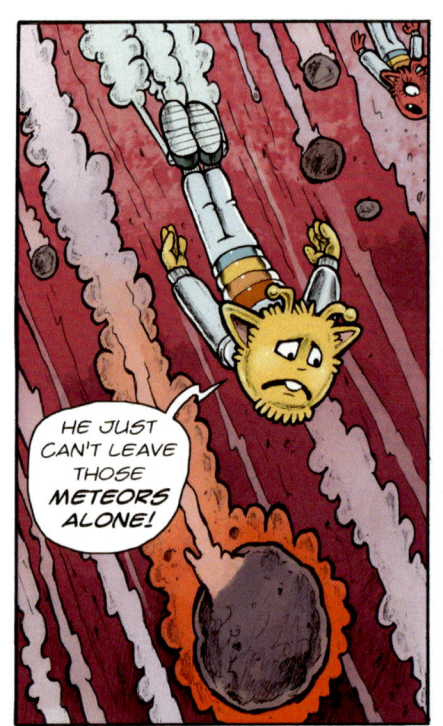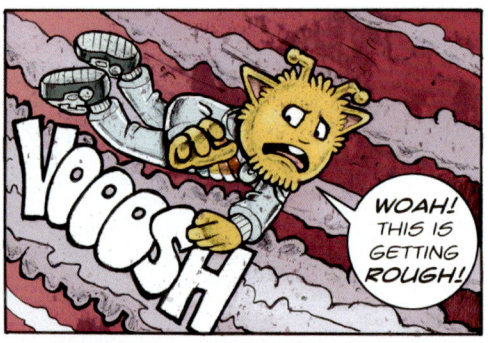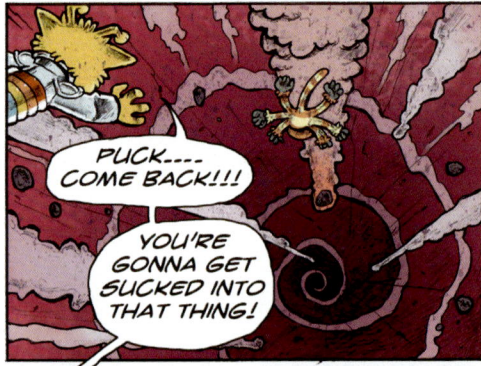

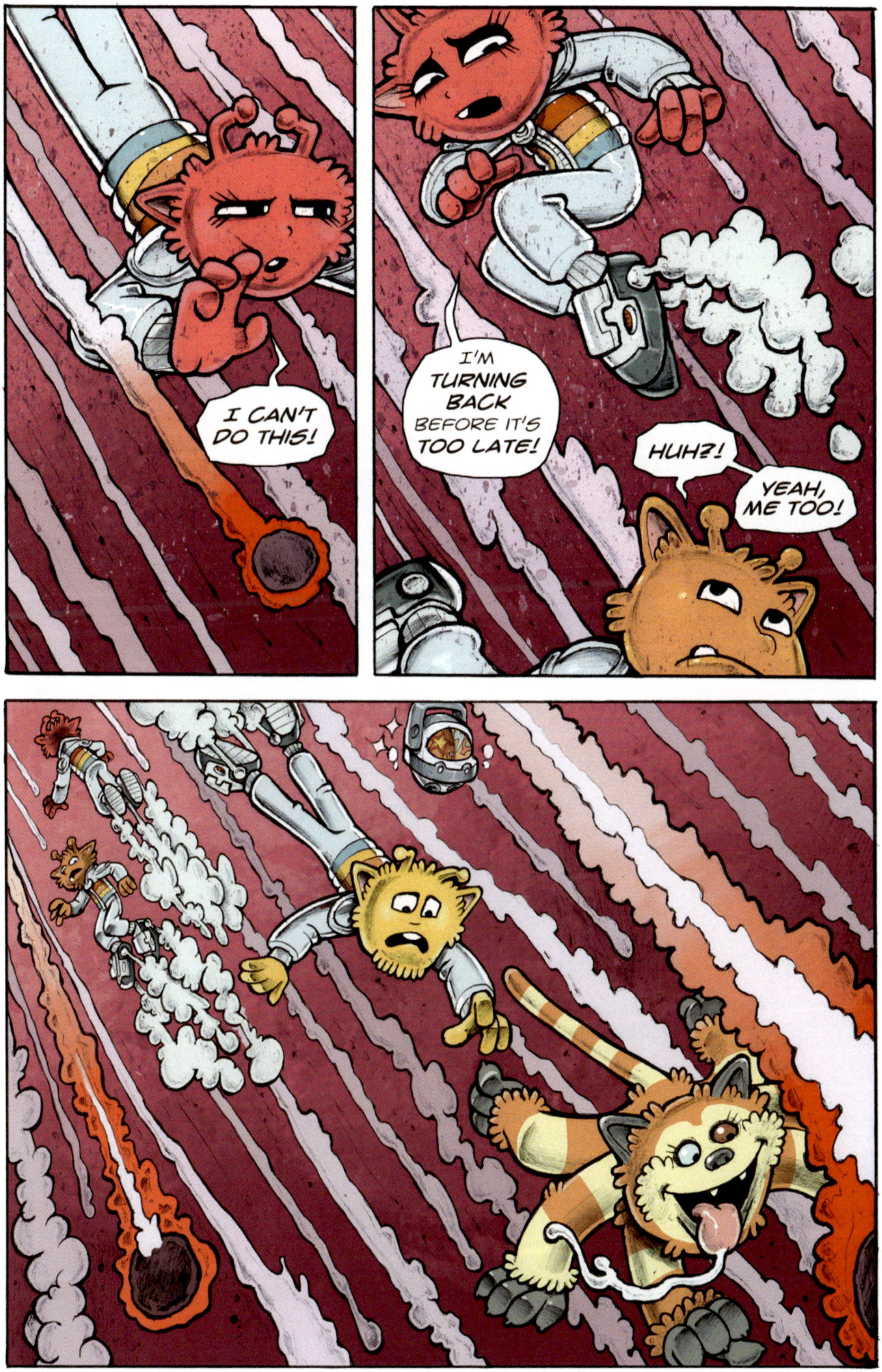

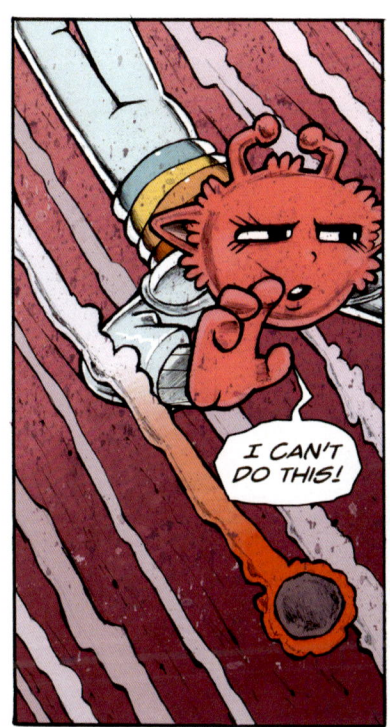
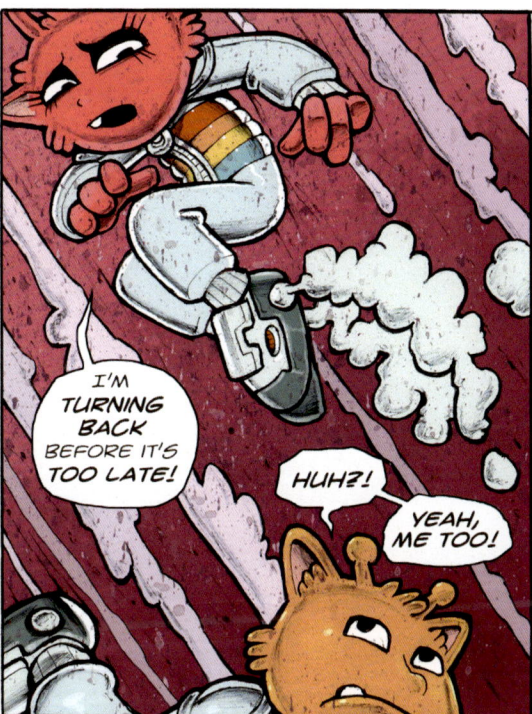

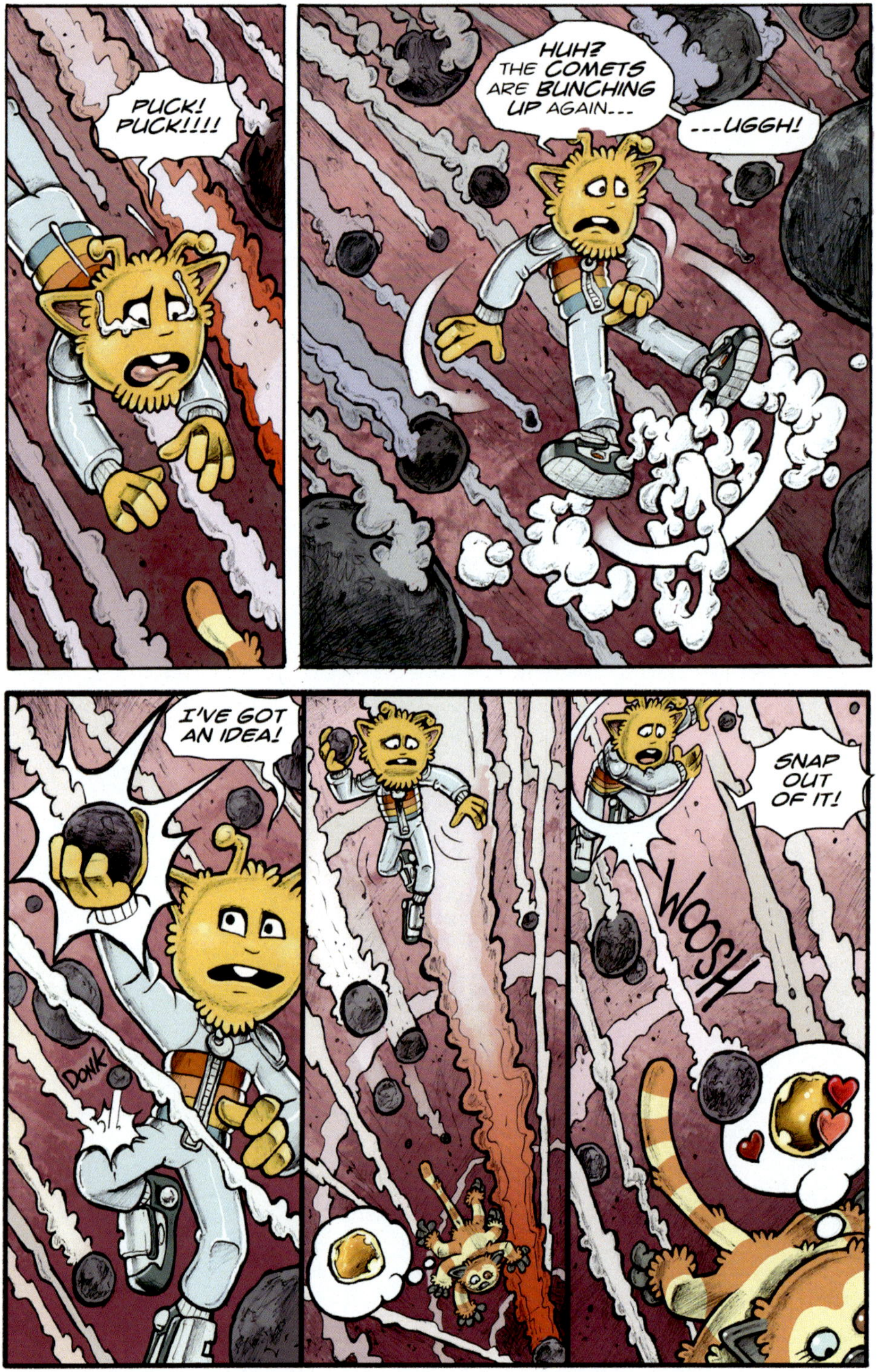

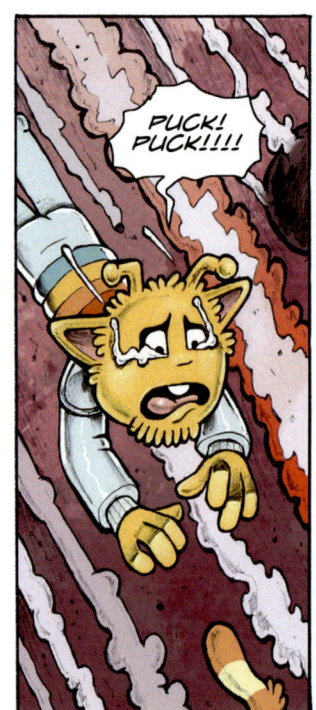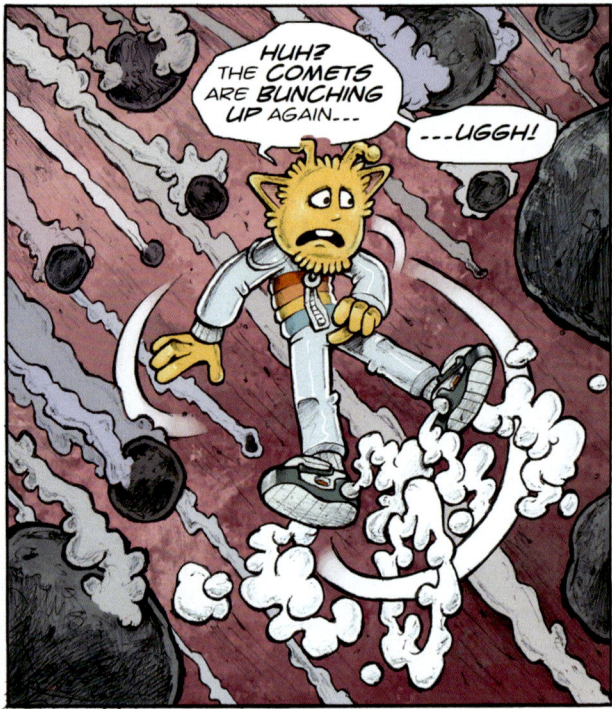

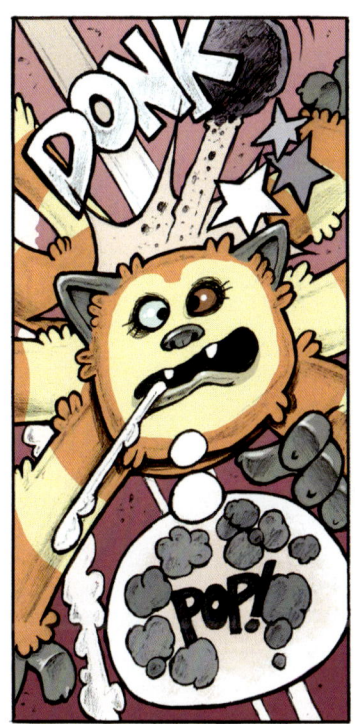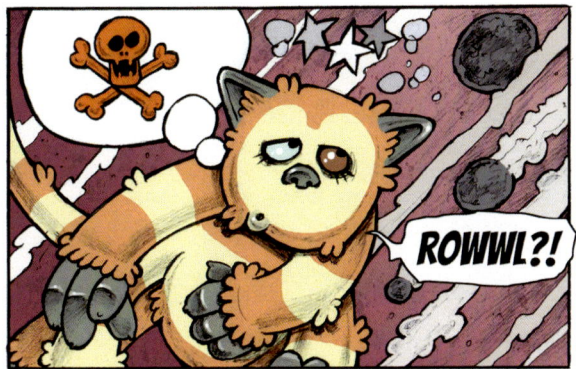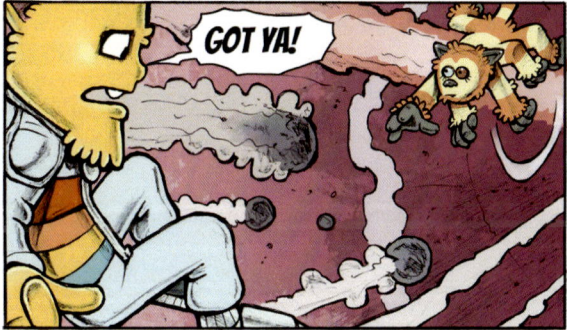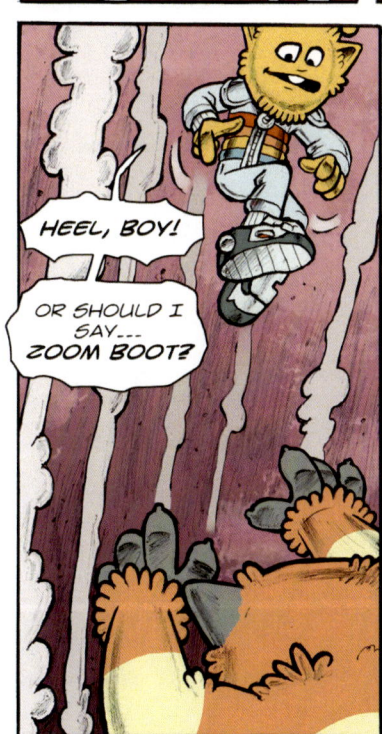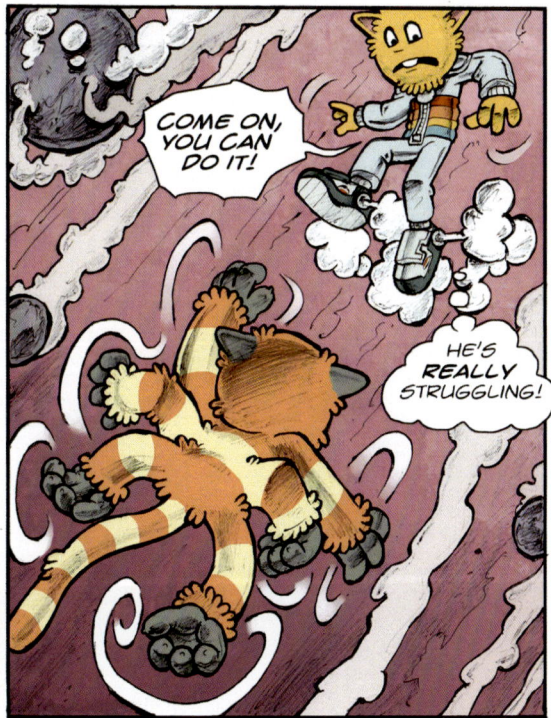

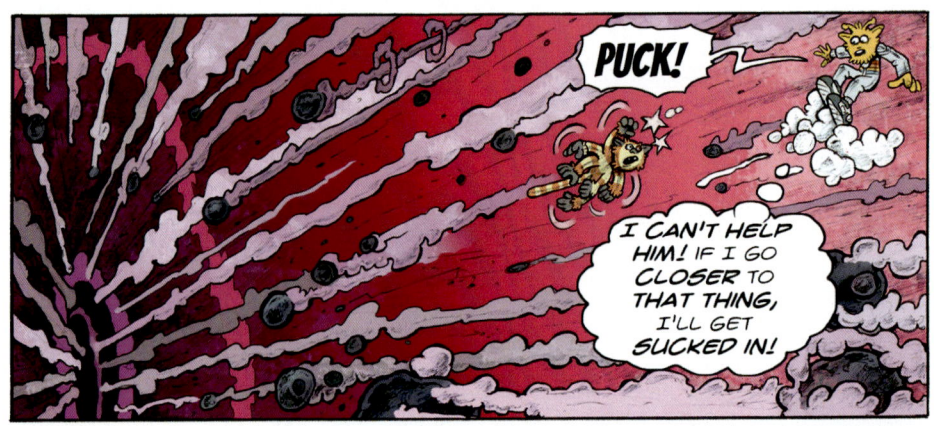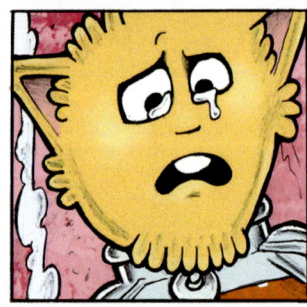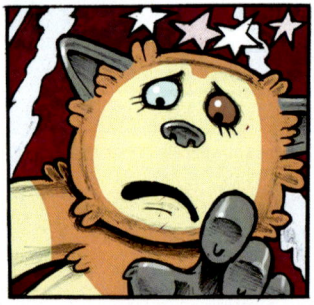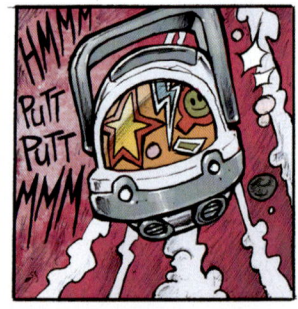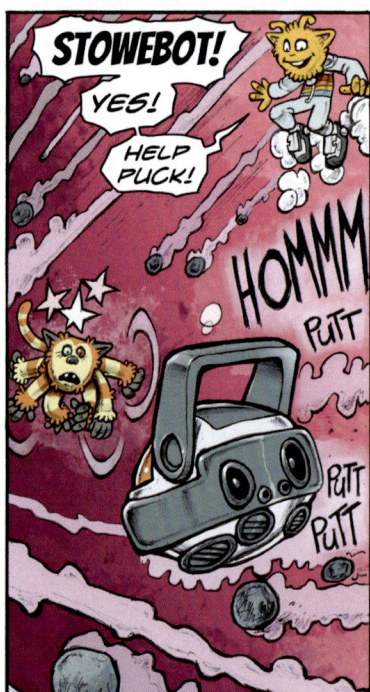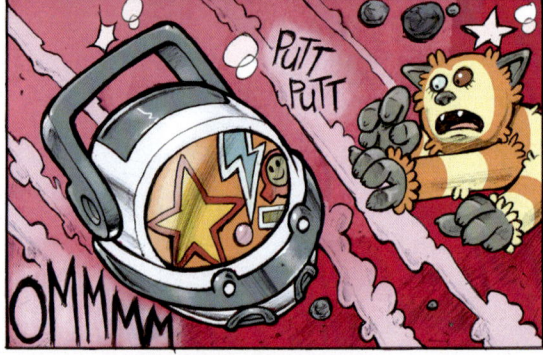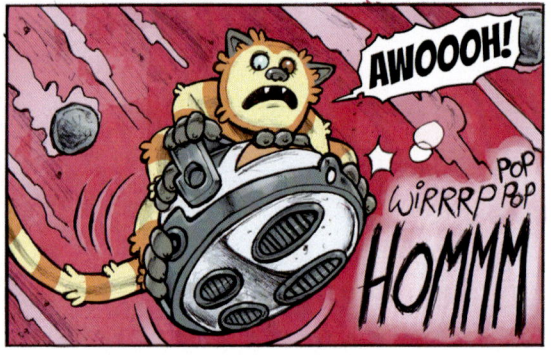

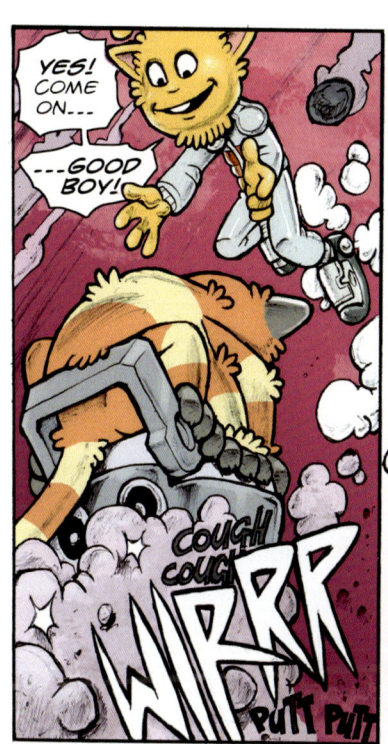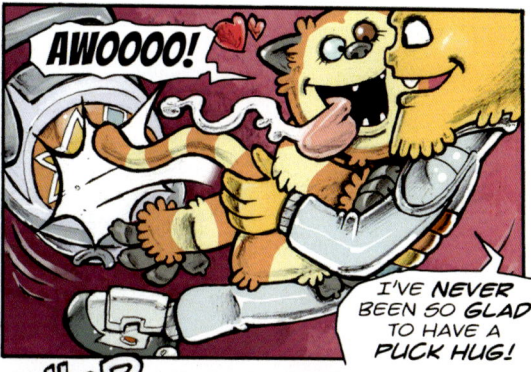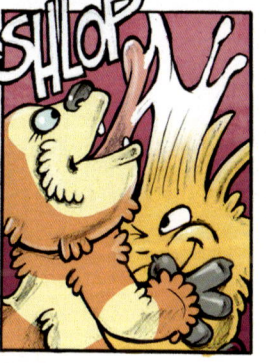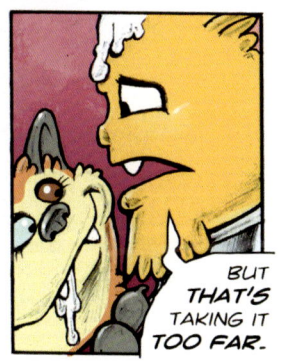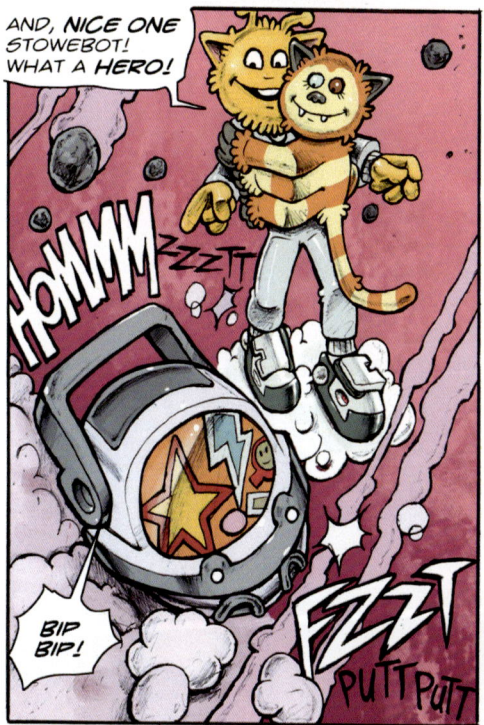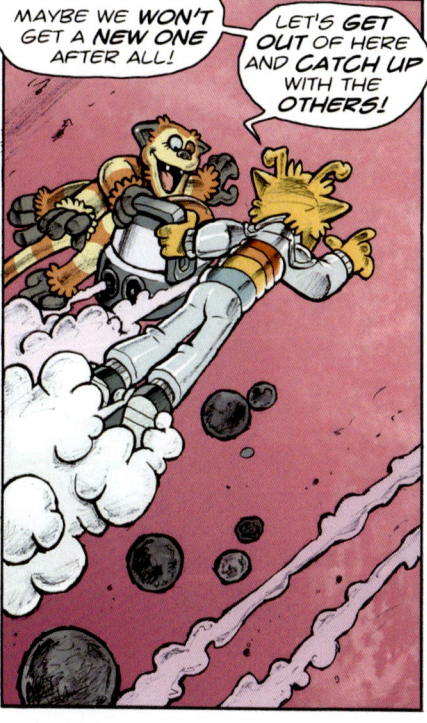

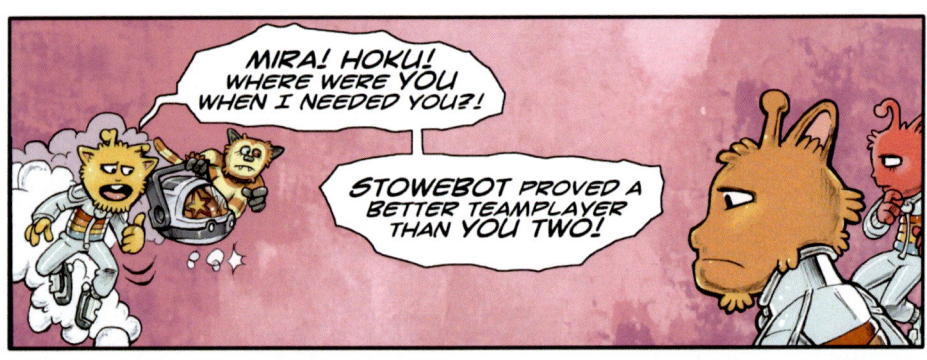
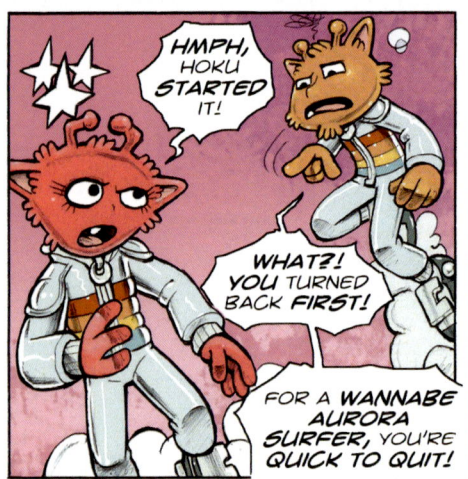
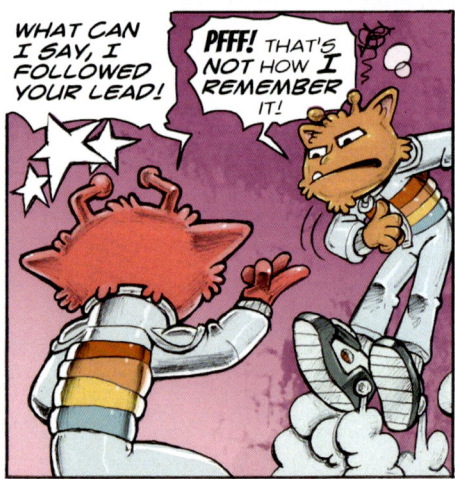
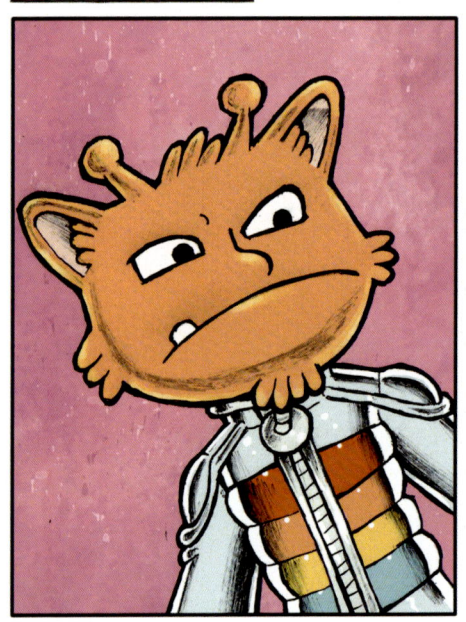
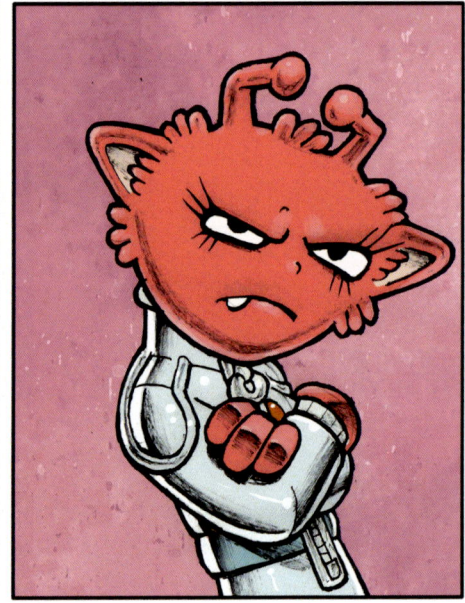

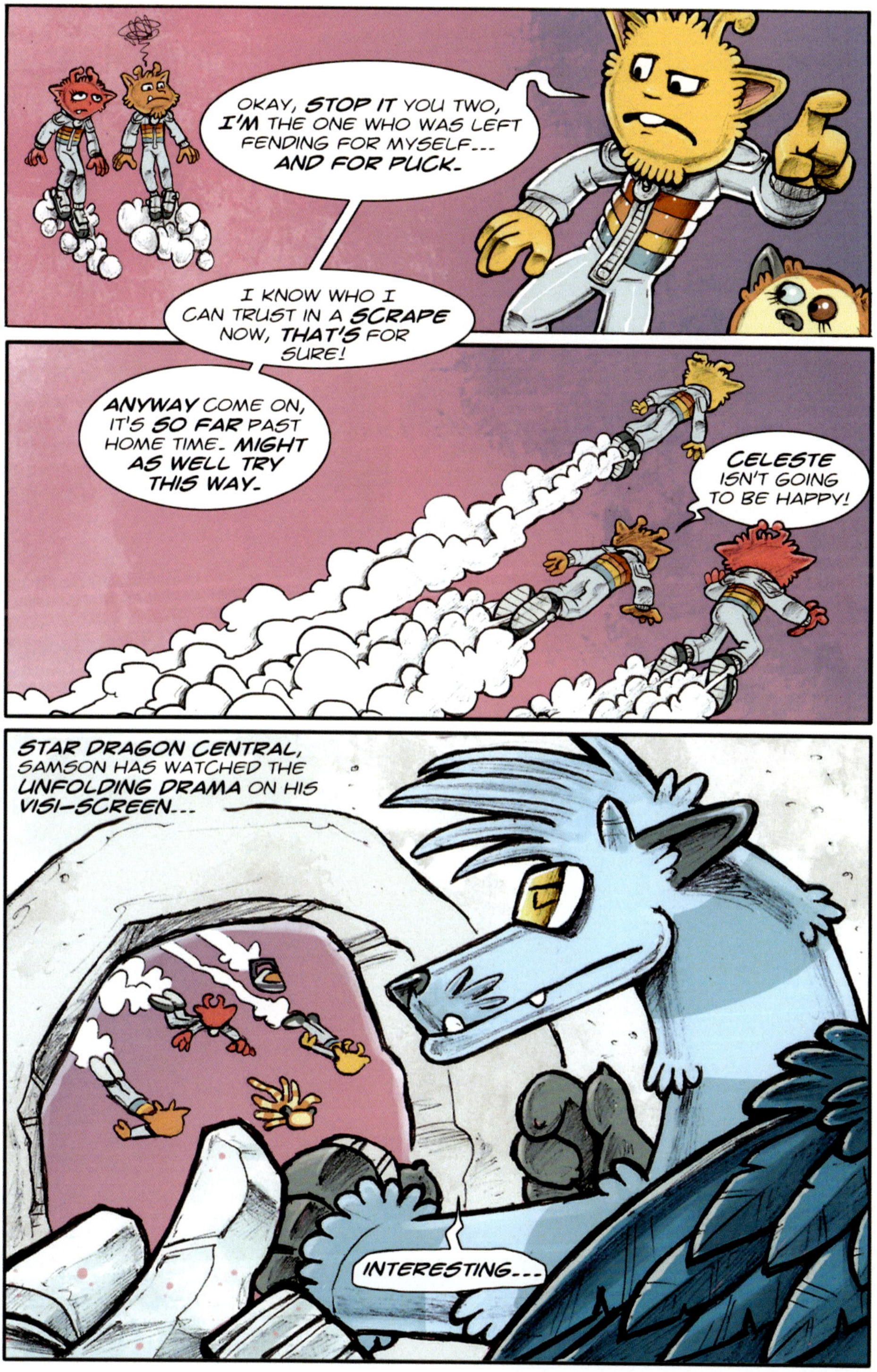

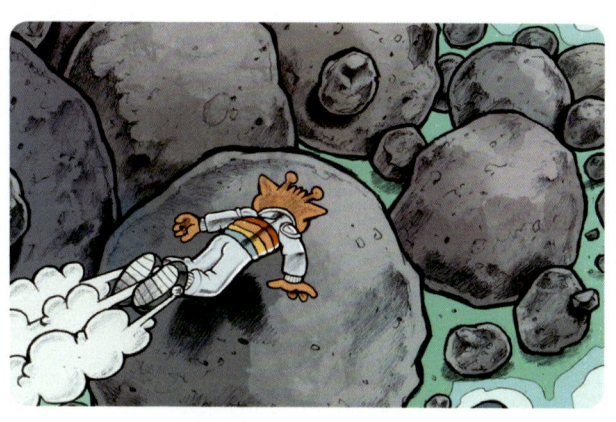

PART TWO

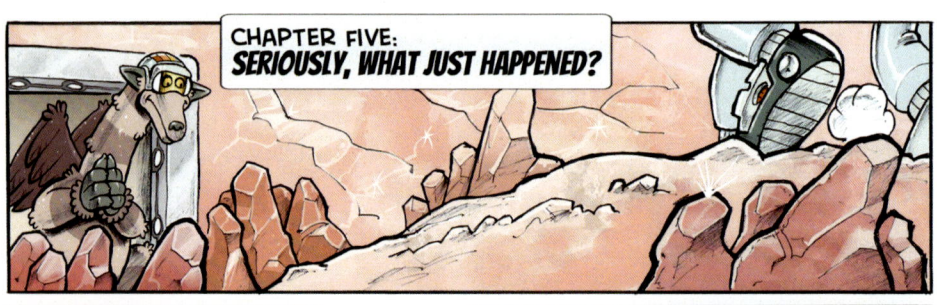
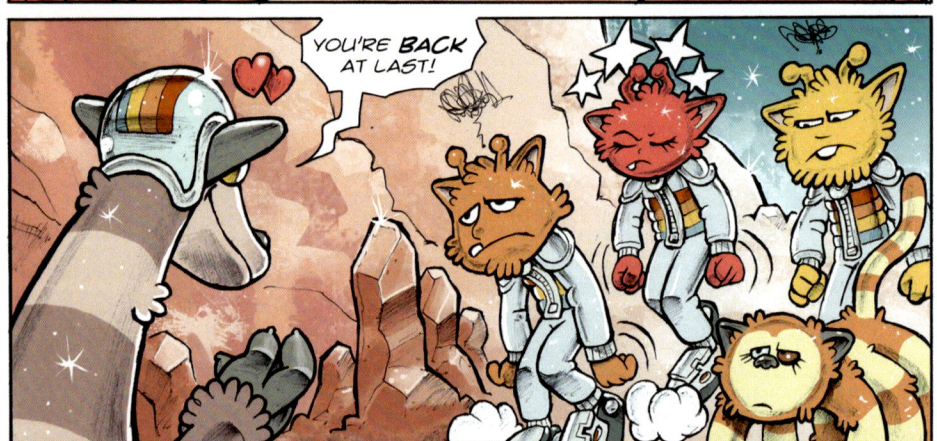
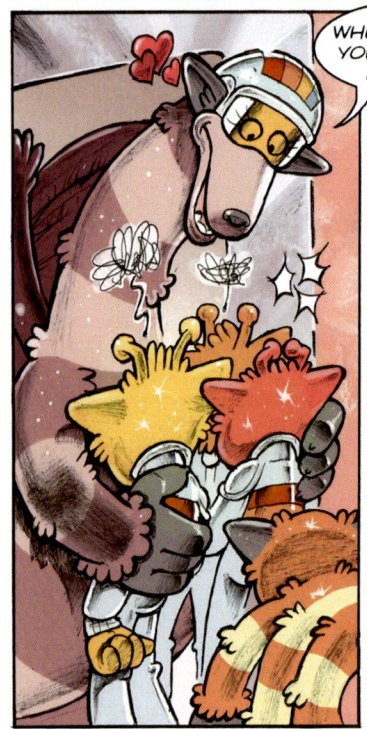
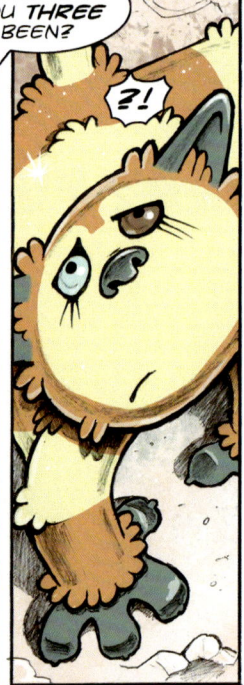
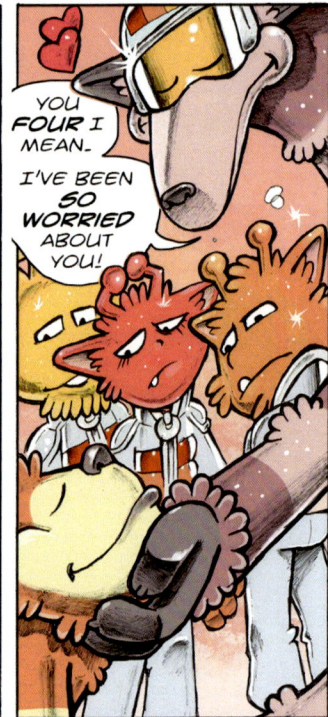

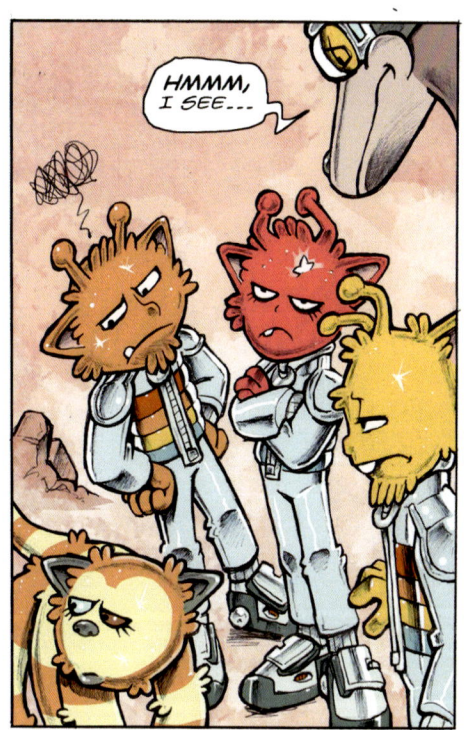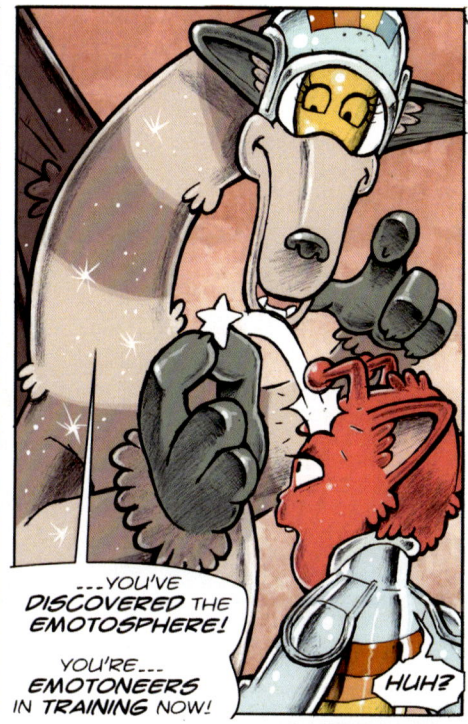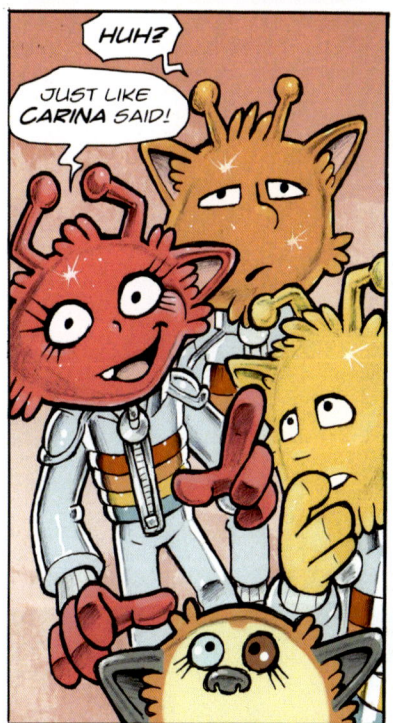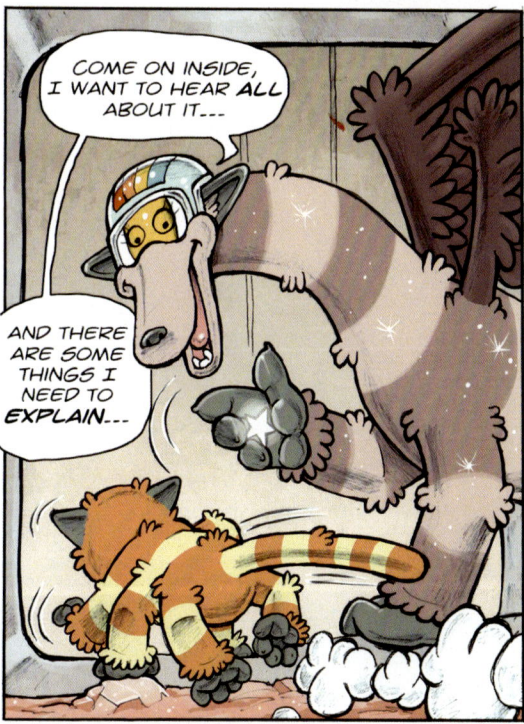

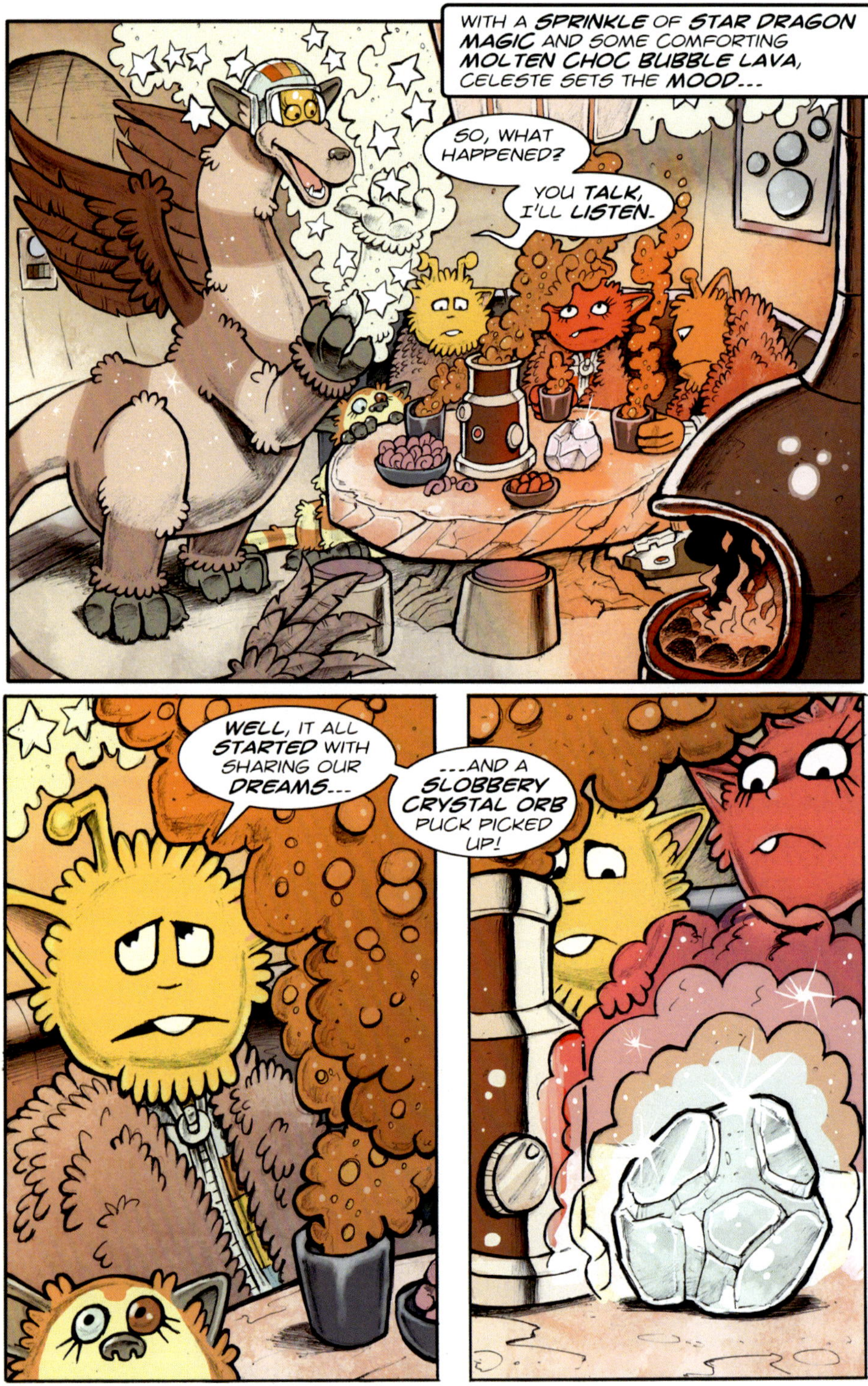

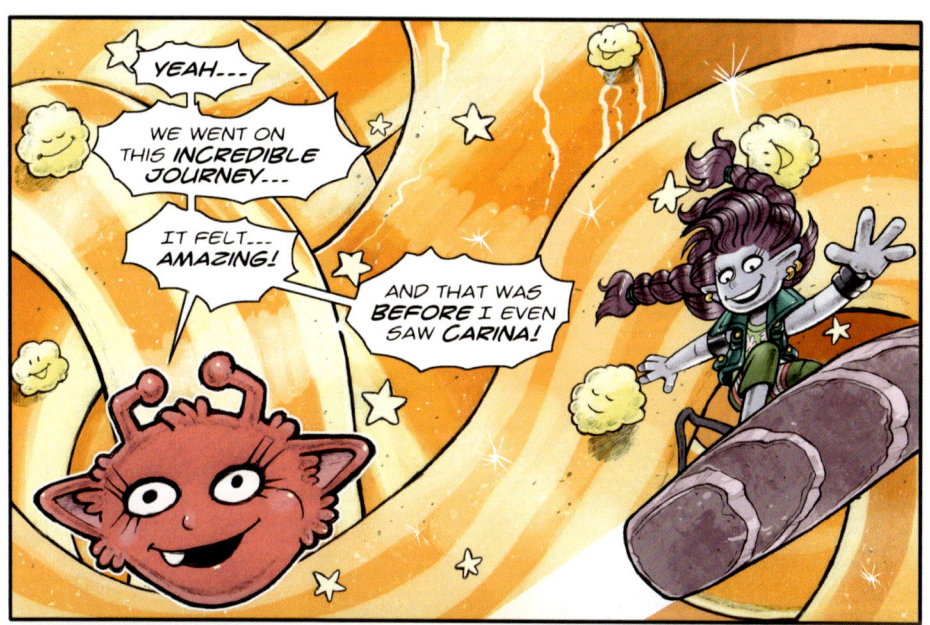

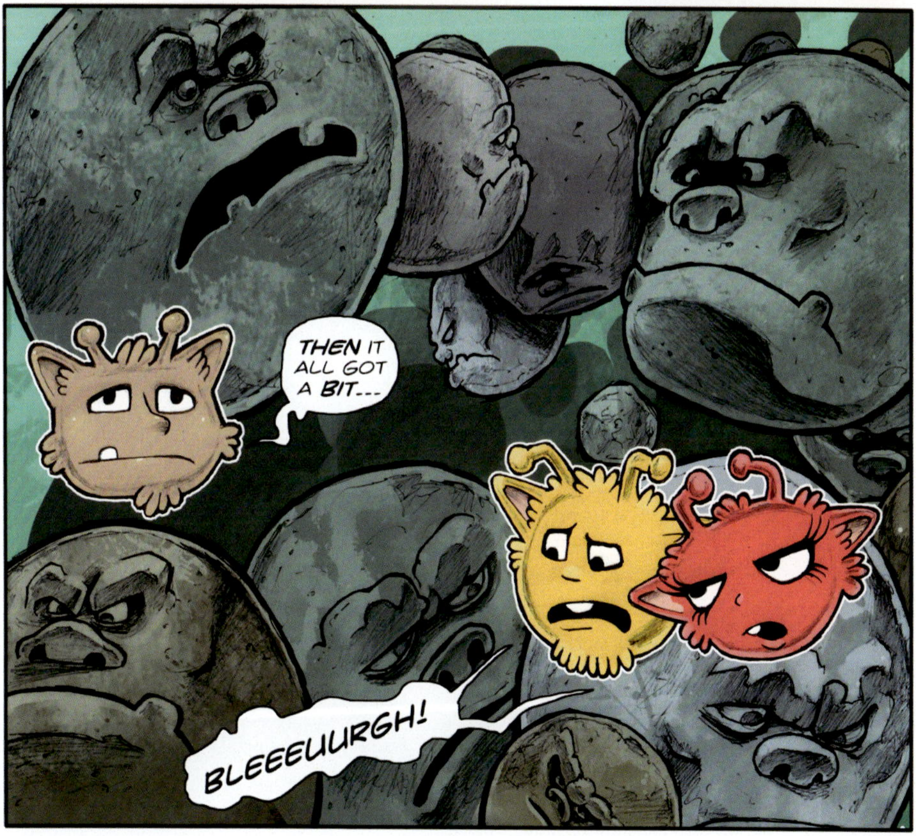

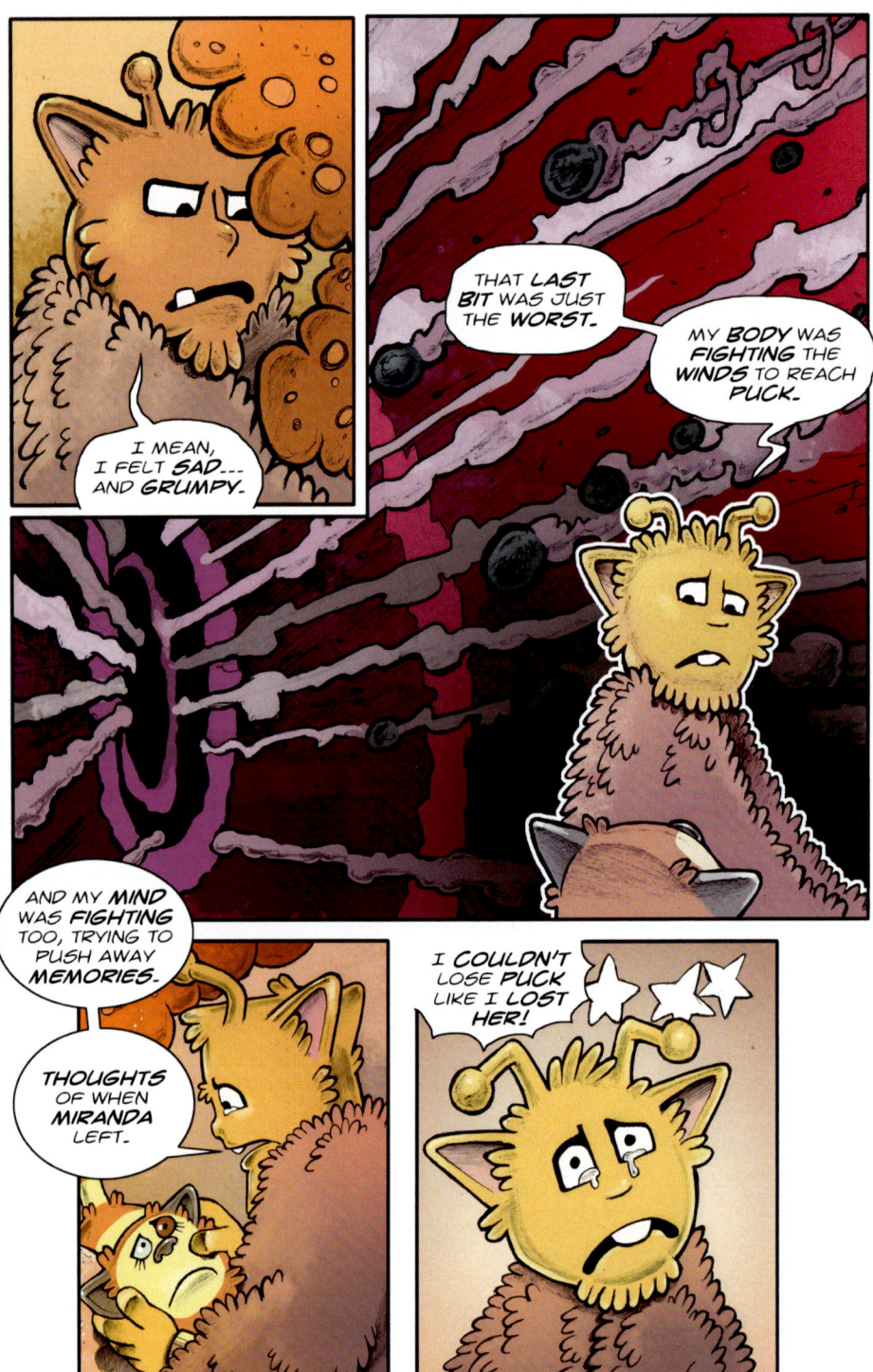

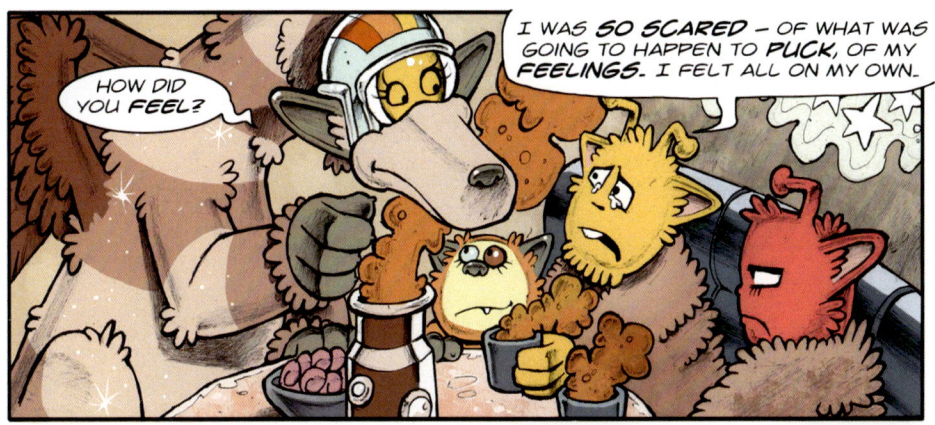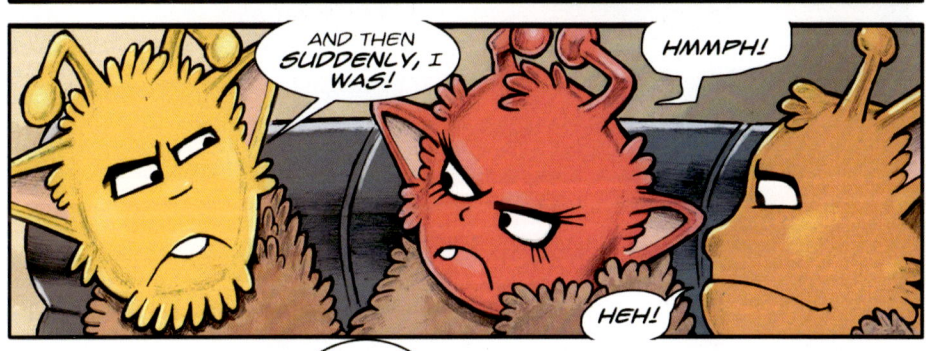

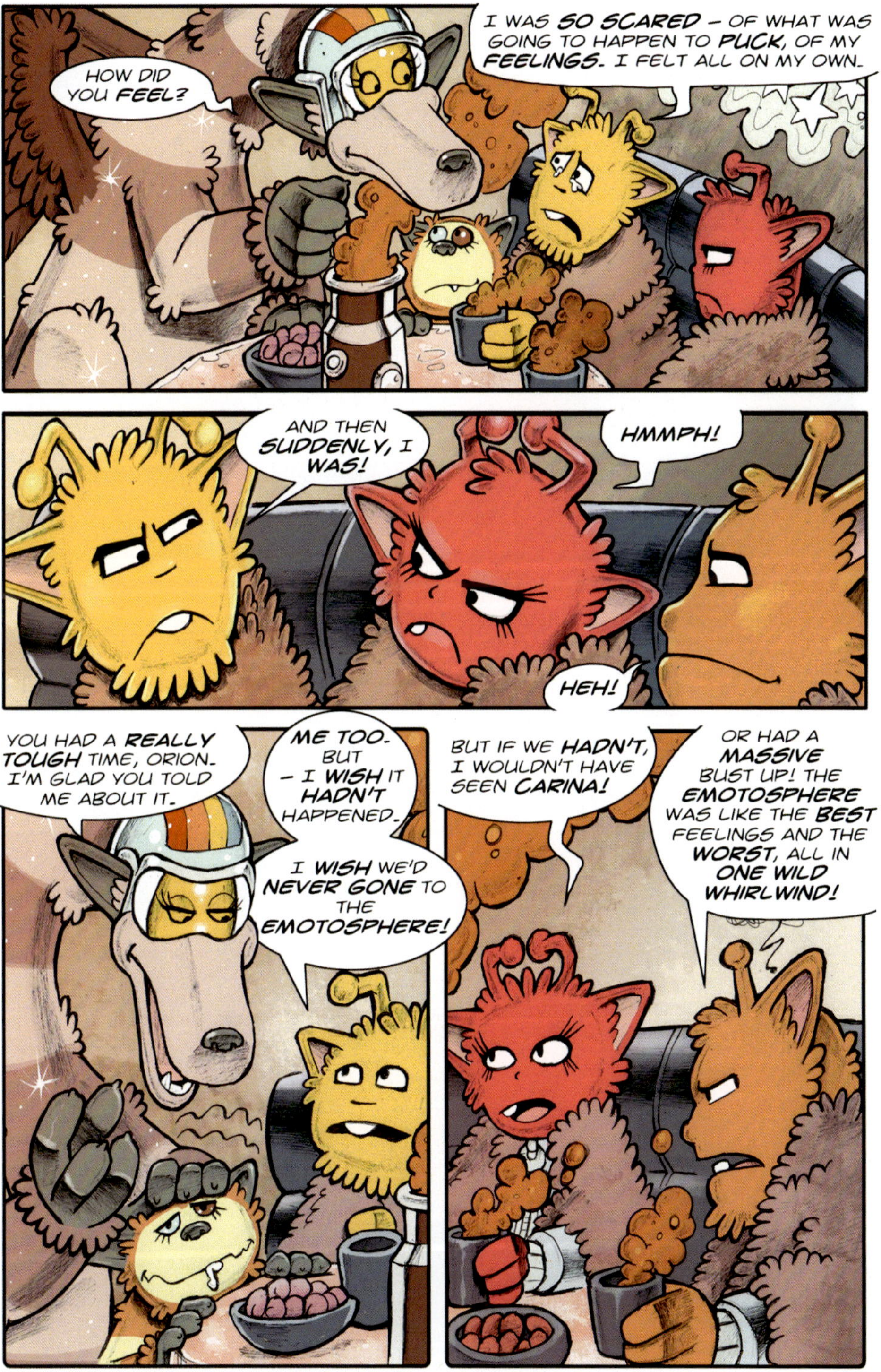

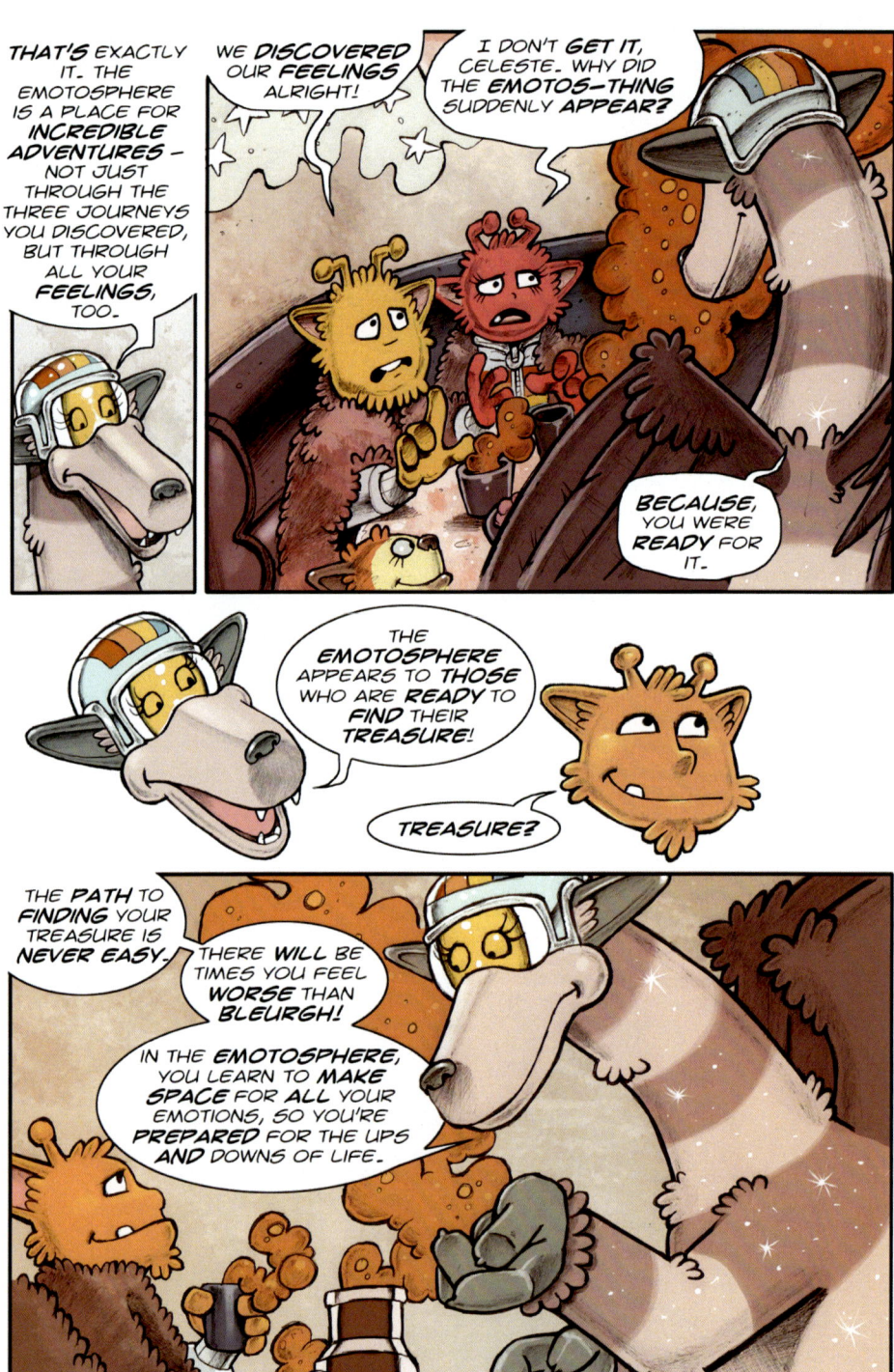

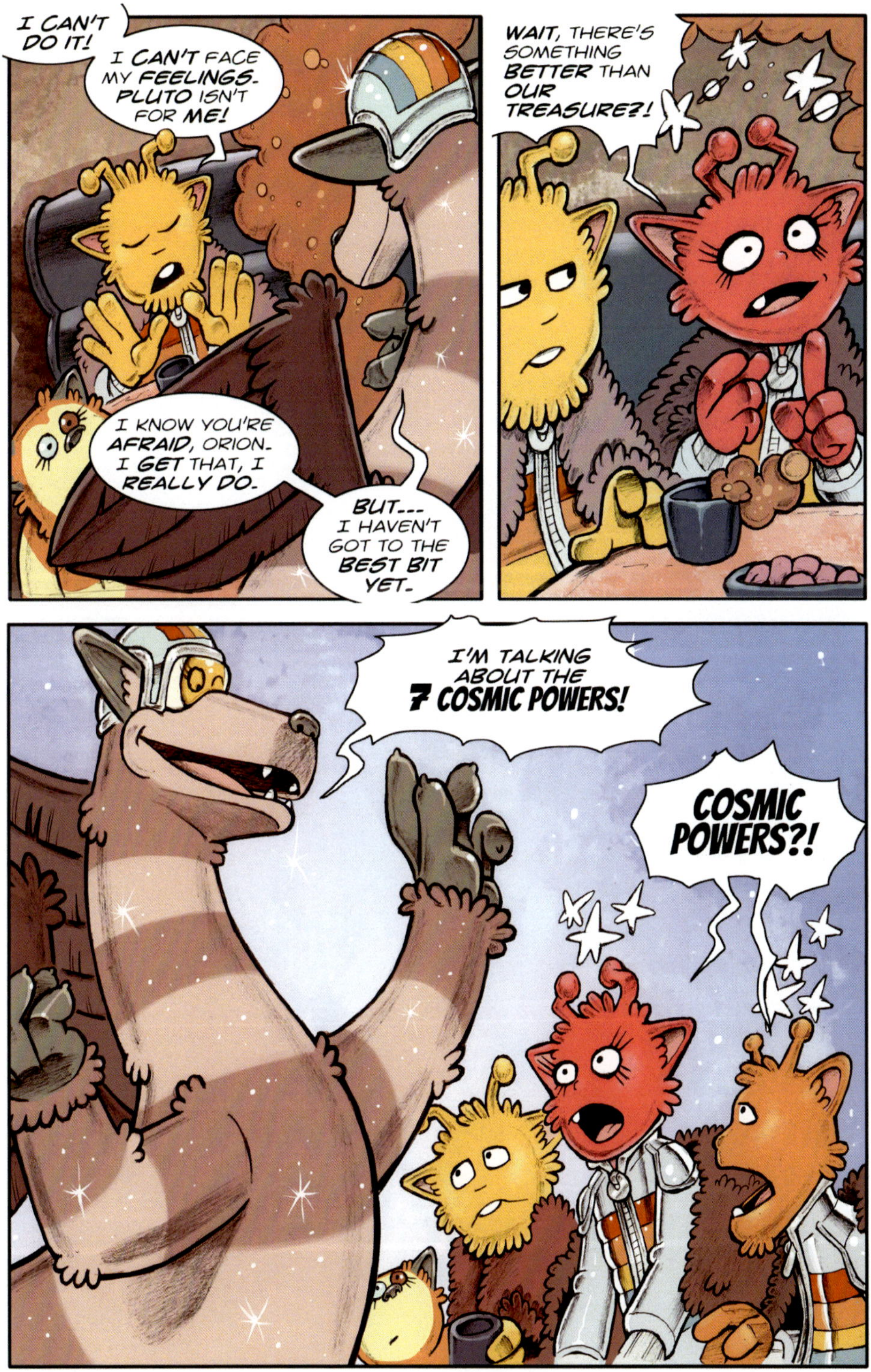

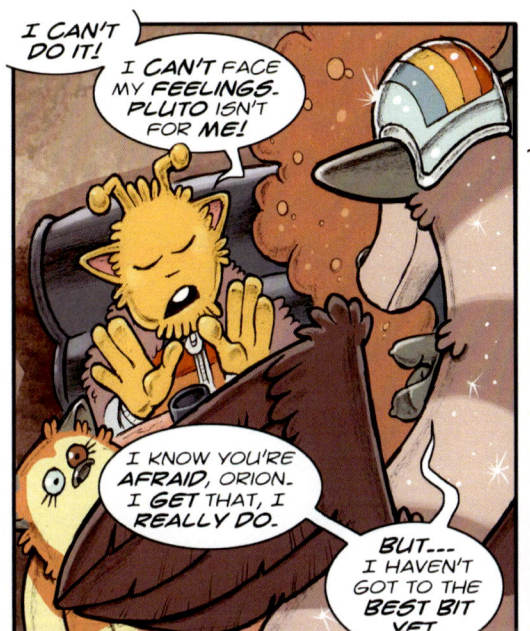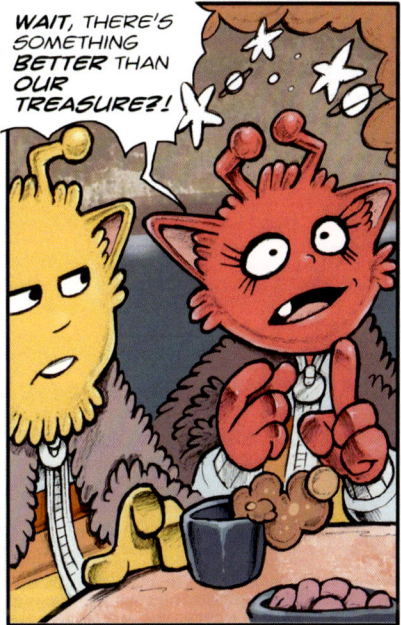

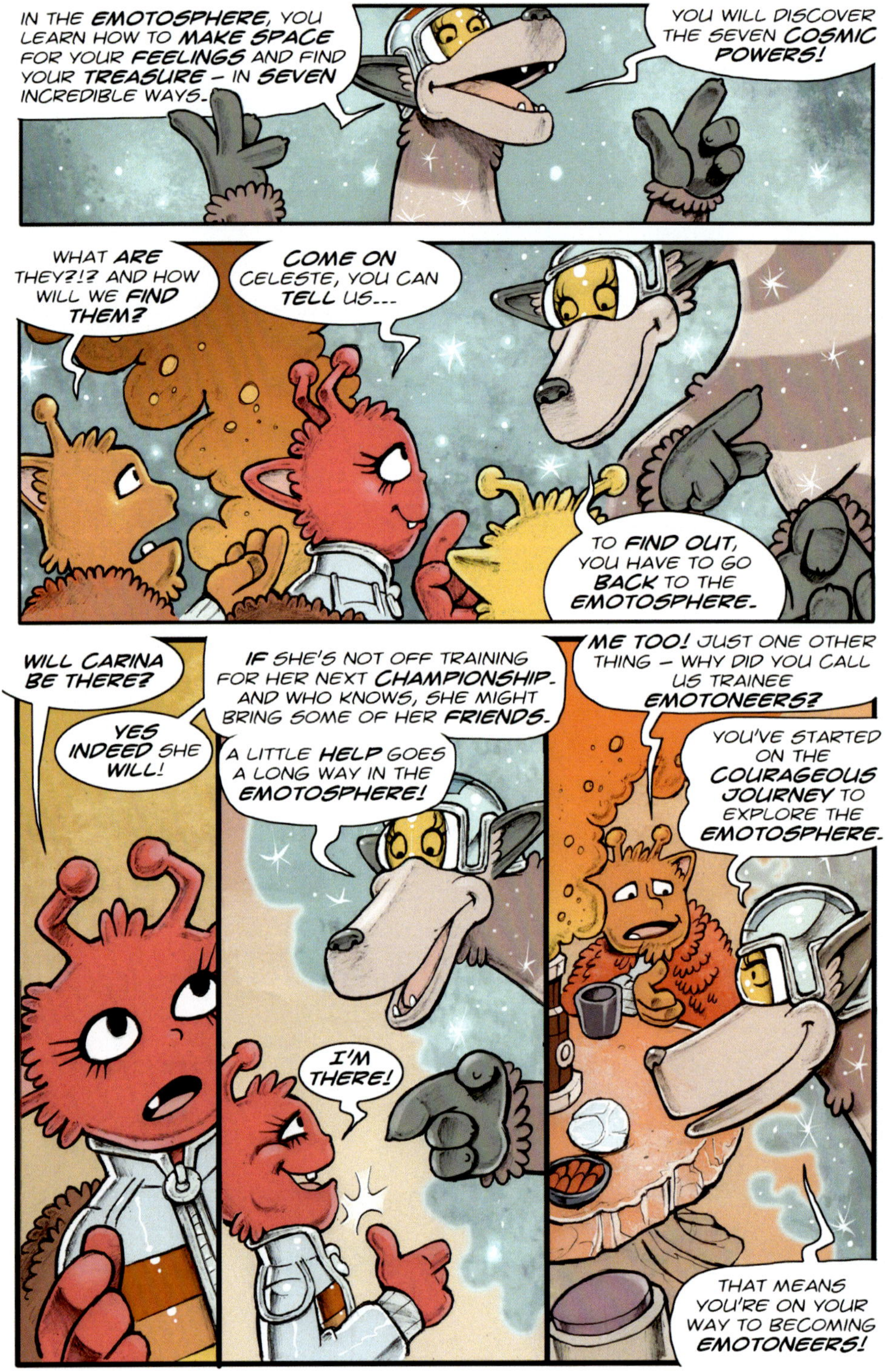

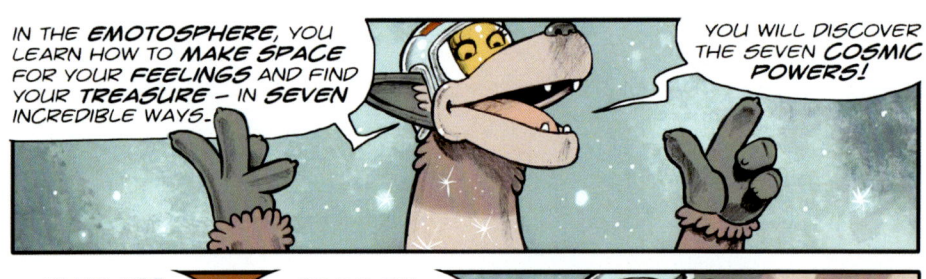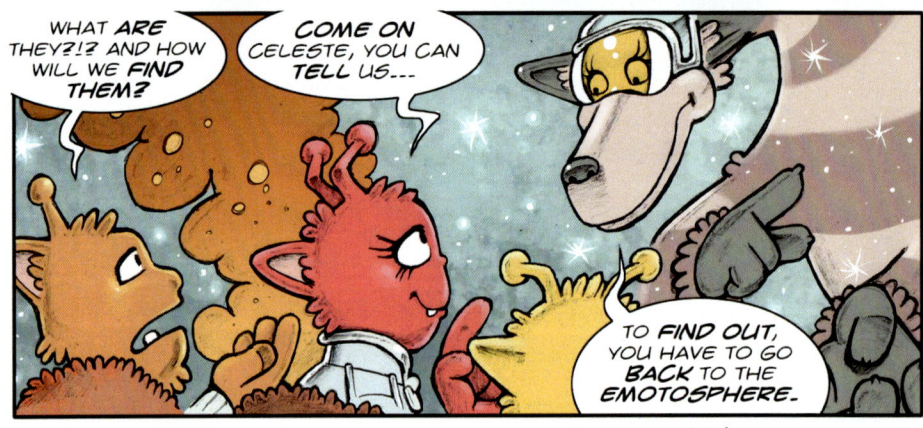

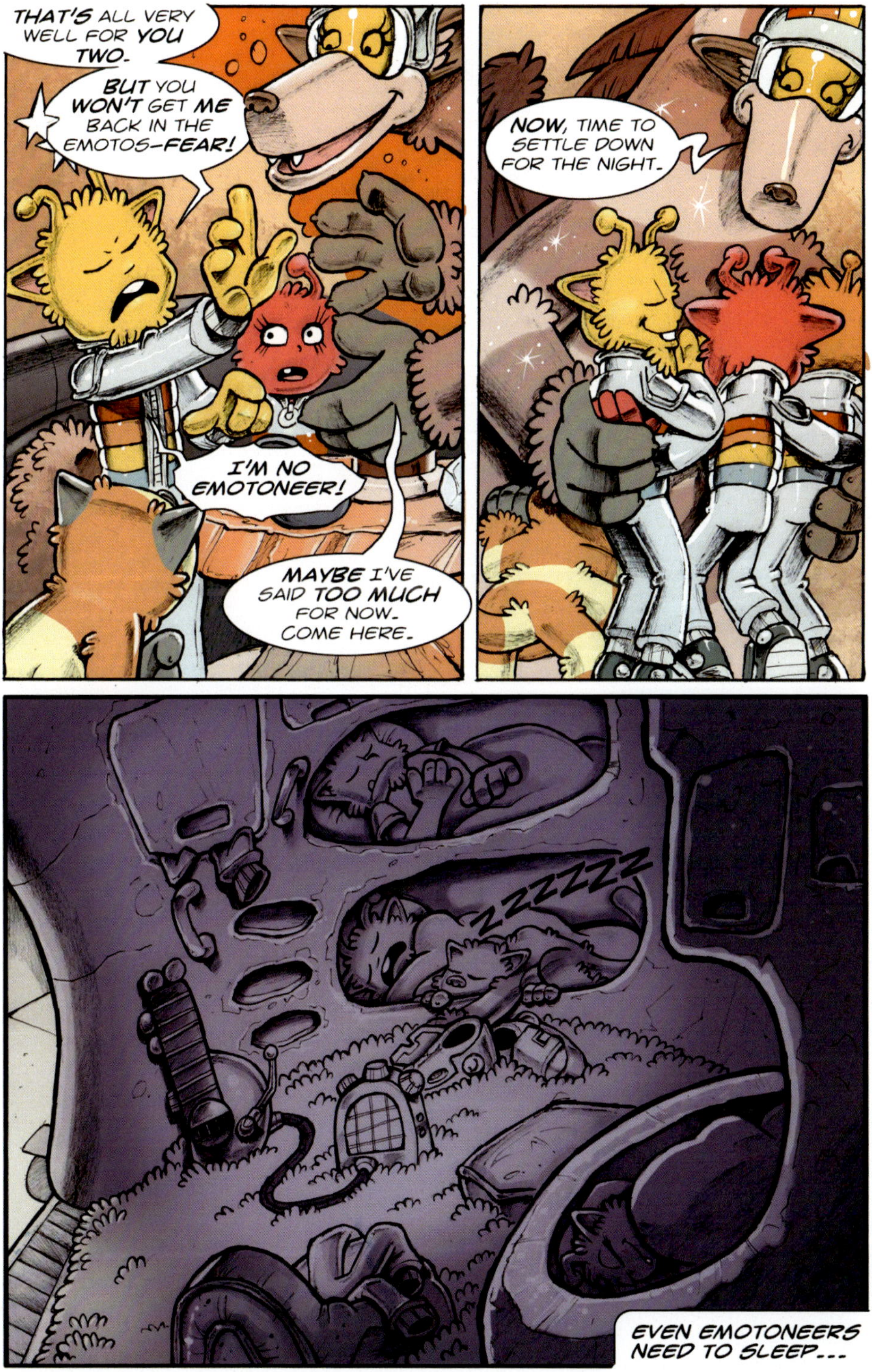

THAT'S ALL VERY WELL FOR *YOU* TWO.

BUT YOU WON'T GET *ME* BACK IN THE EMOTOS—*FEAR*!

I'M NO EMOTONEER!

MAYBE I'VE SAID *TOO MUCH* FOR NOW... COME HERE.

NOW, TIME TO SETTLE DOWN FOR THE NIGHT.

EVEN EMOTONEERS NEED TO SLEEP...

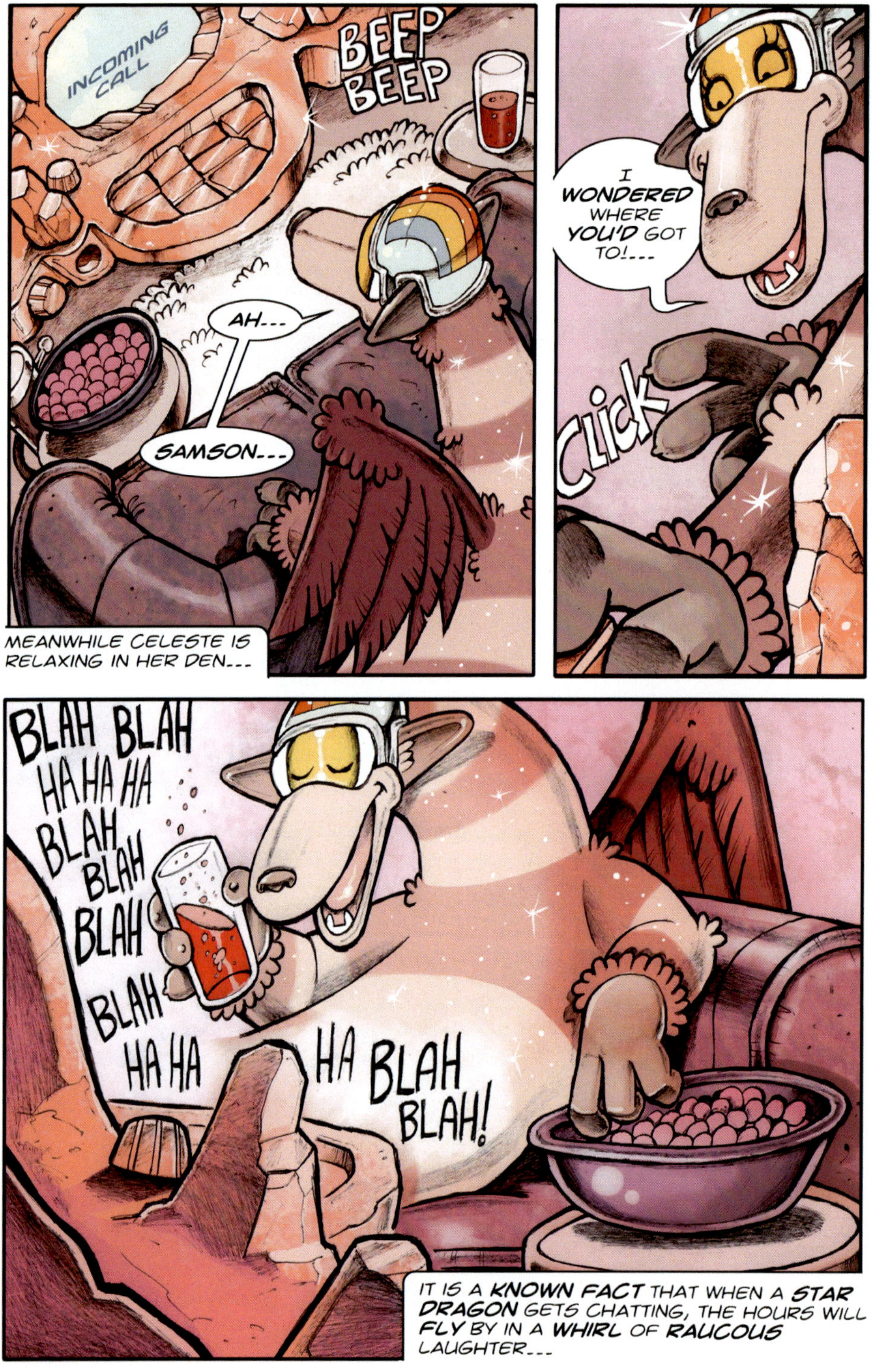

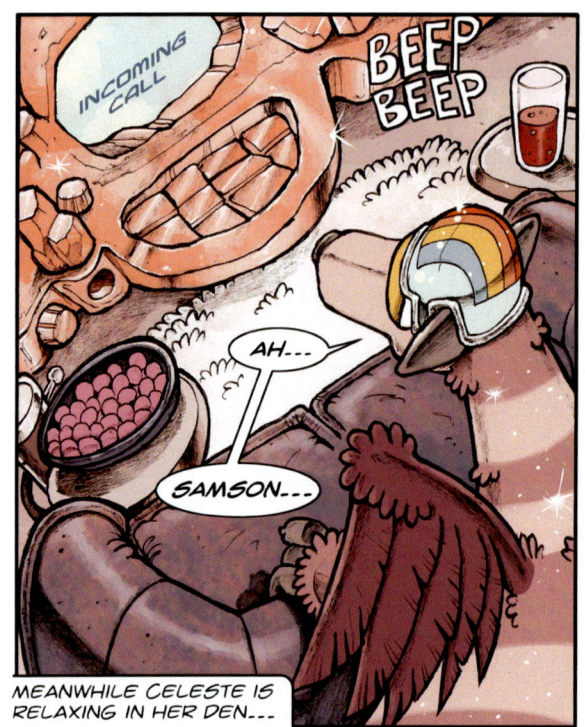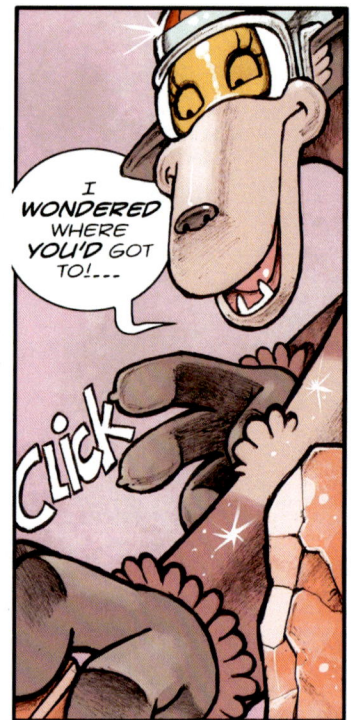

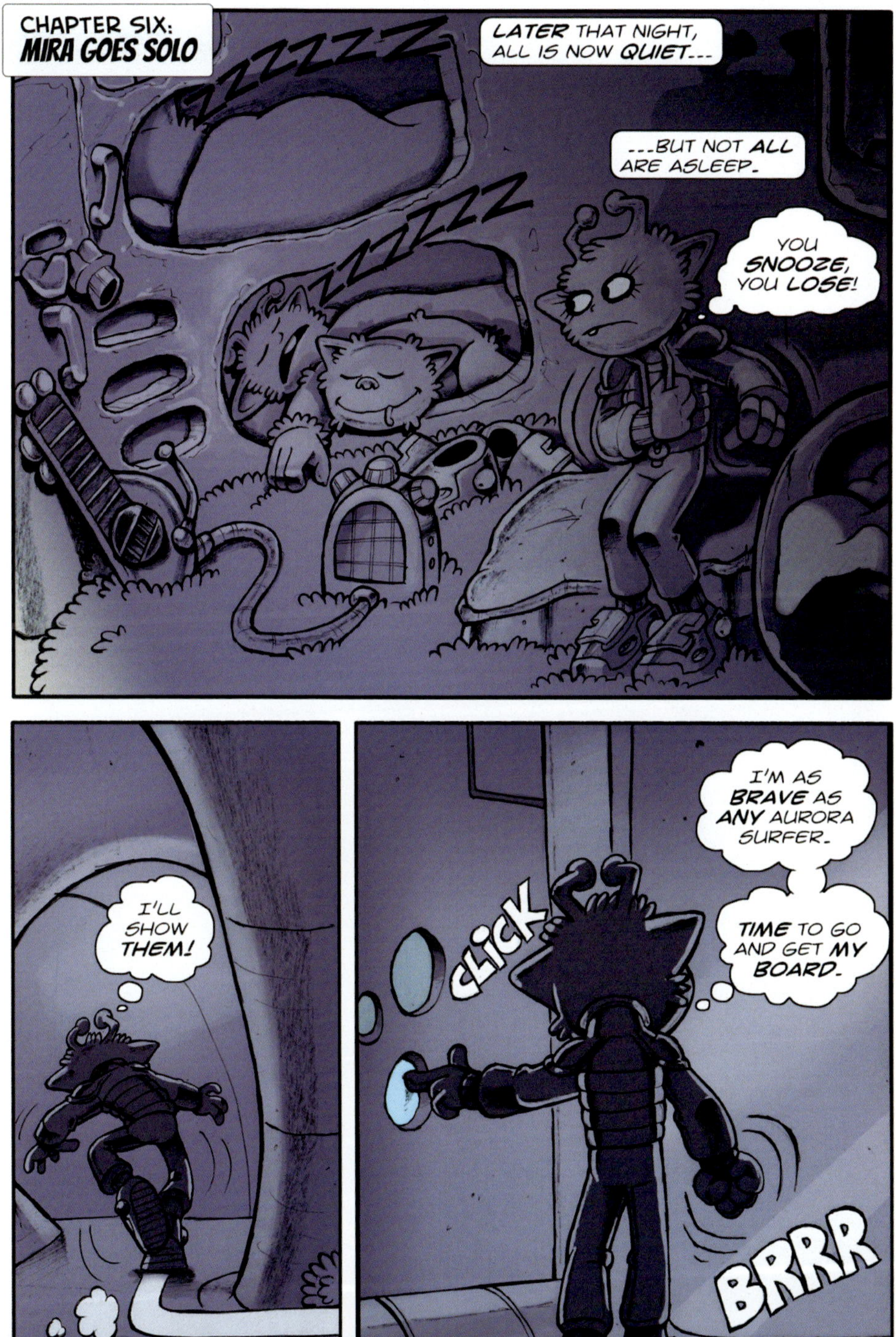

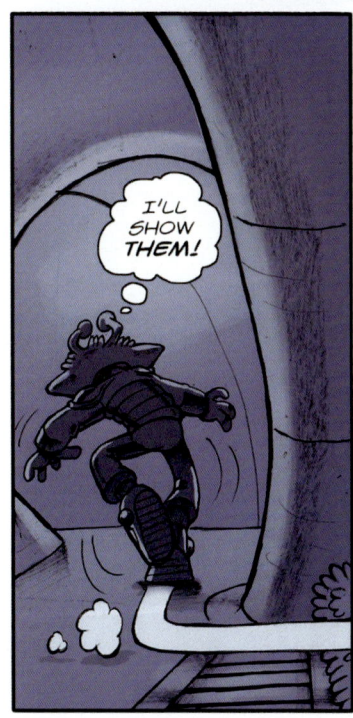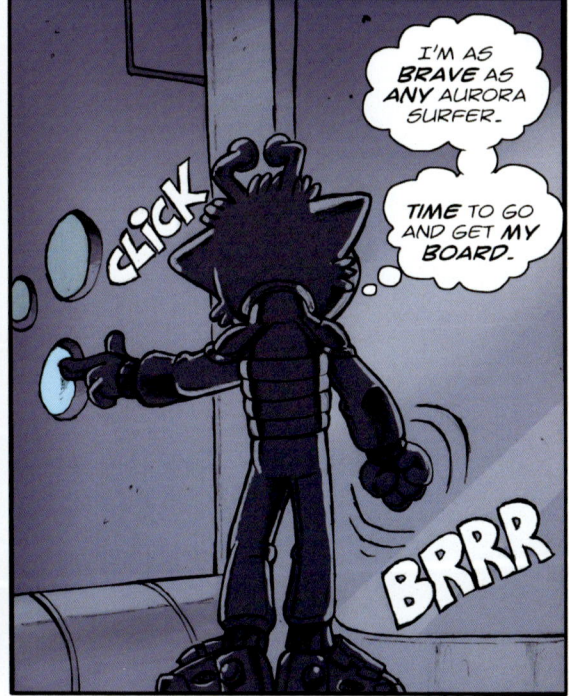

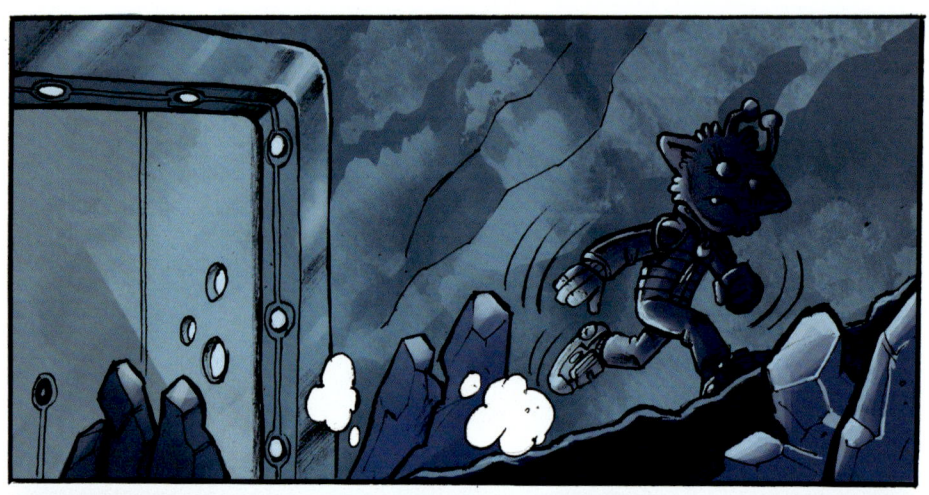
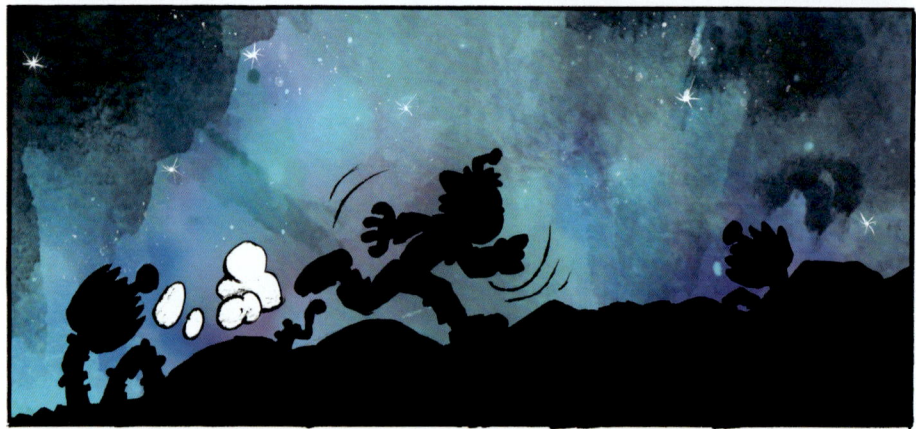
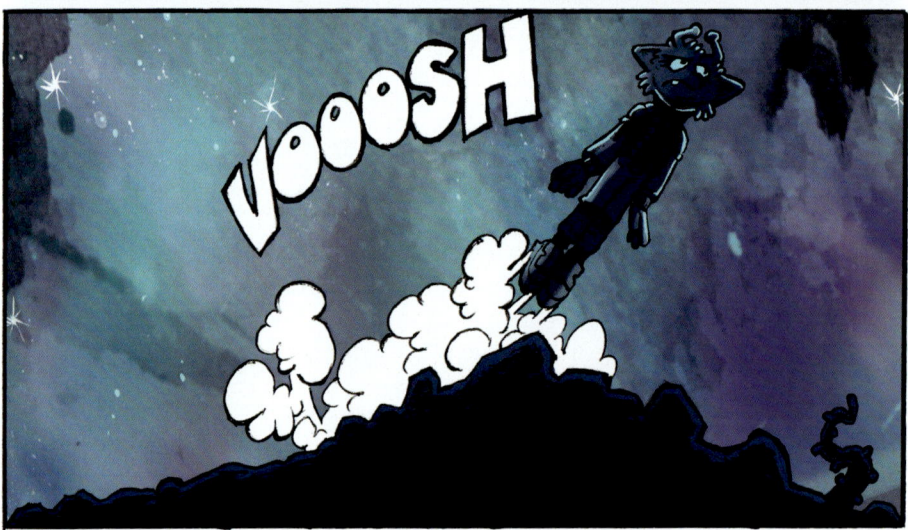

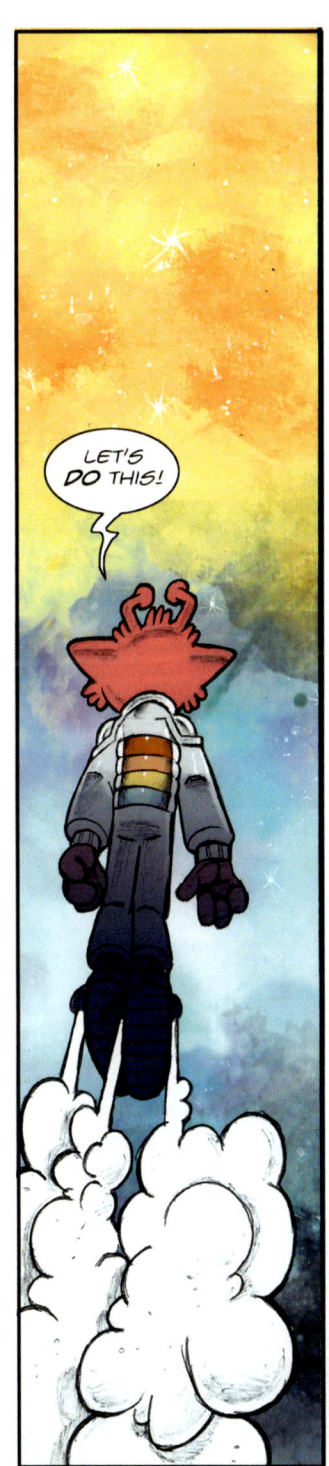

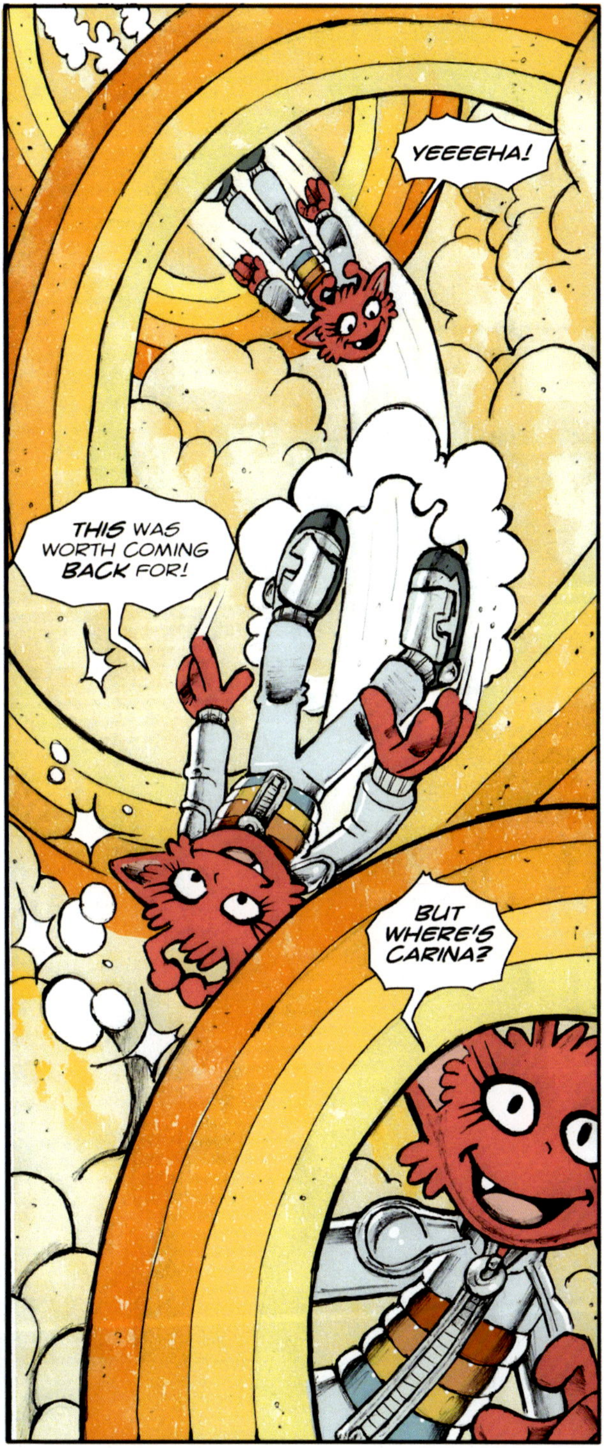

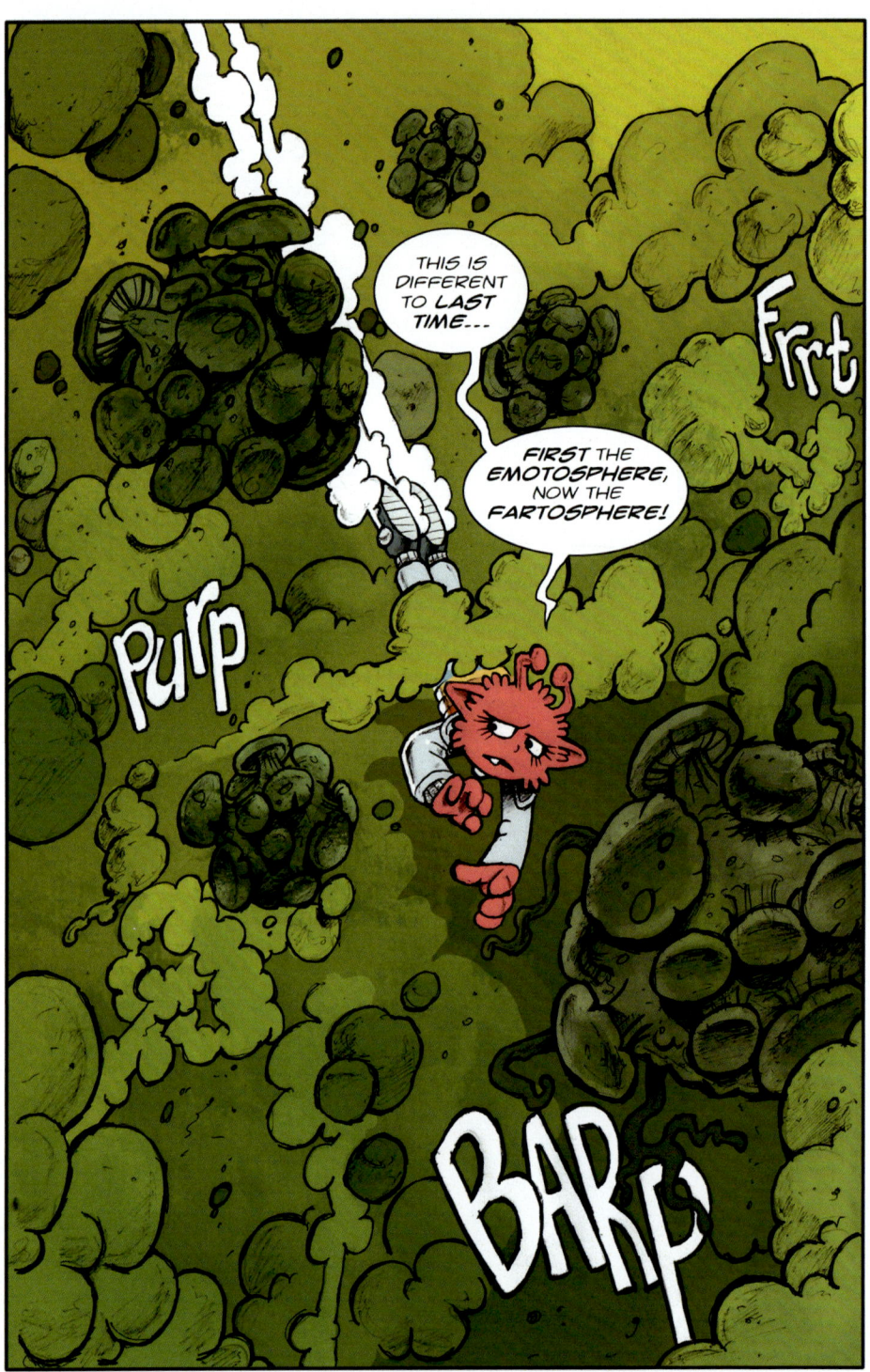

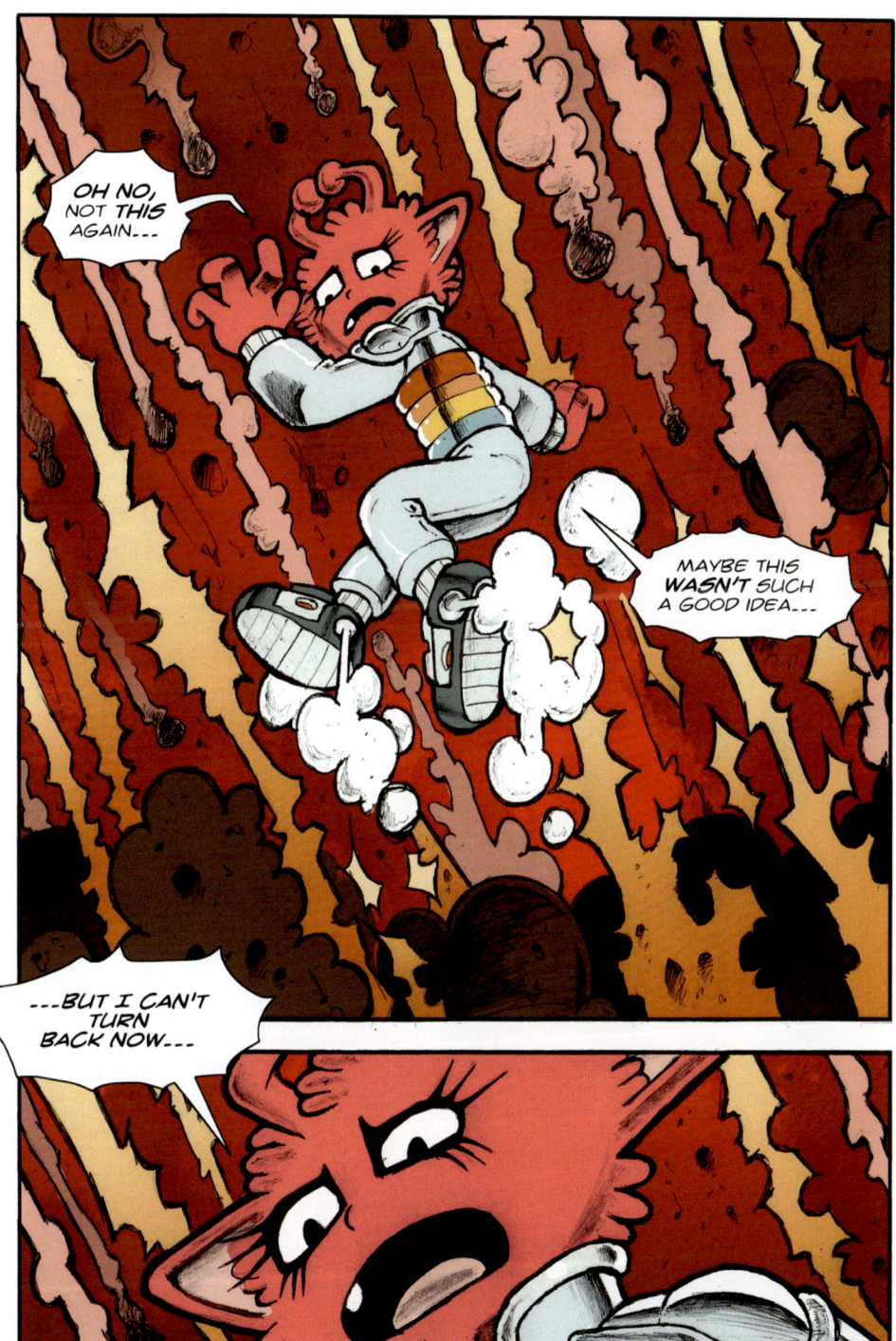

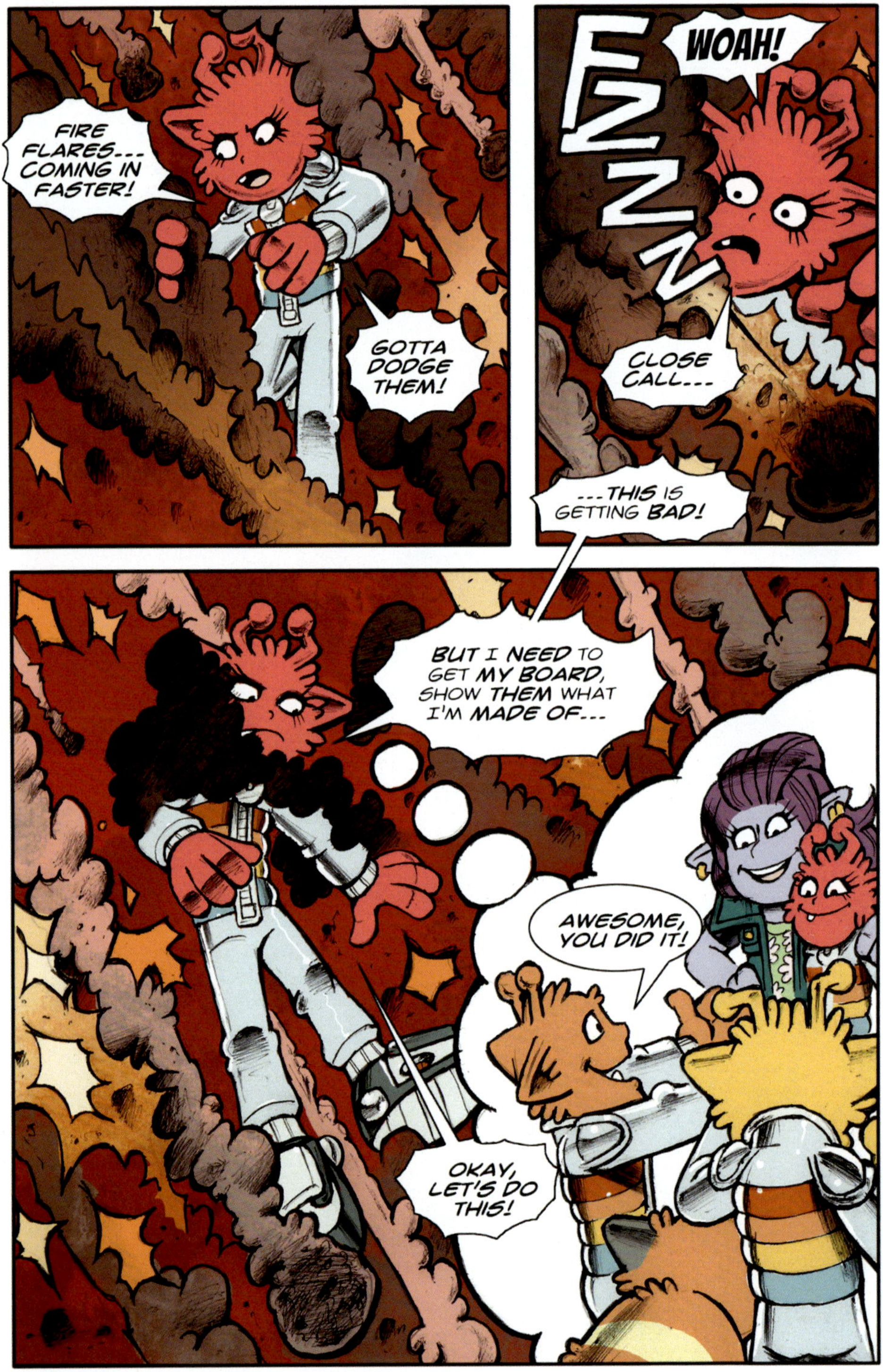

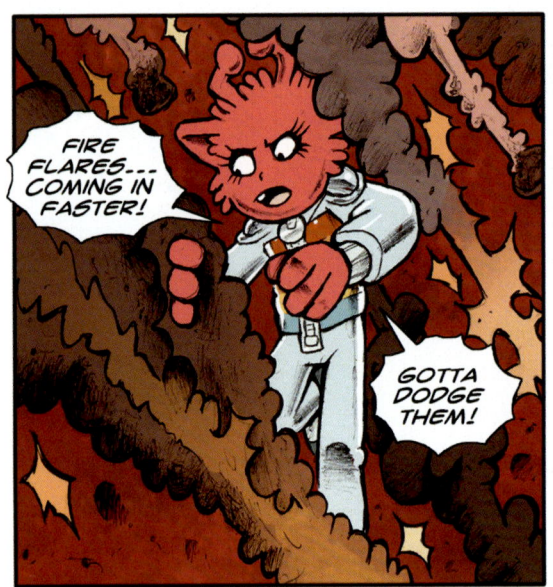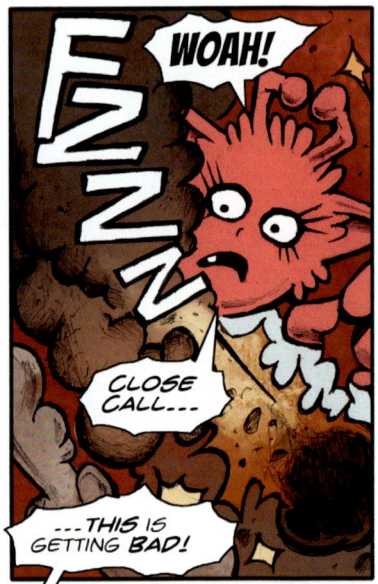

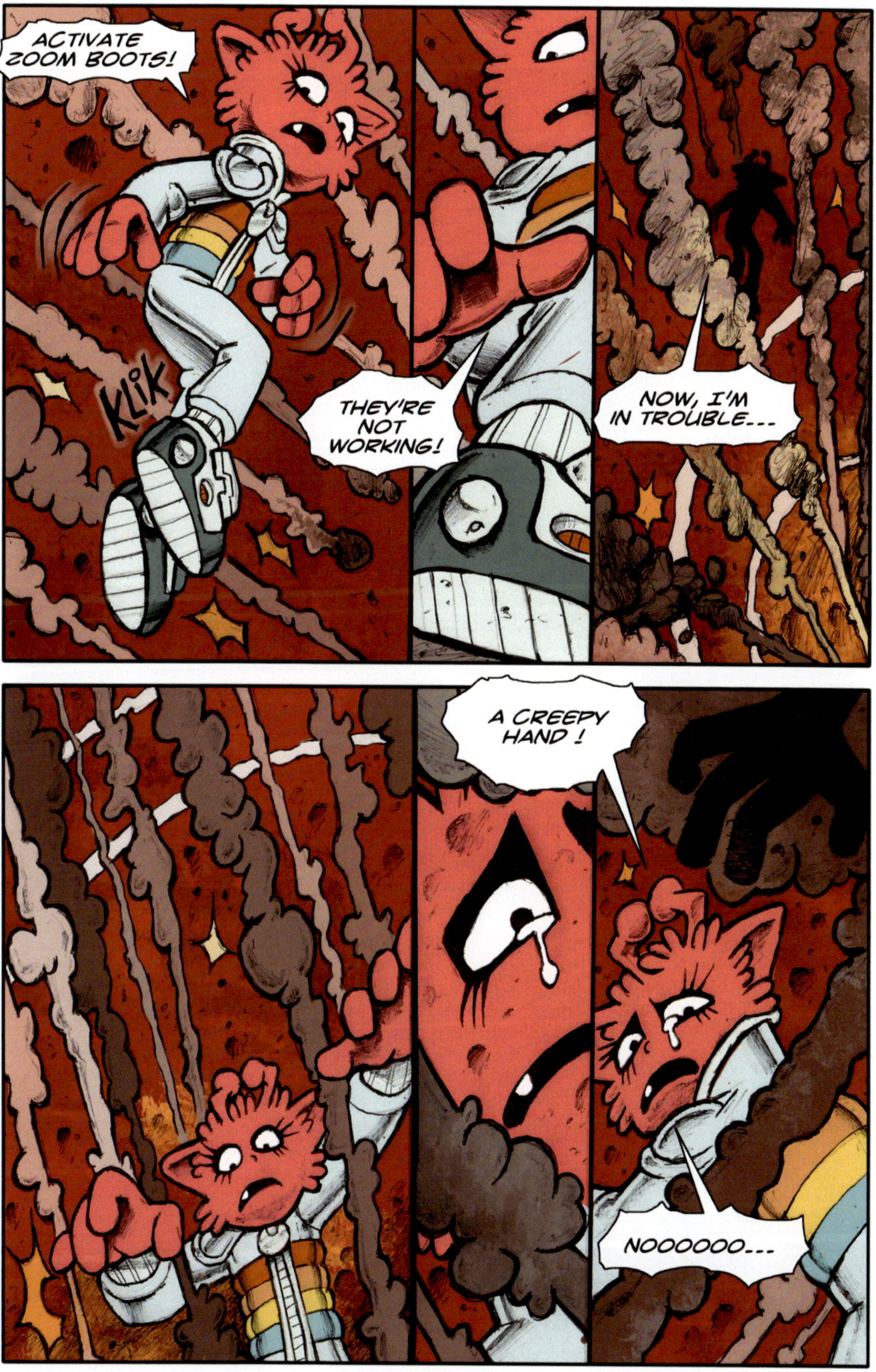

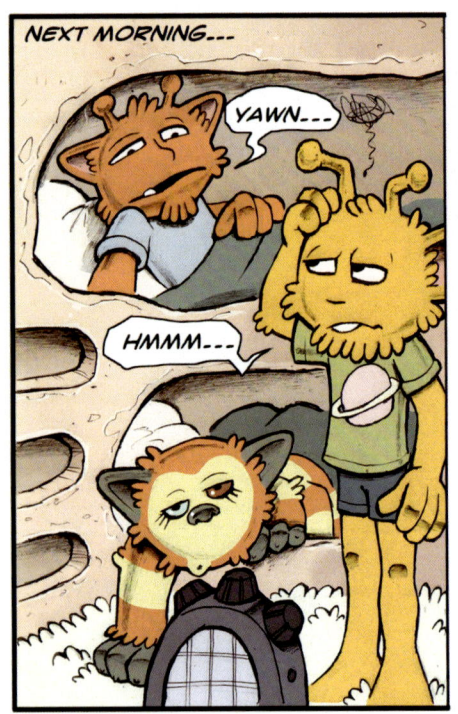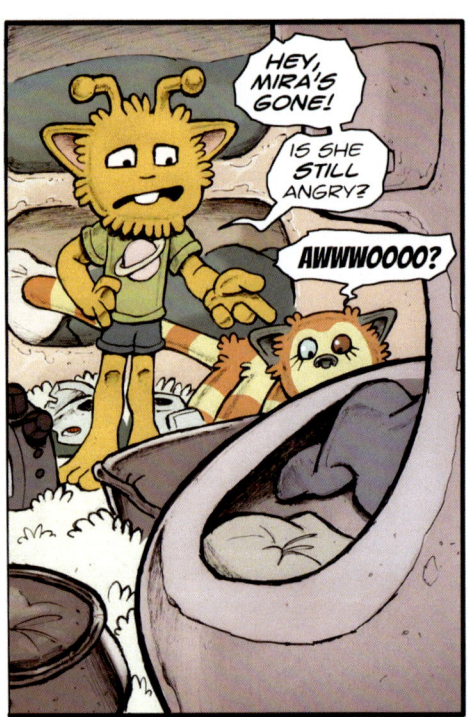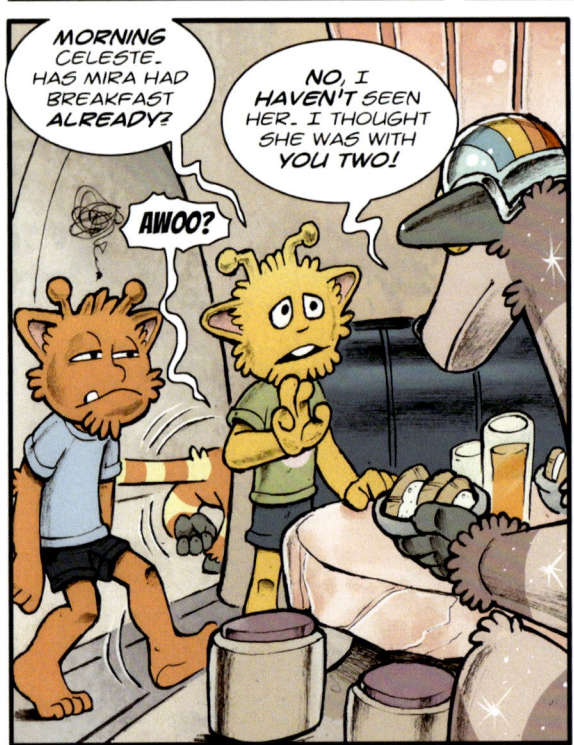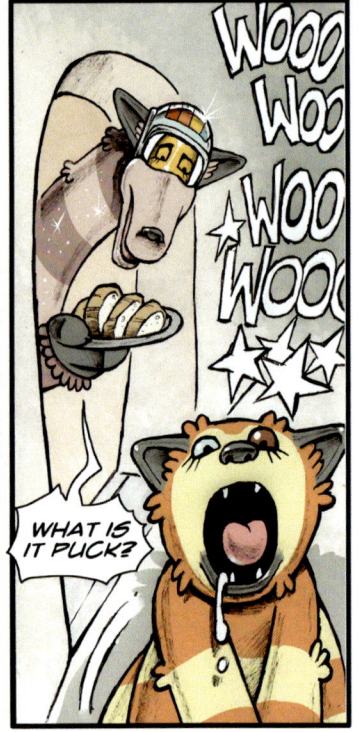

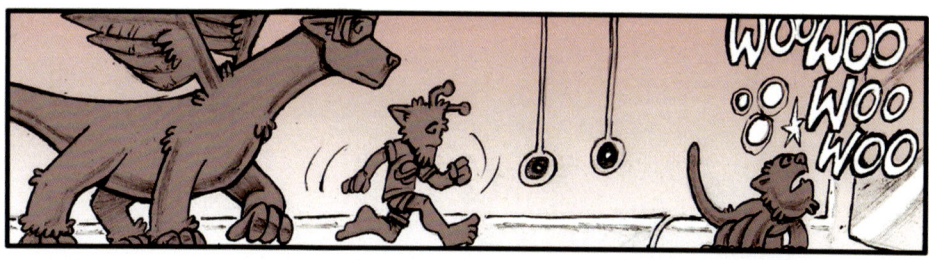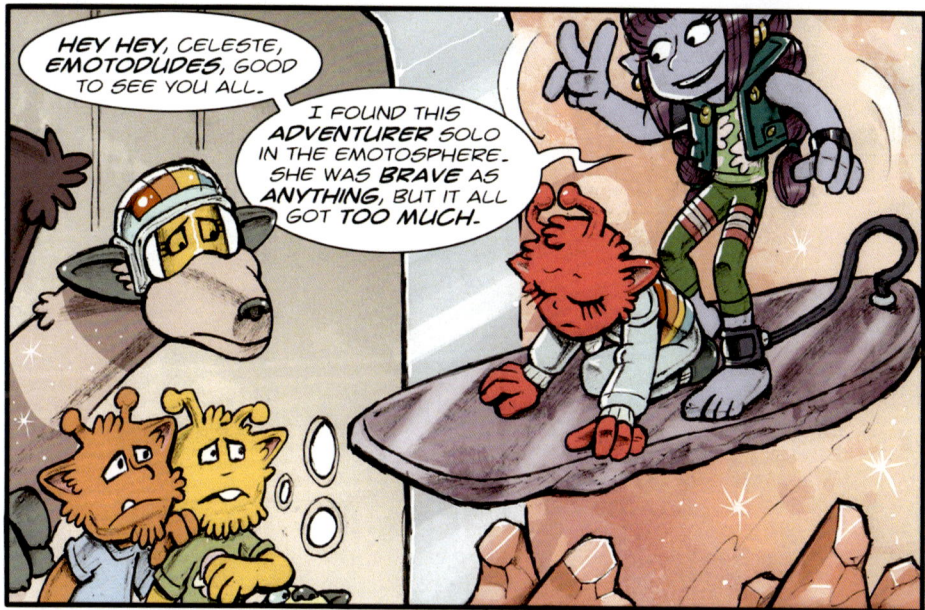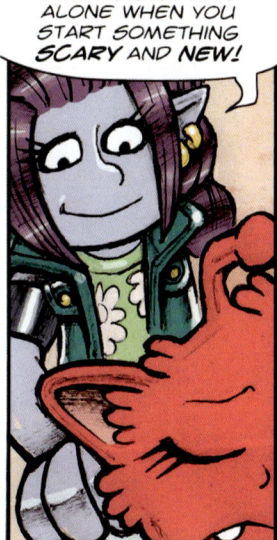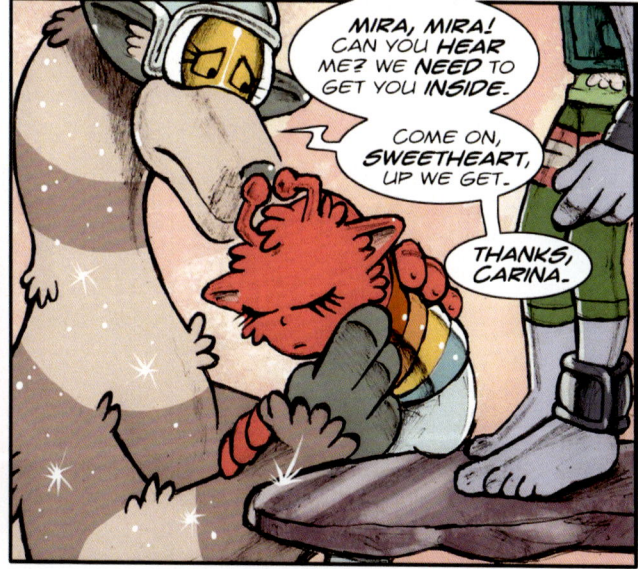

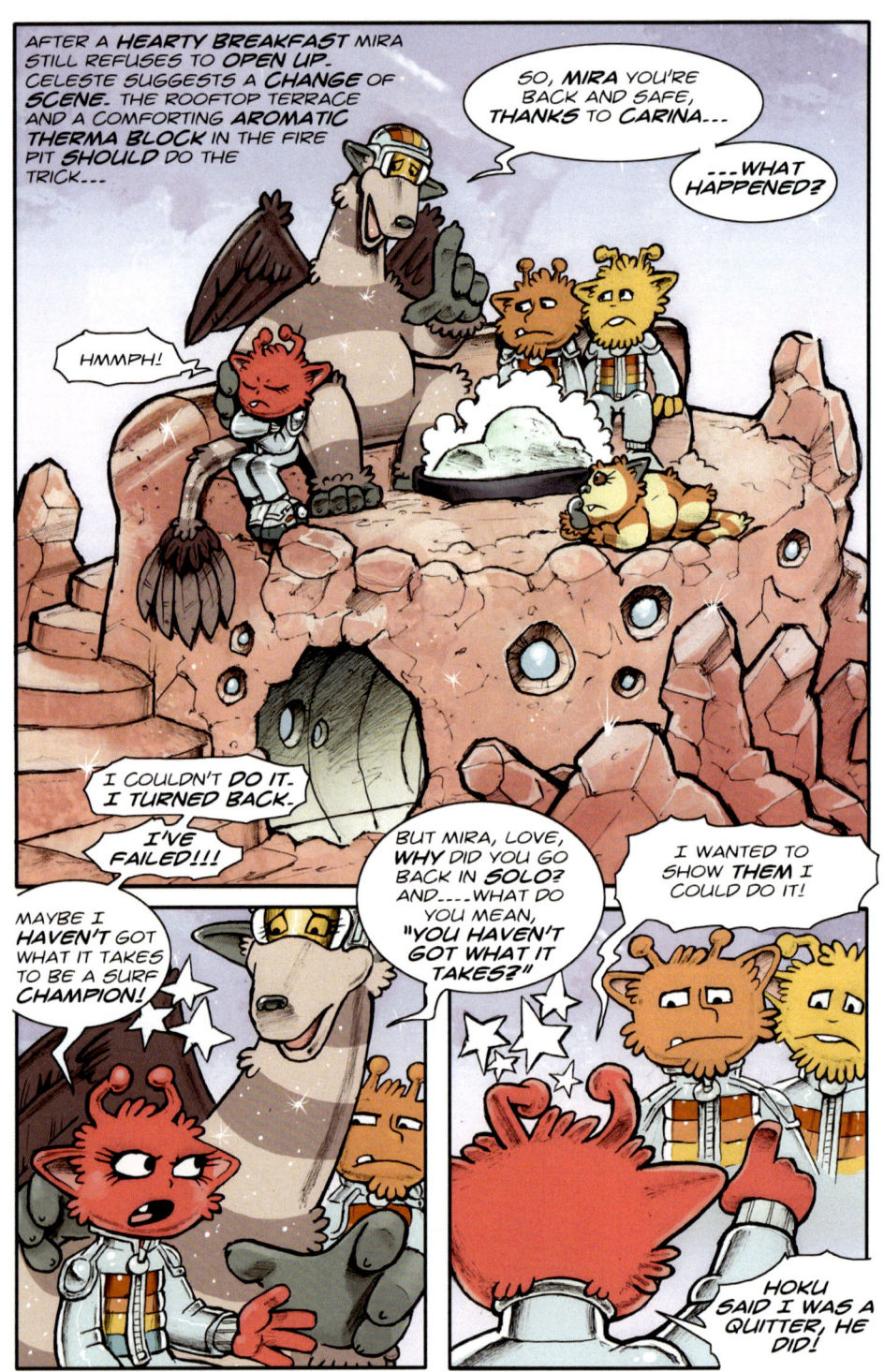

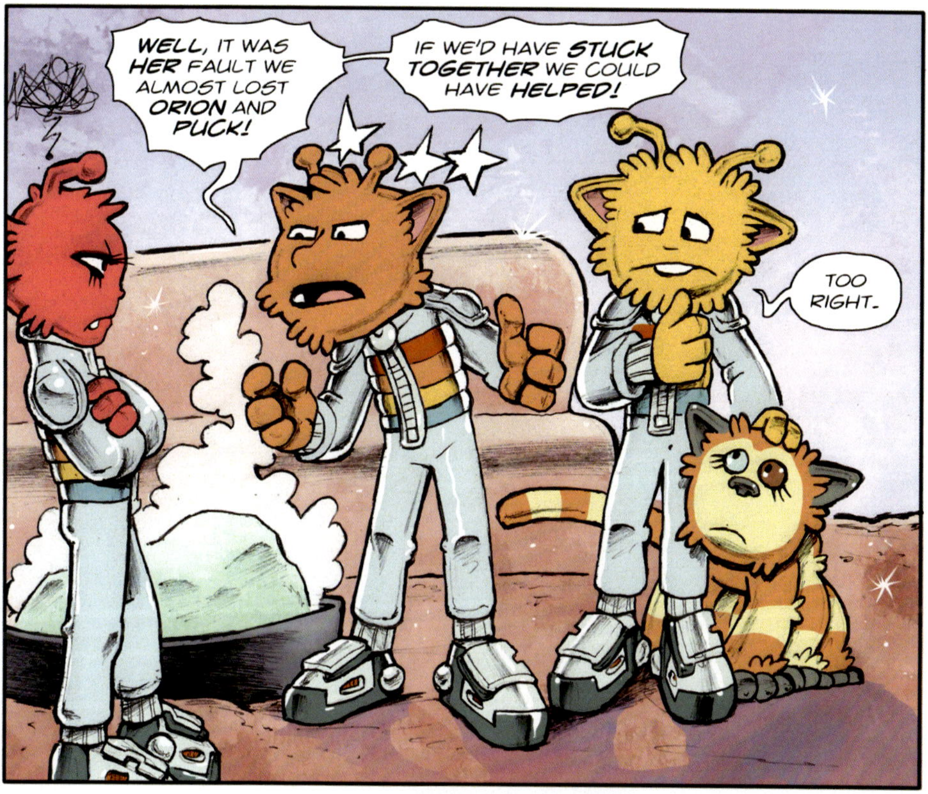

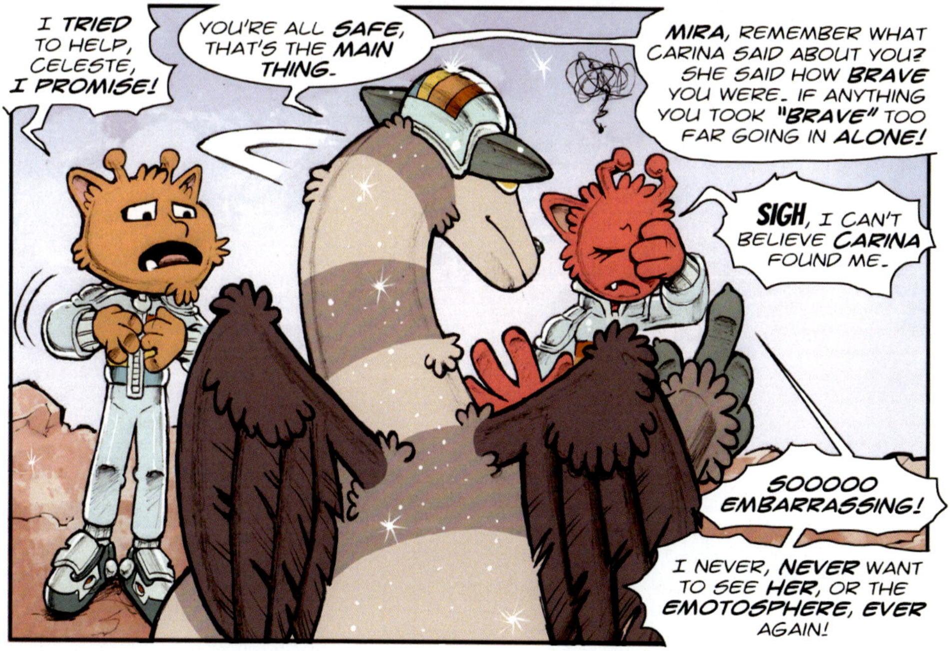

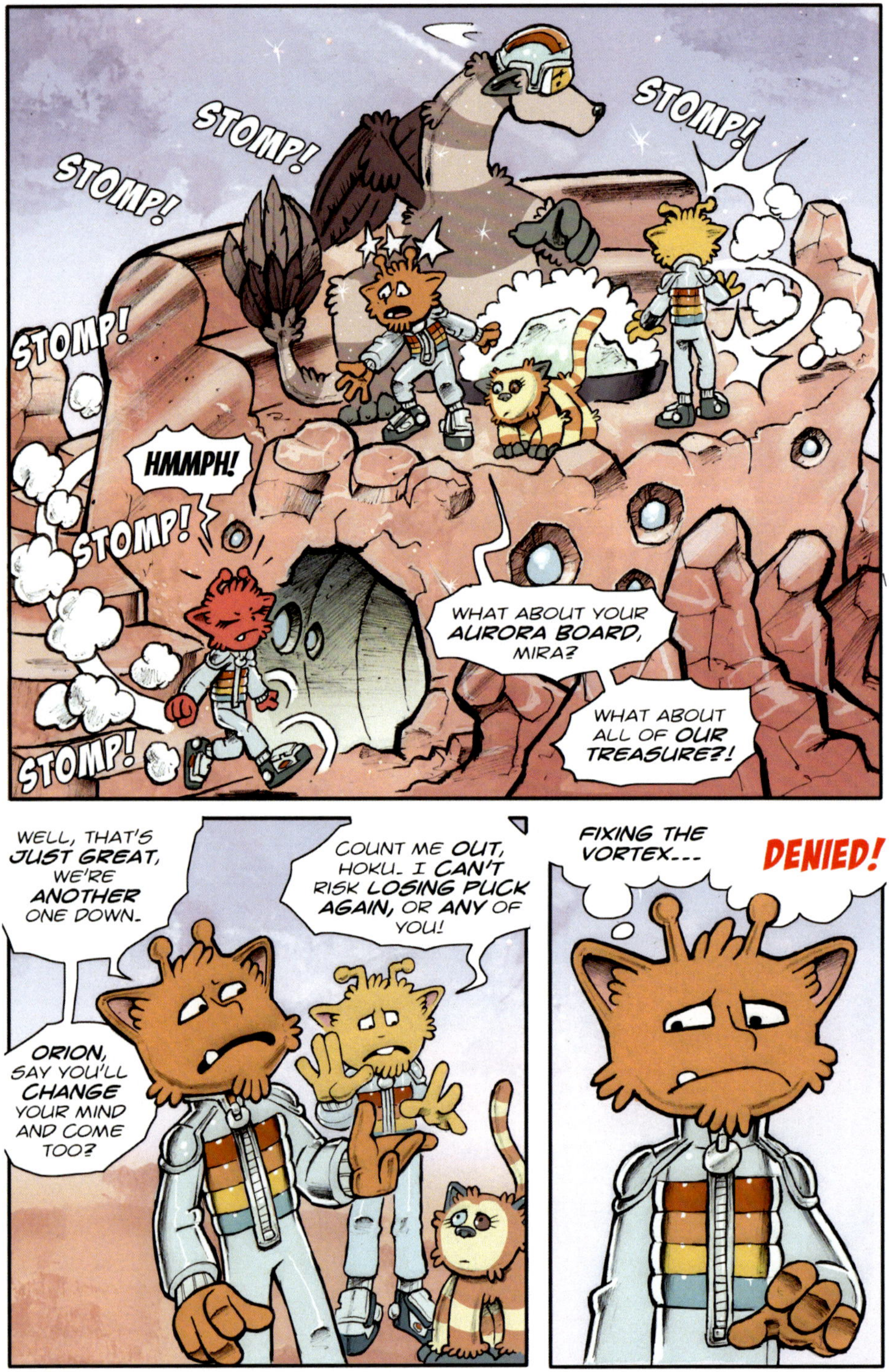

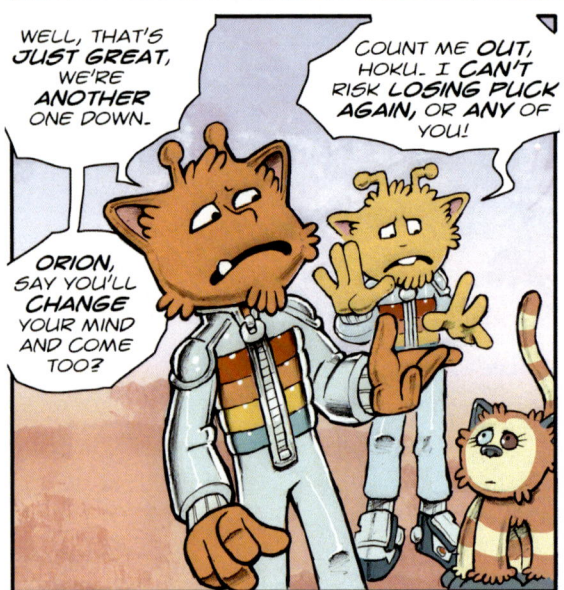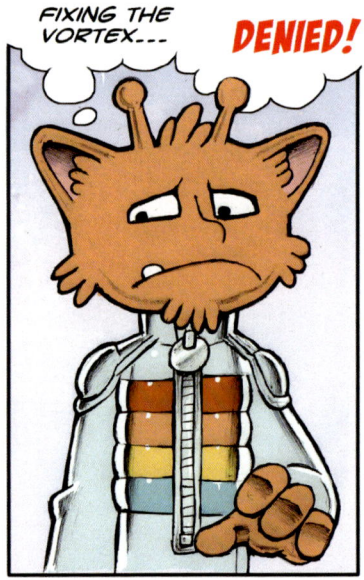

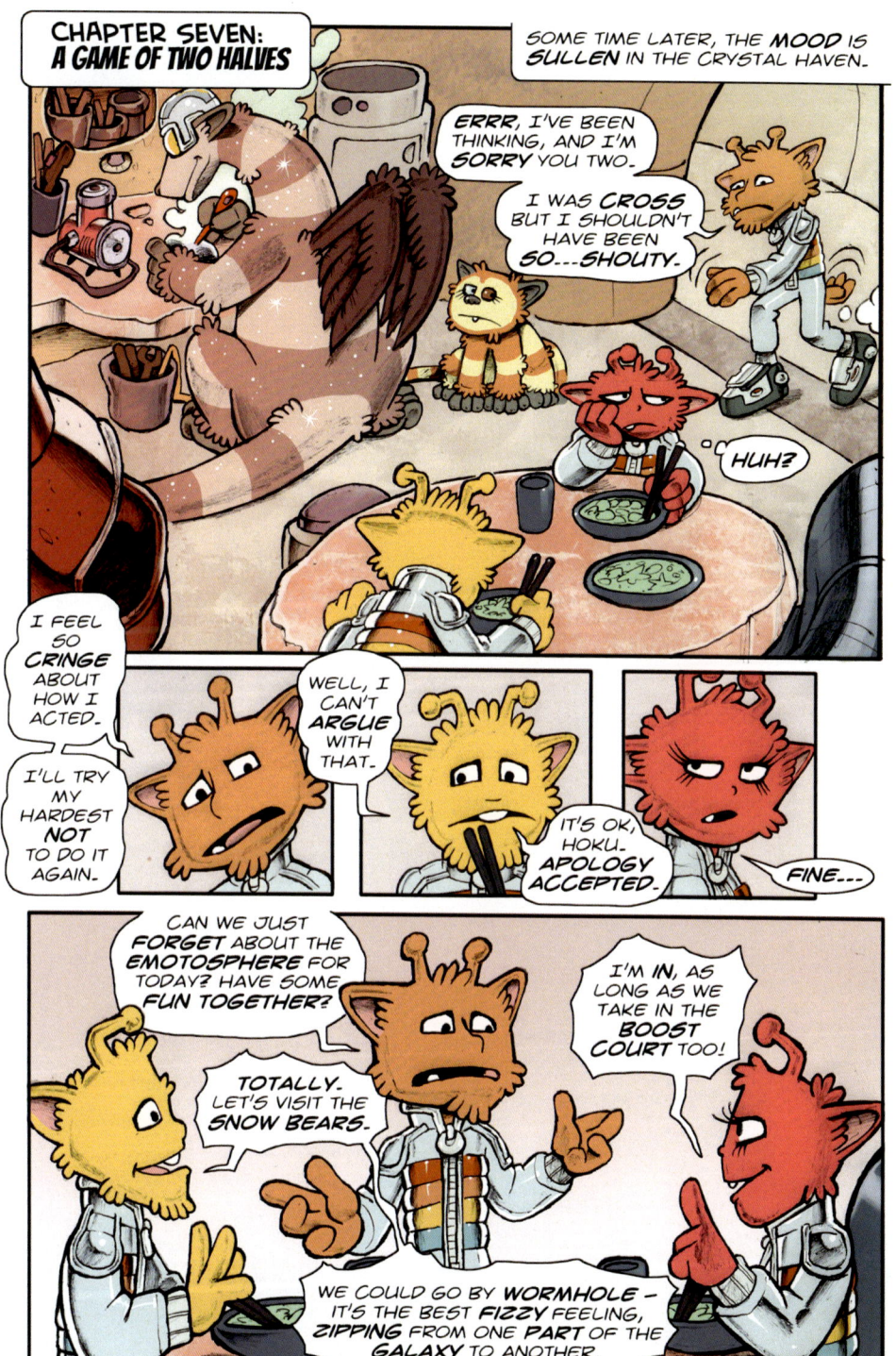

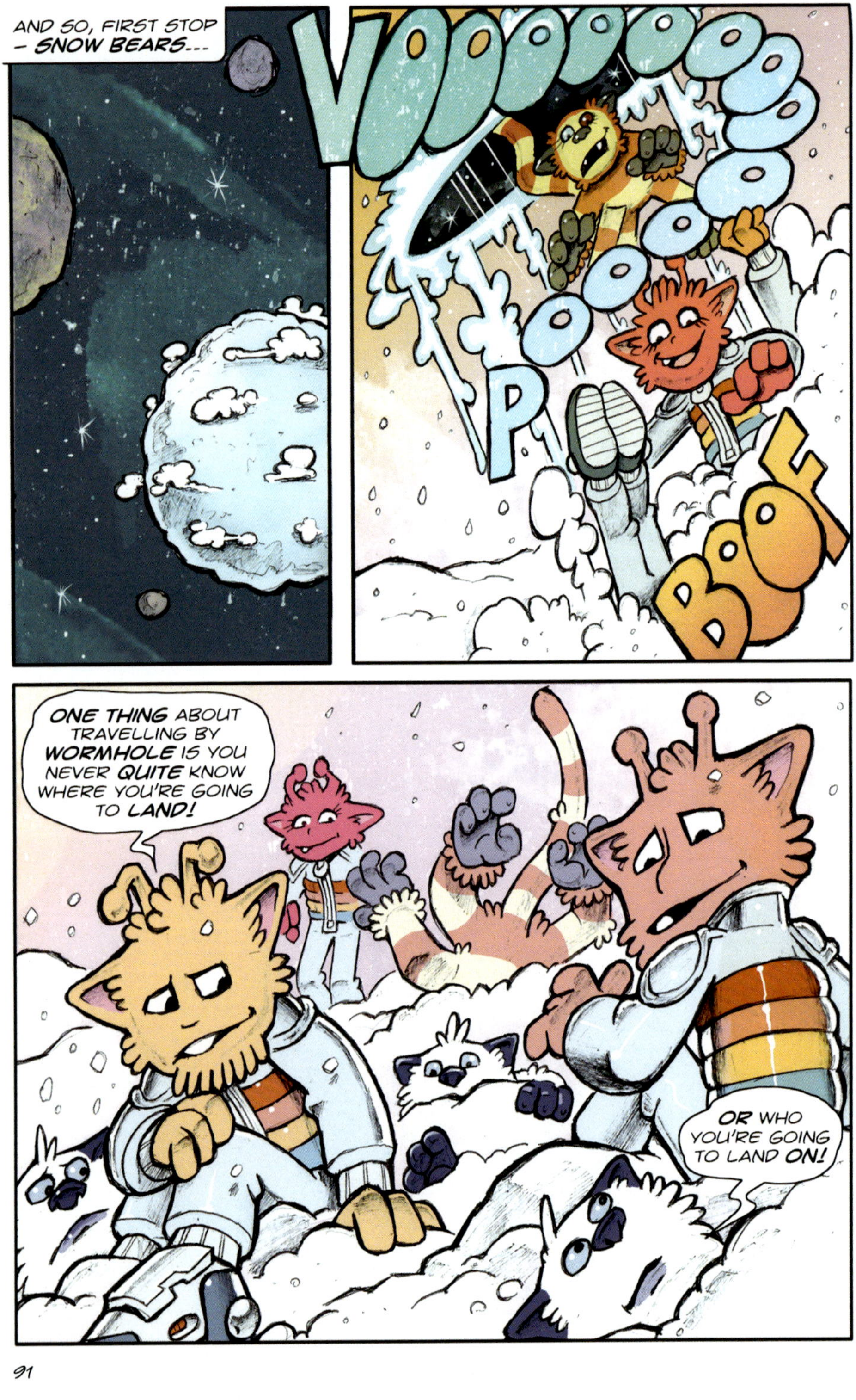

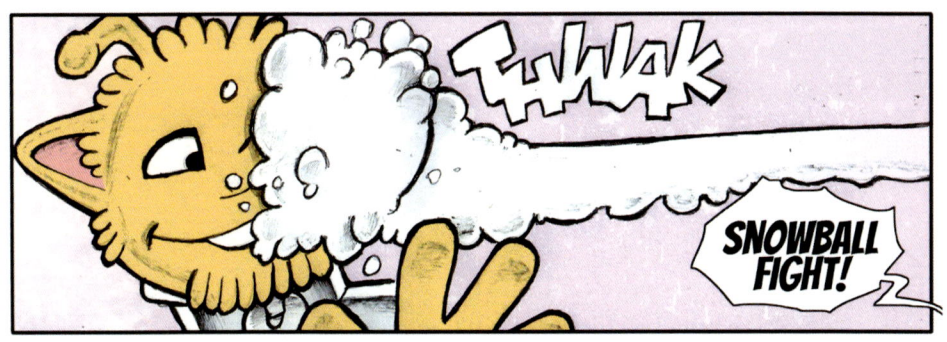

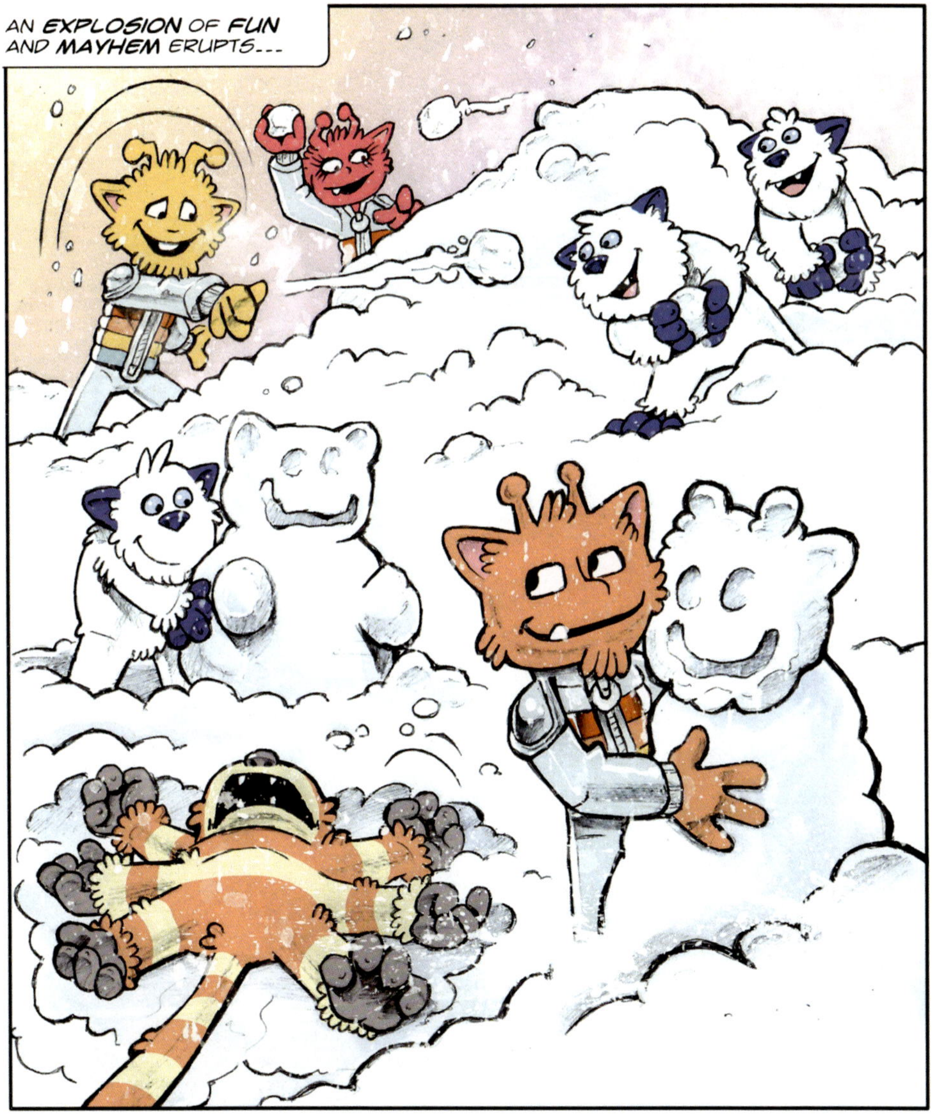

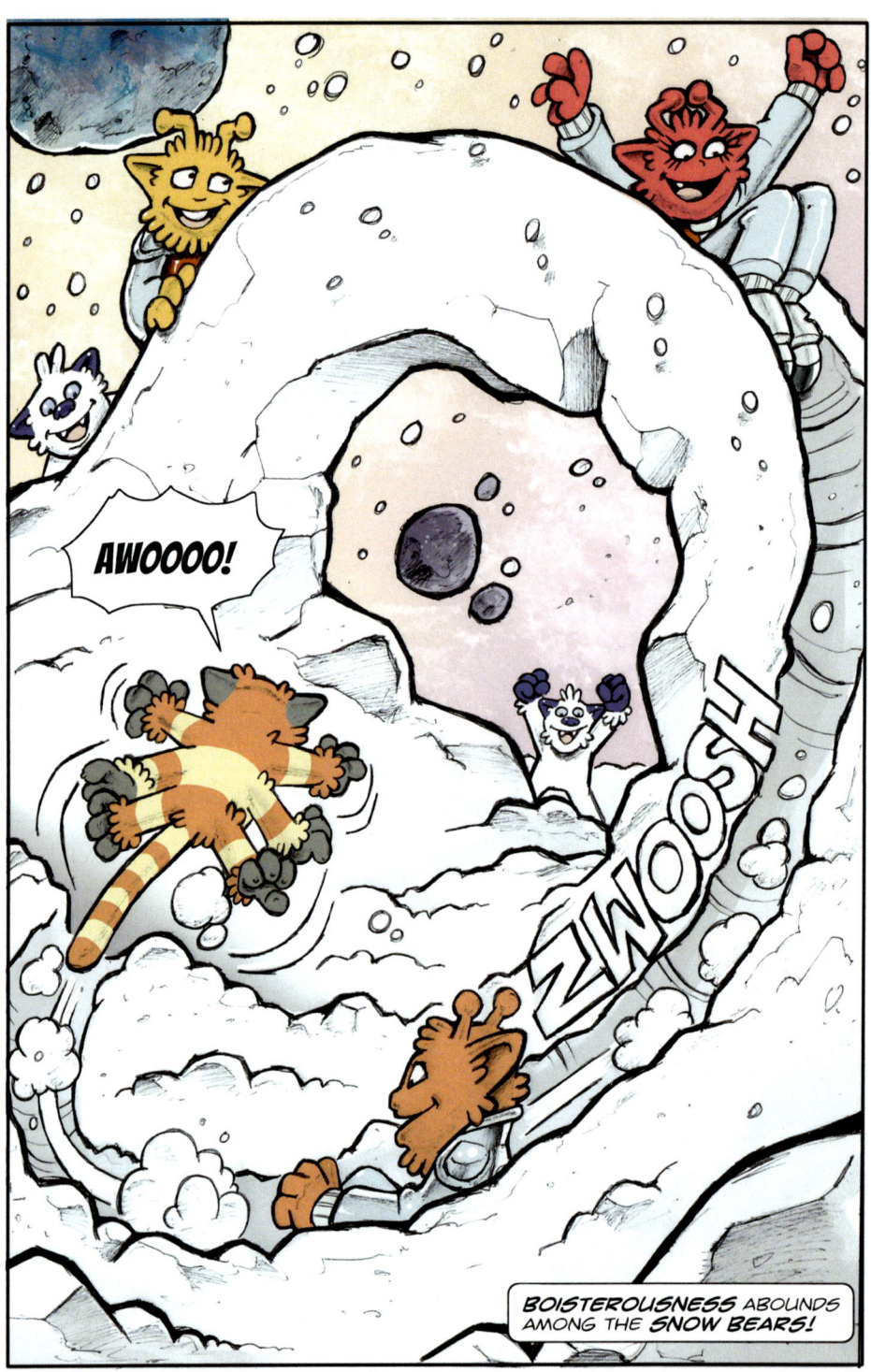

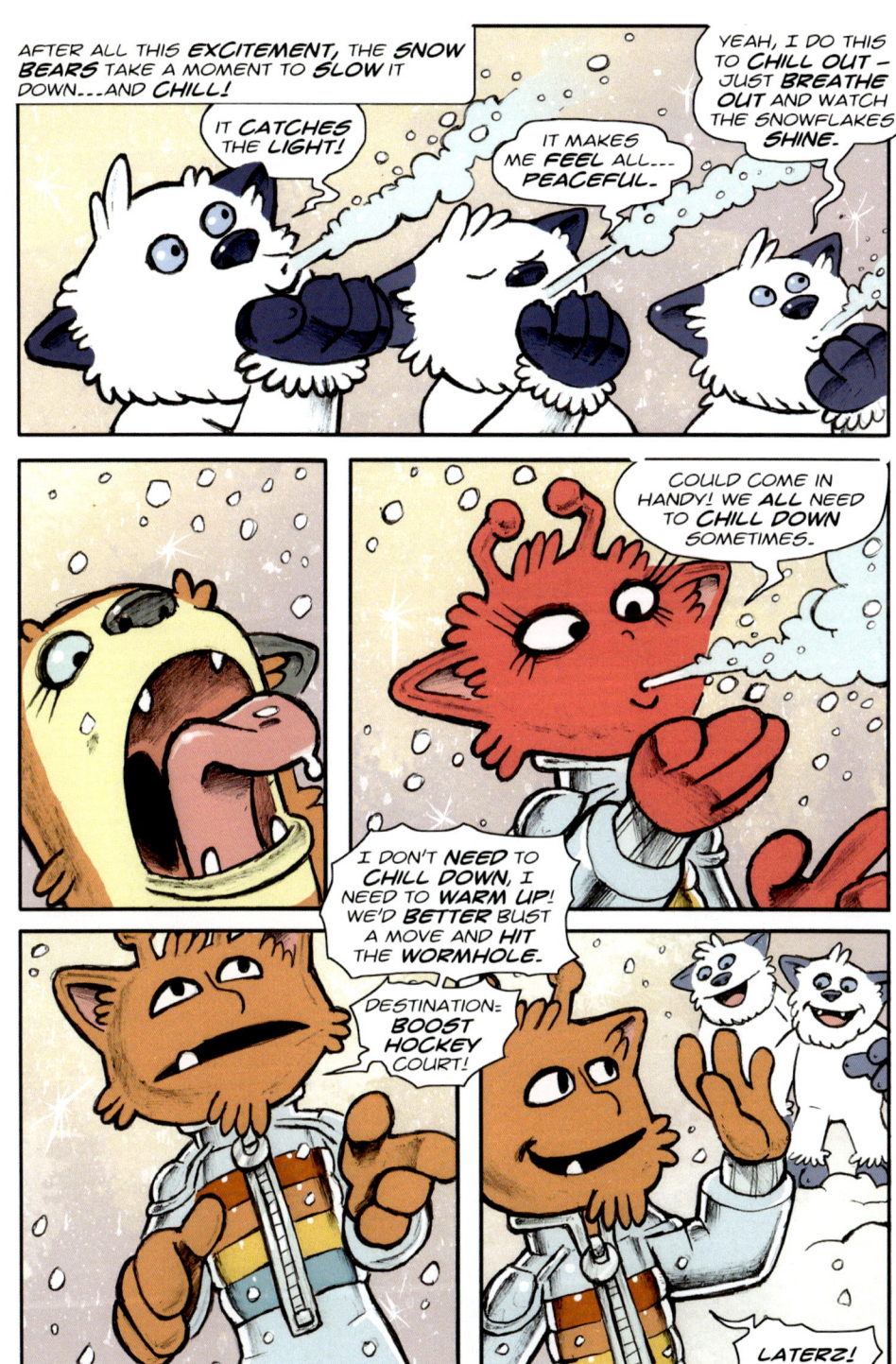

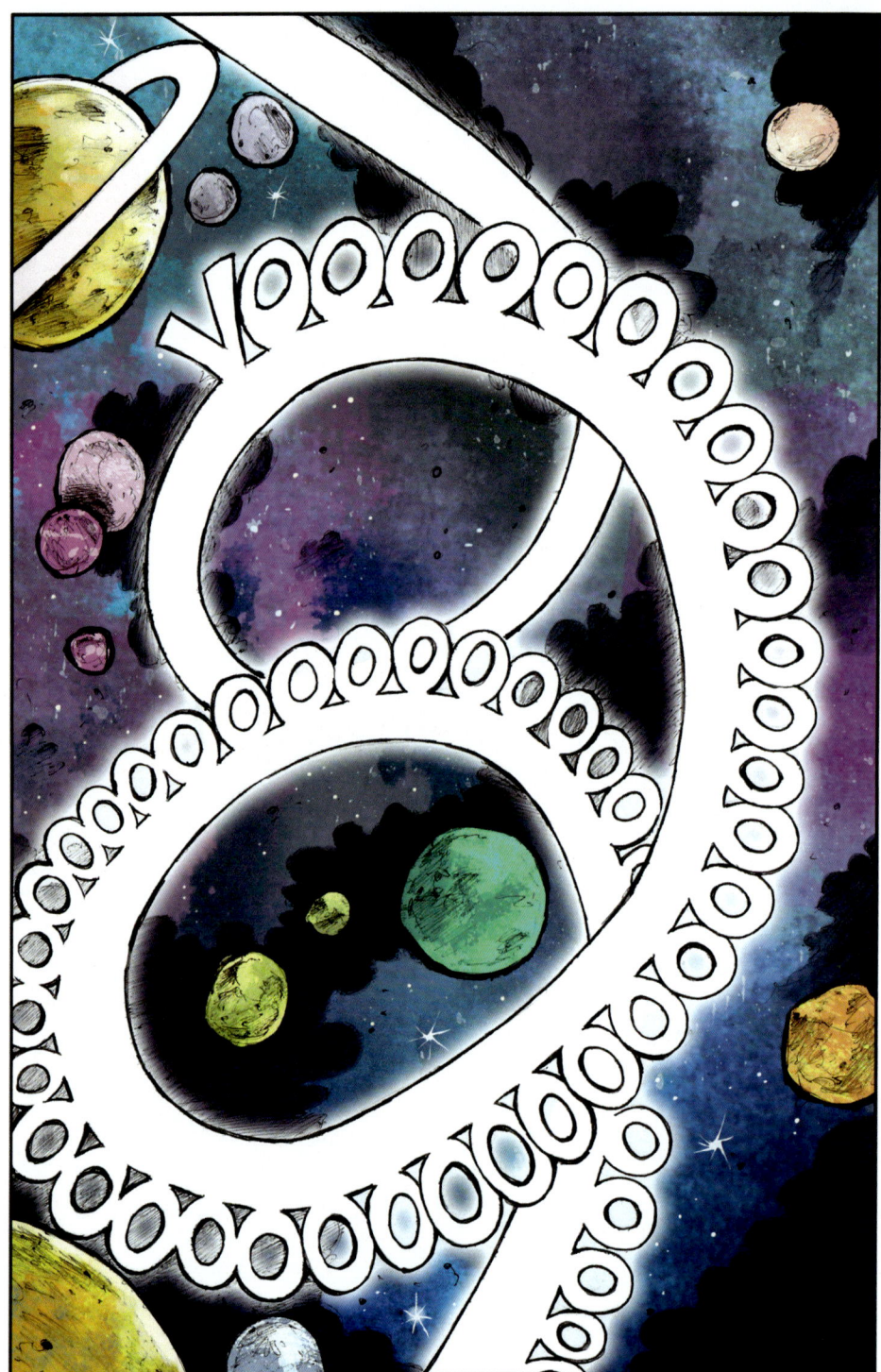

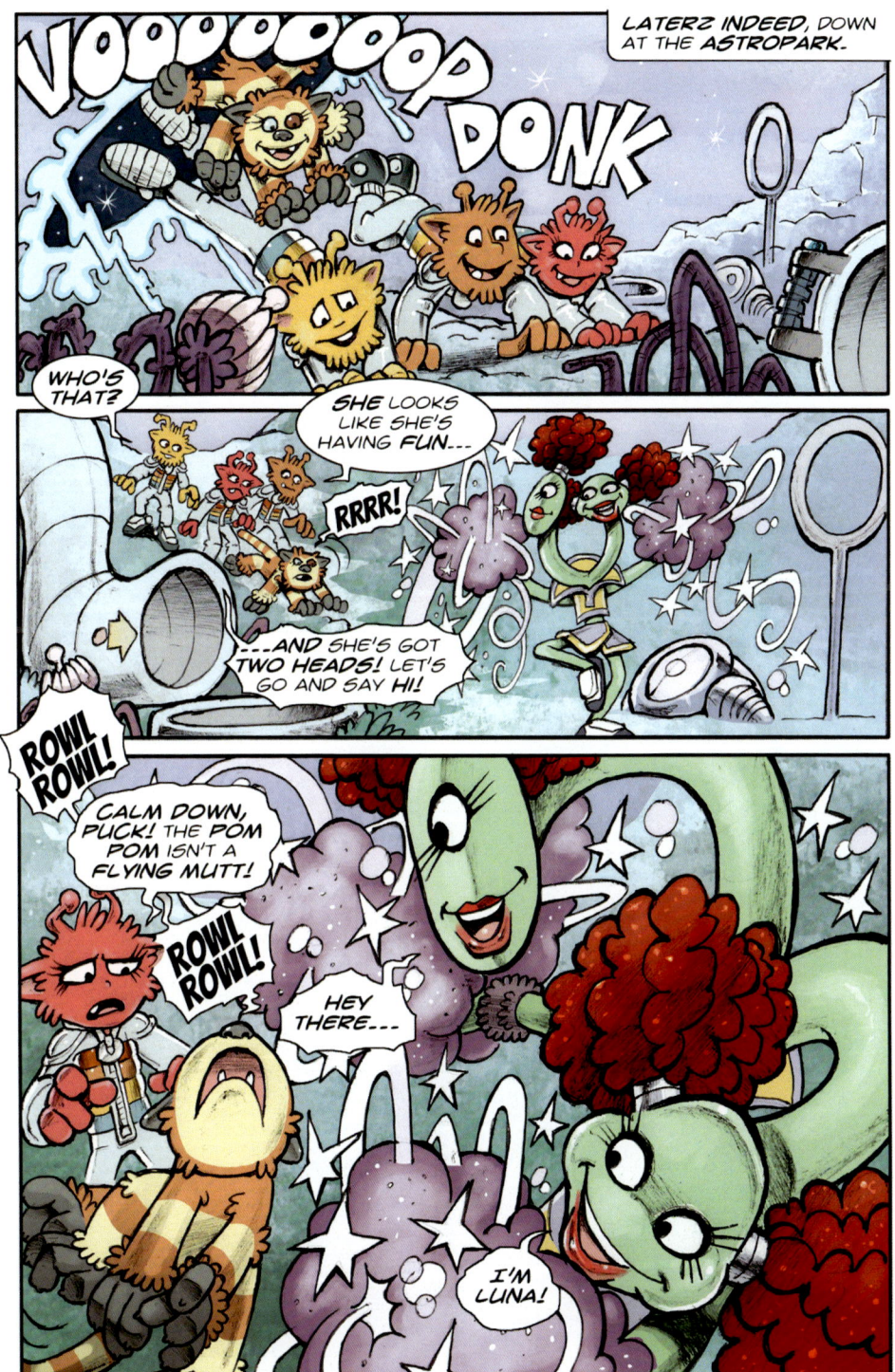

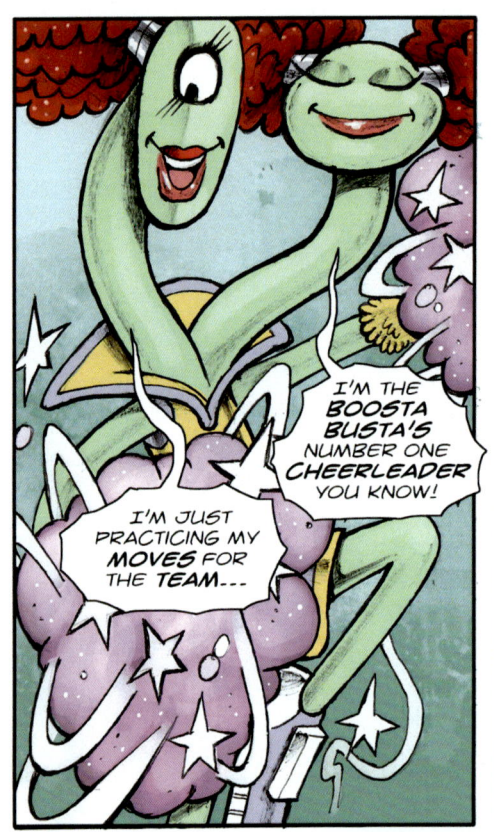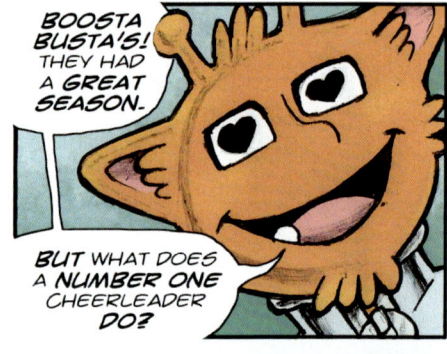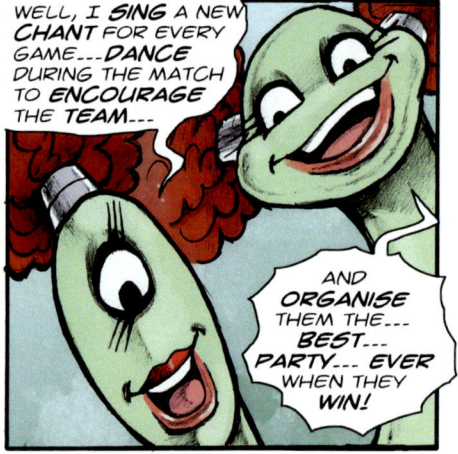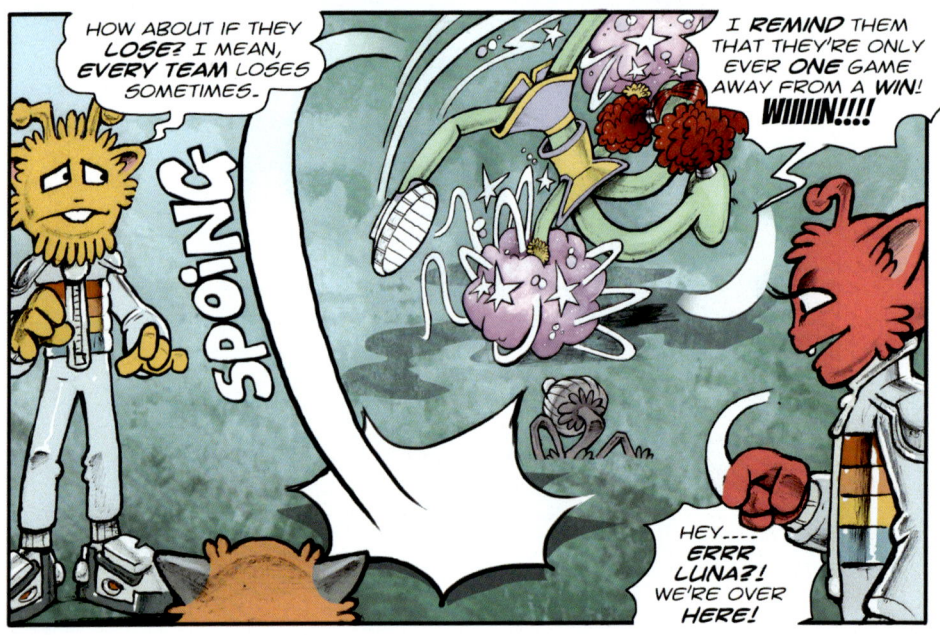

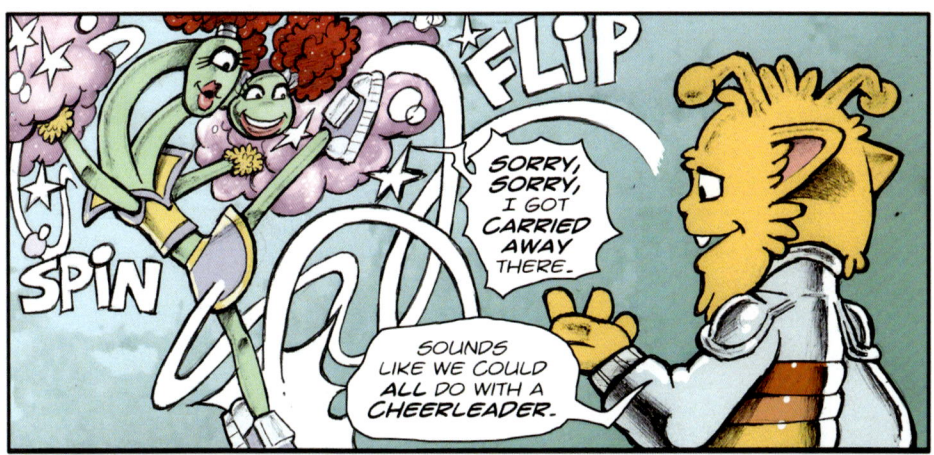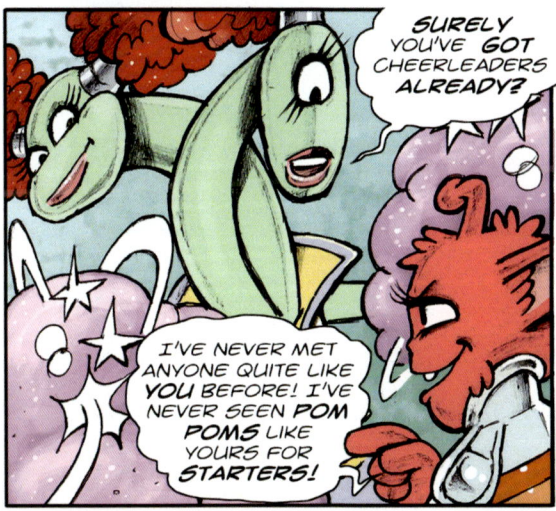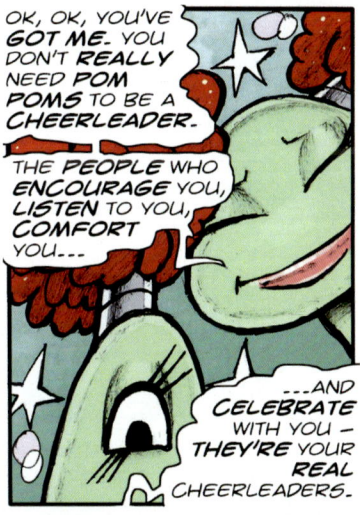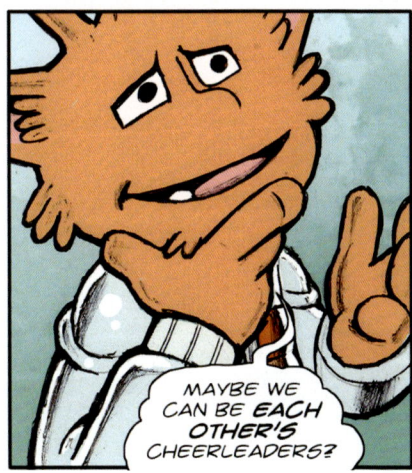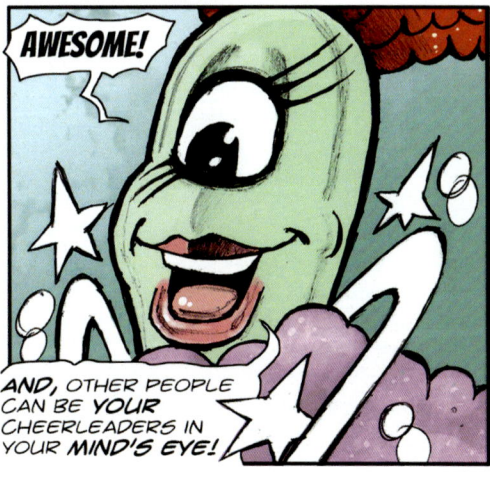

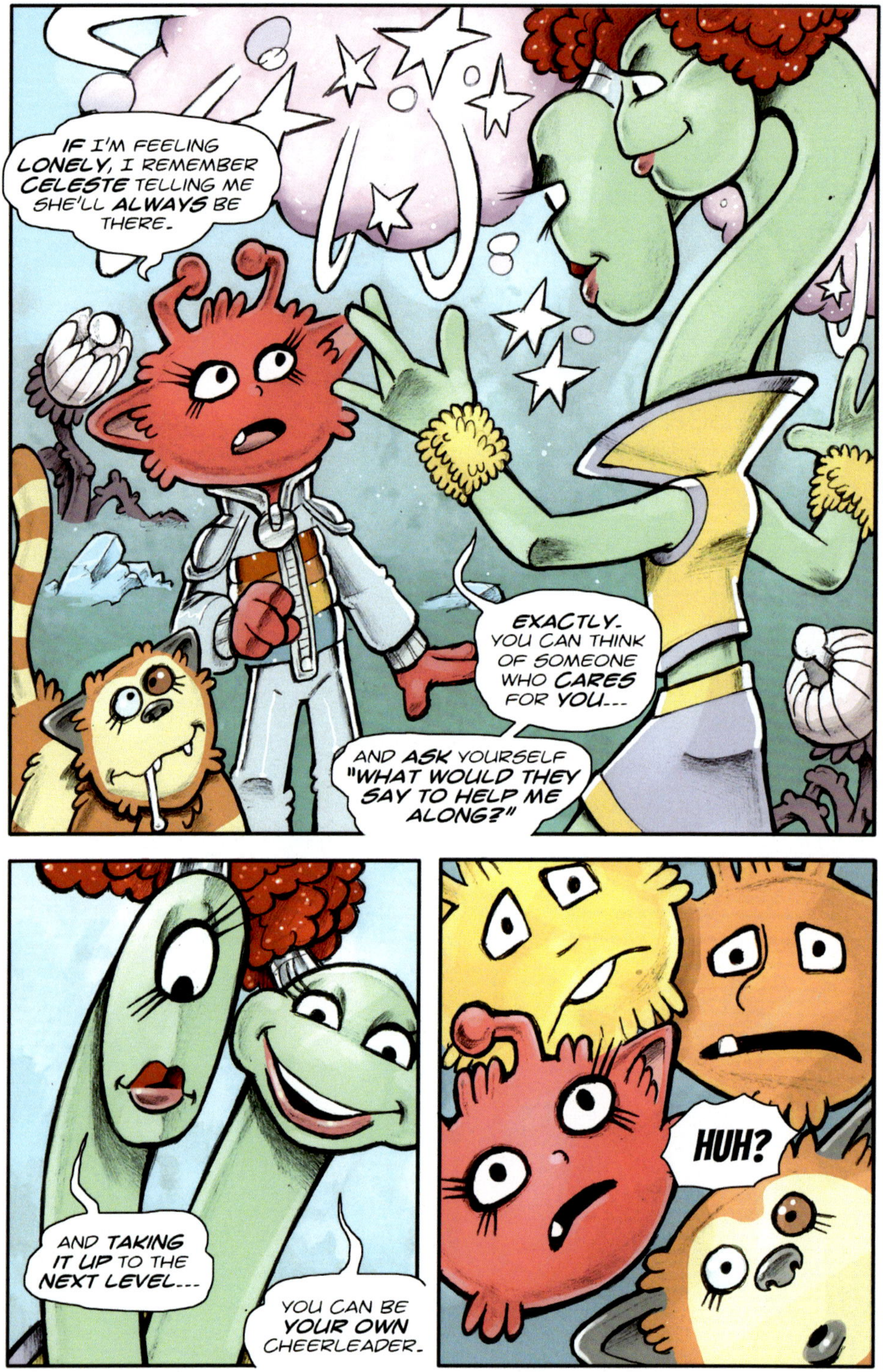

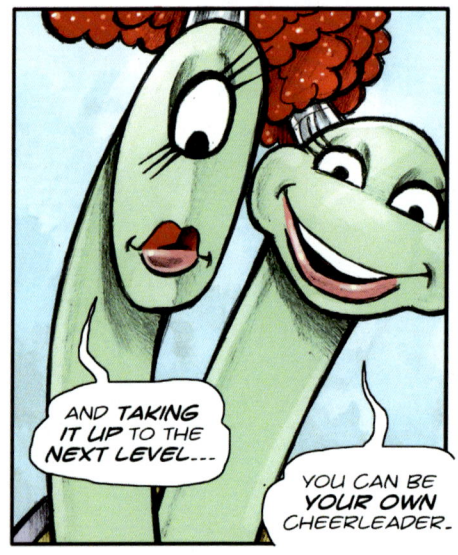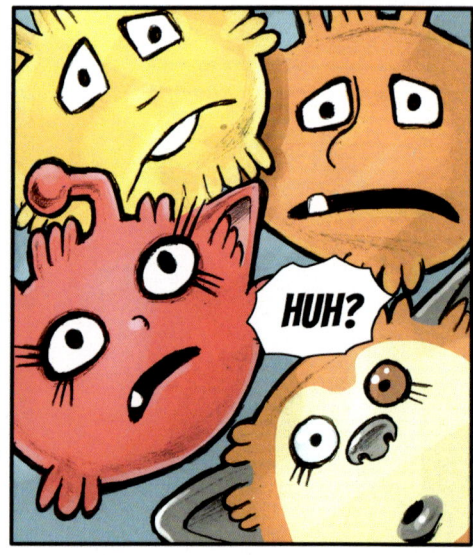

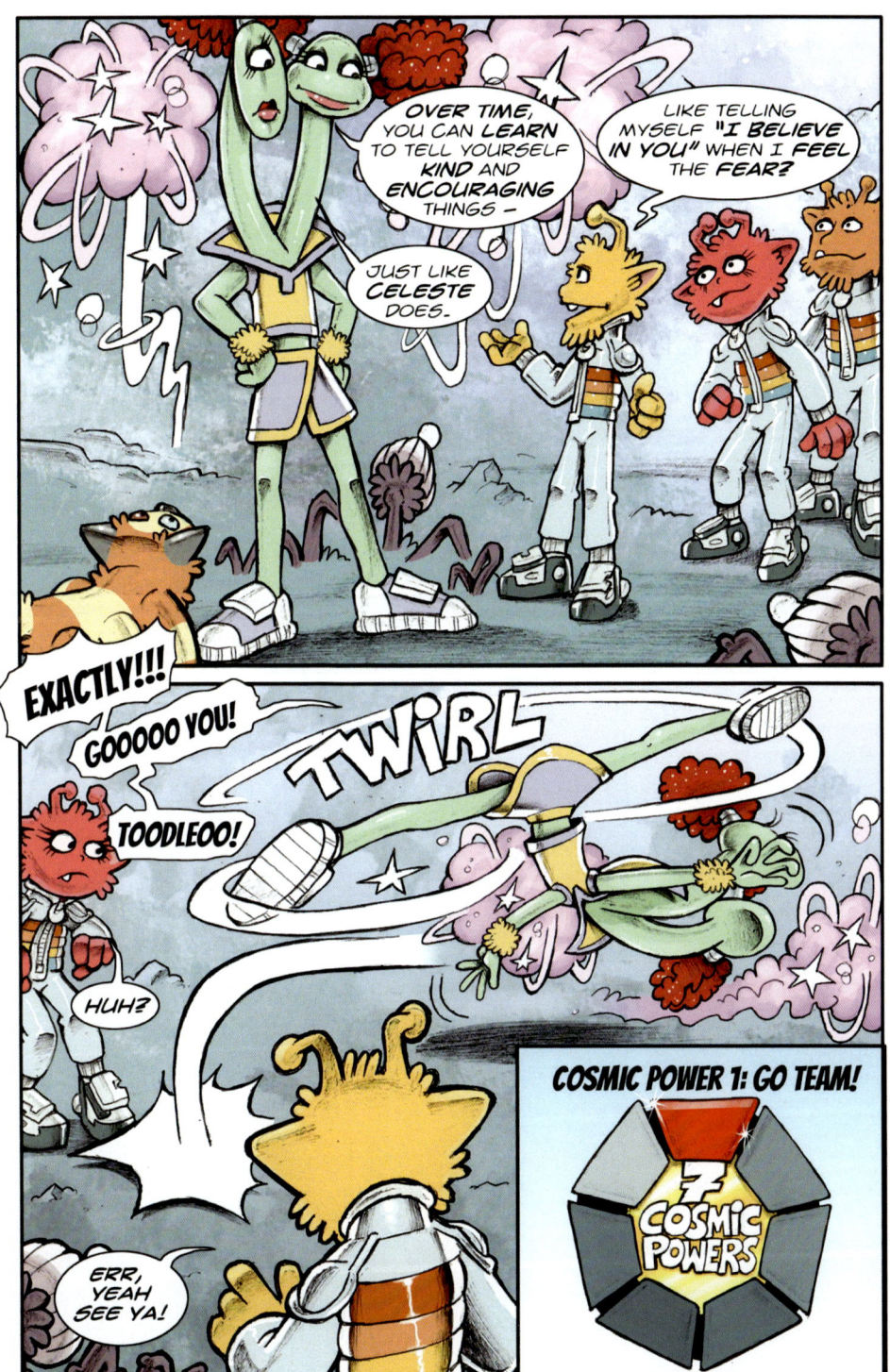

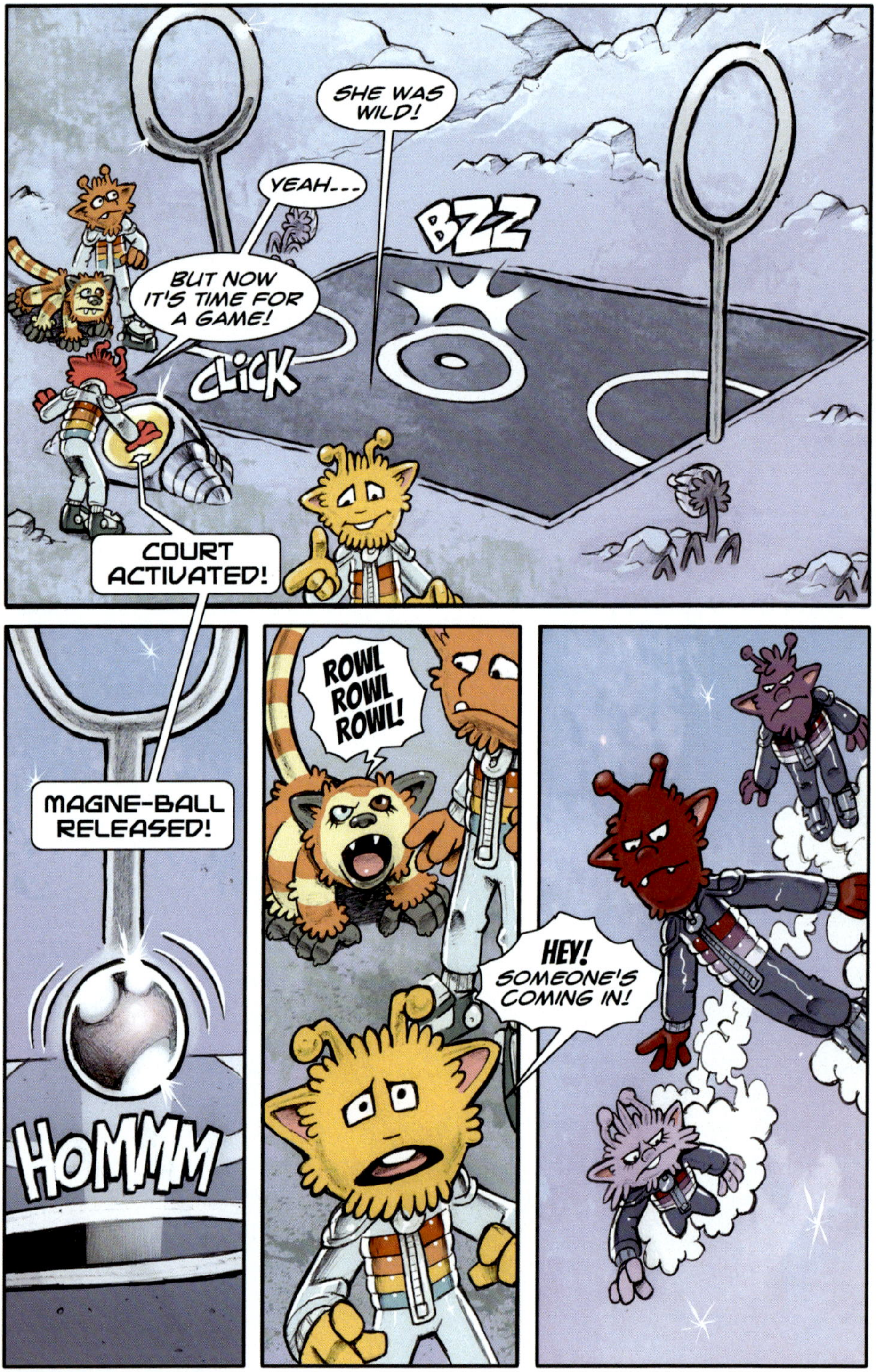

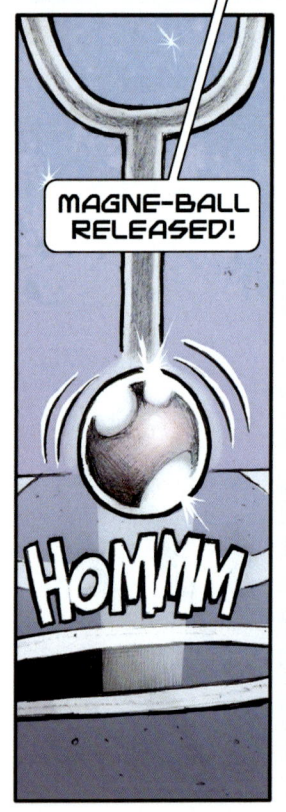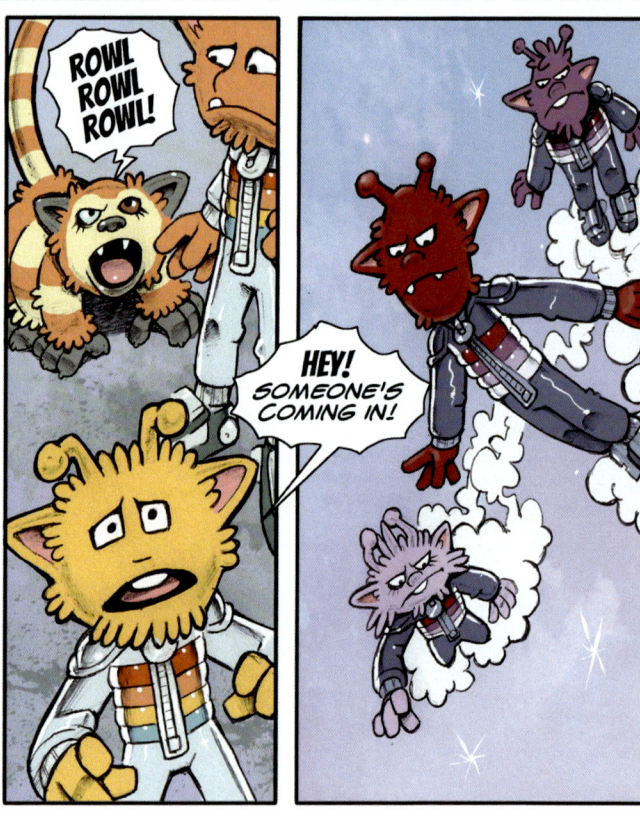

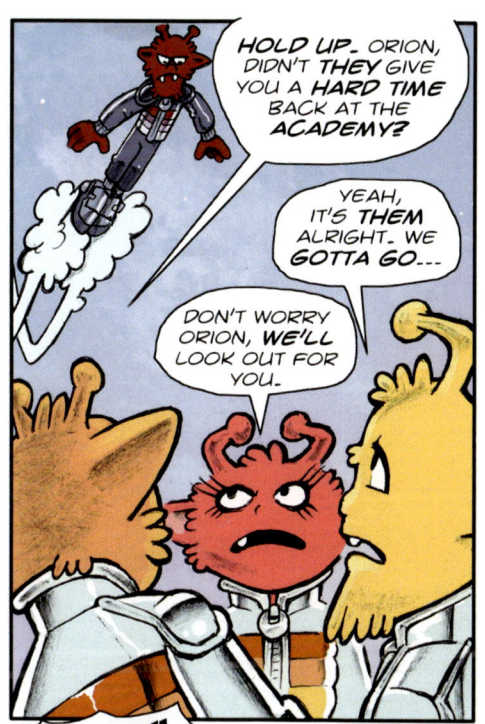
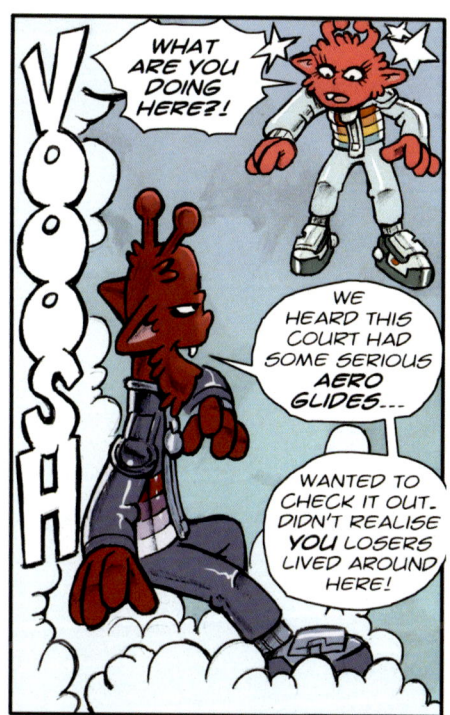
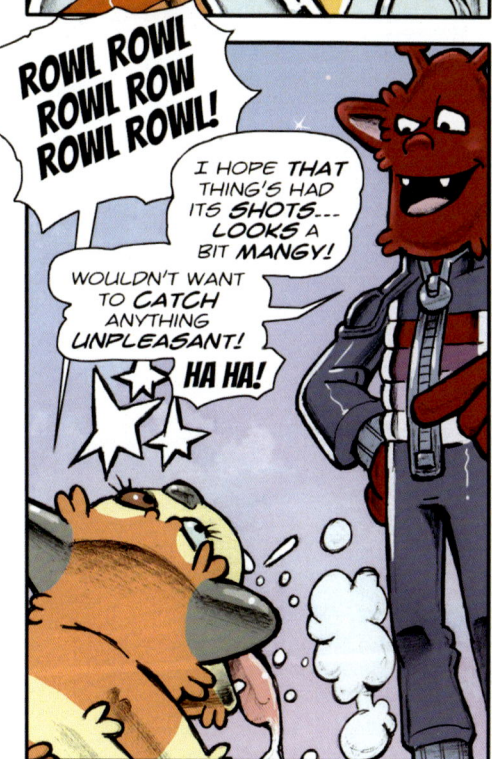
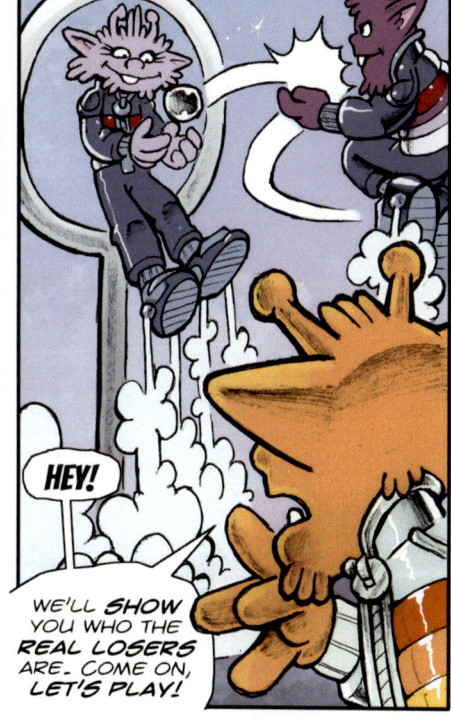

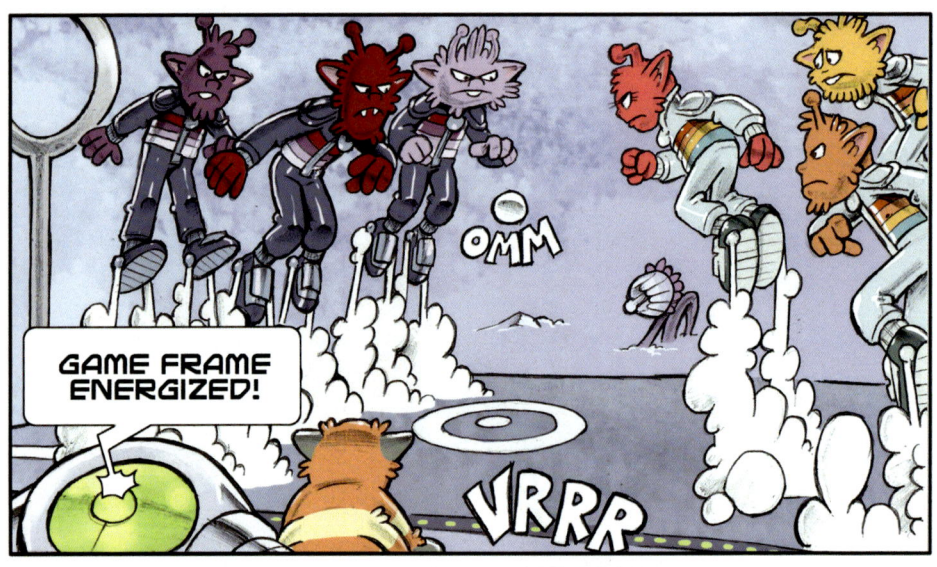
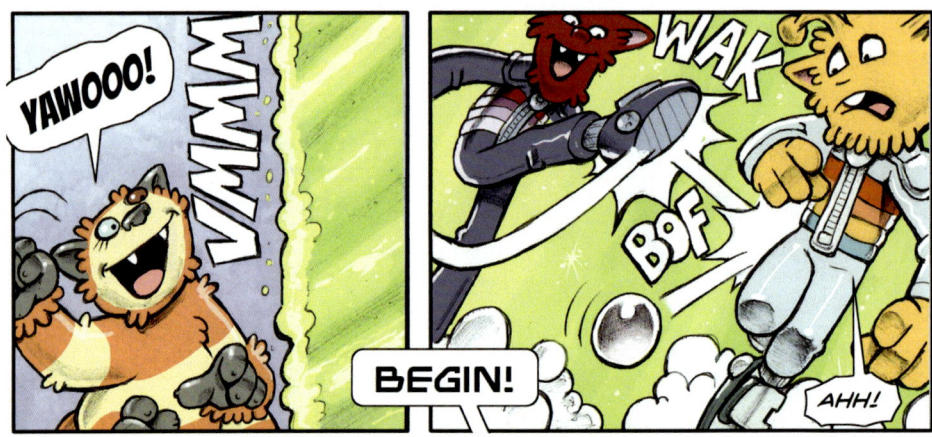
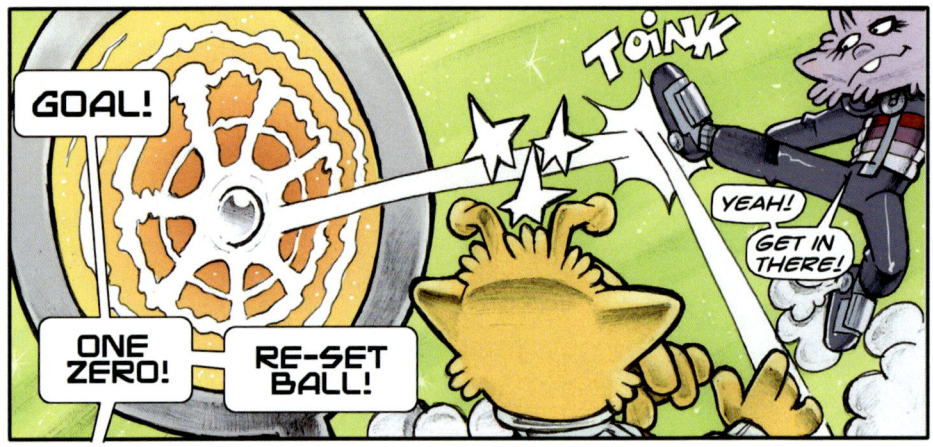

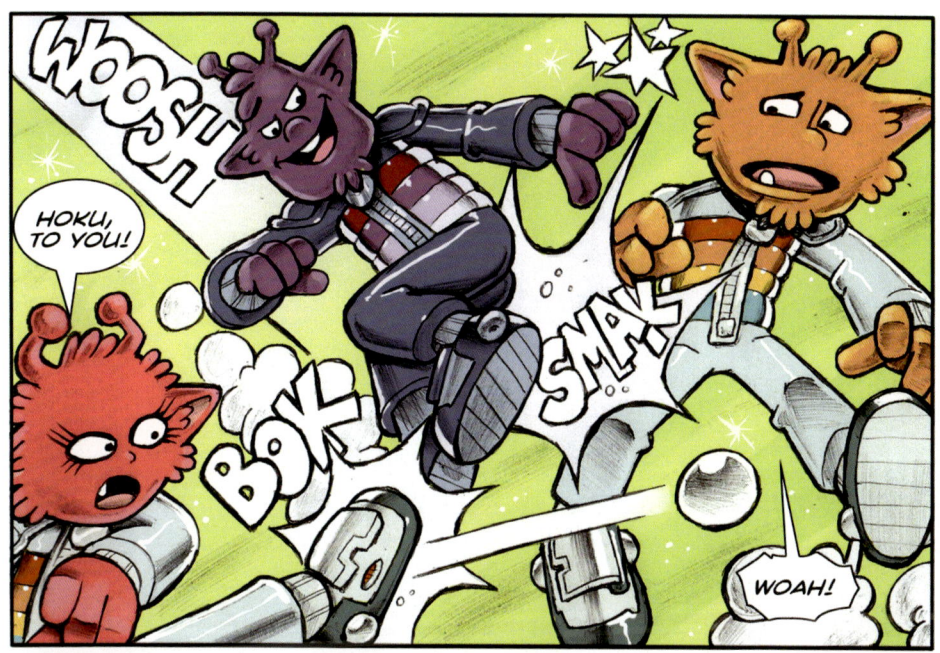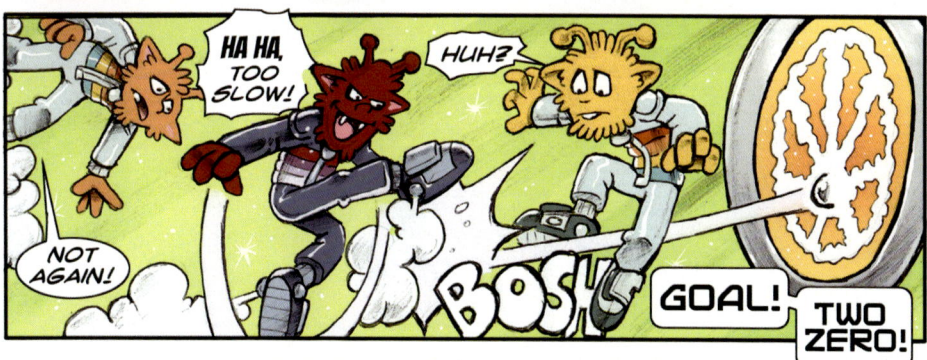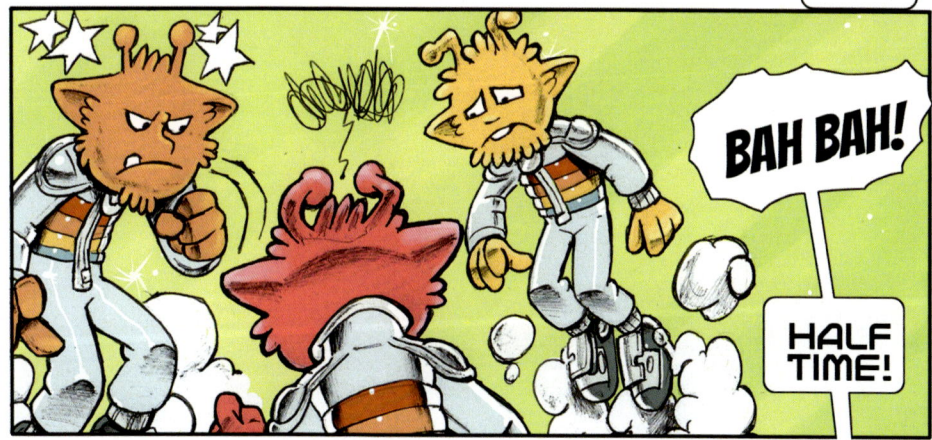

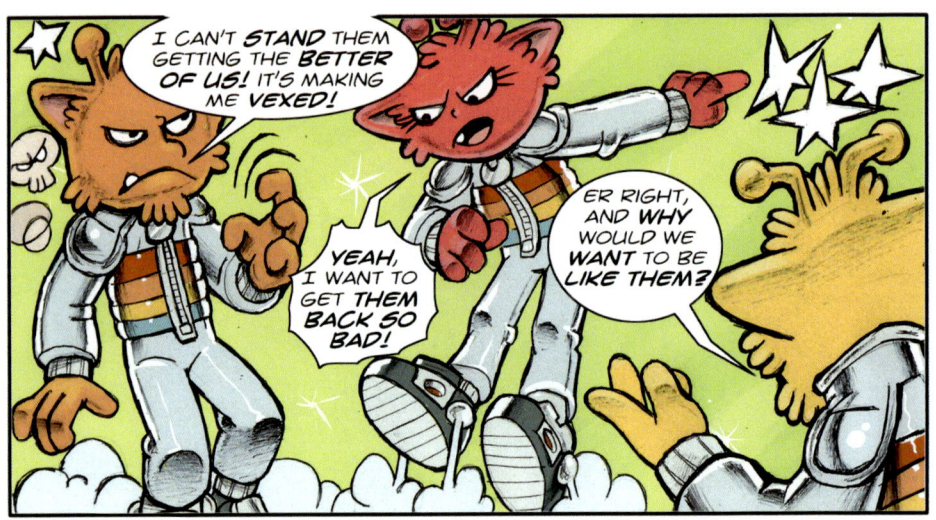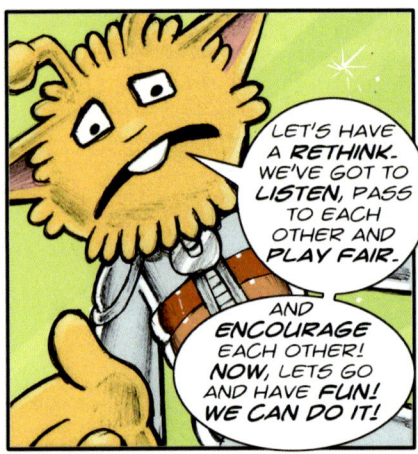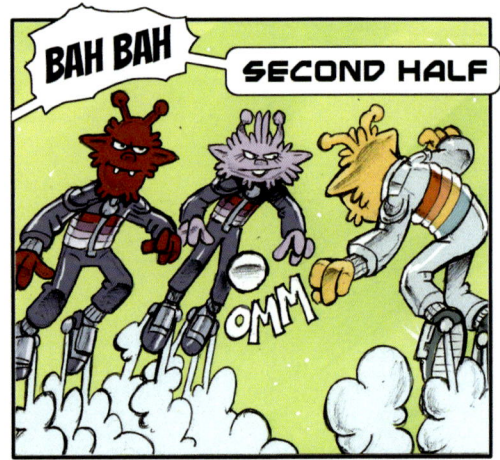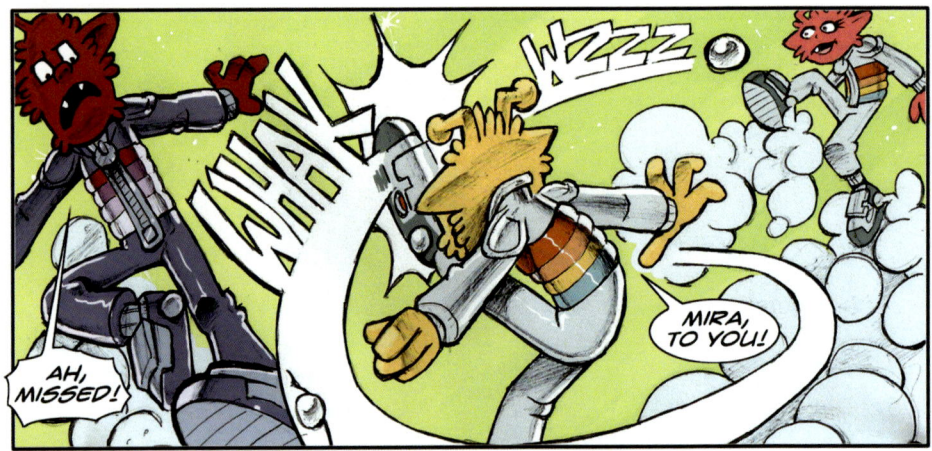

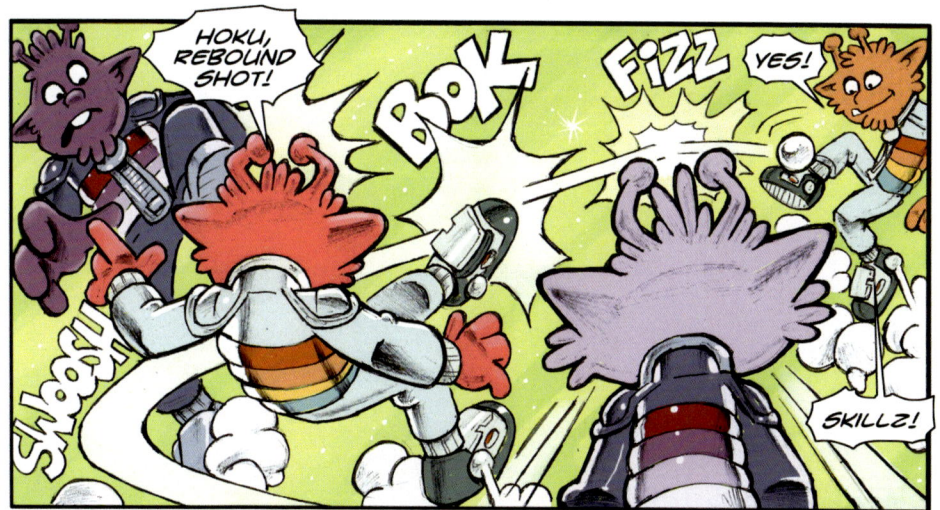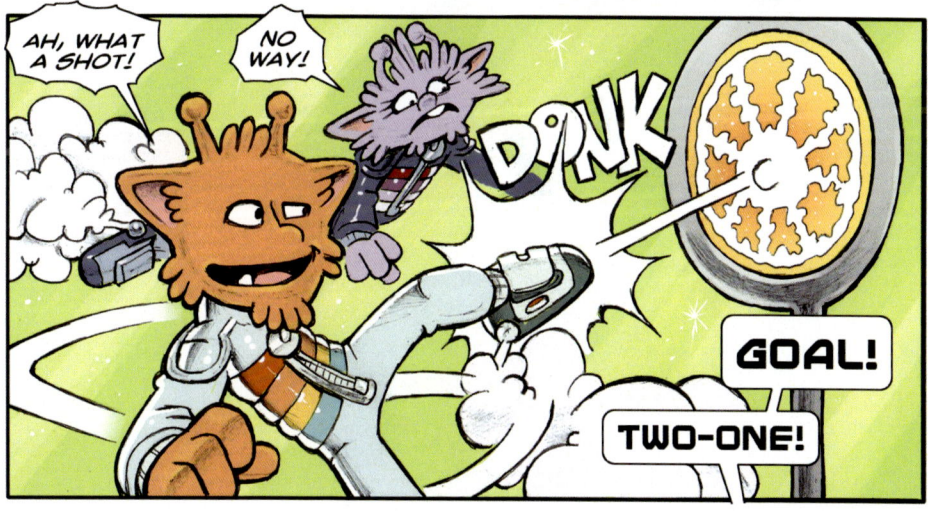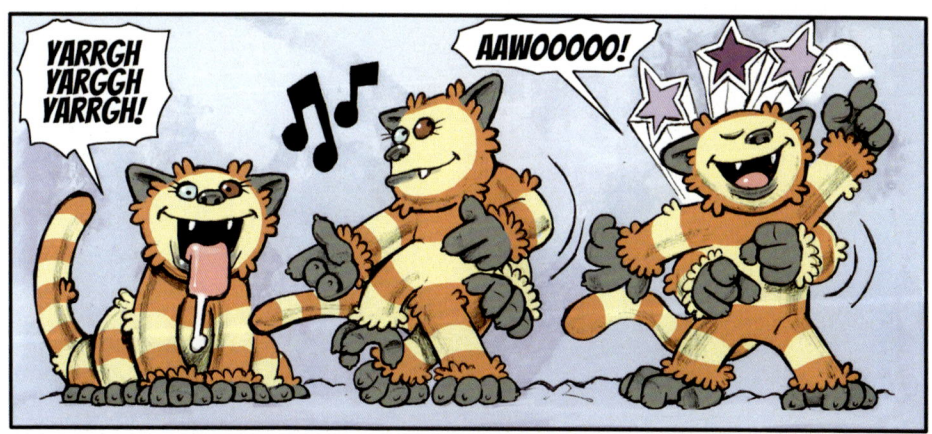

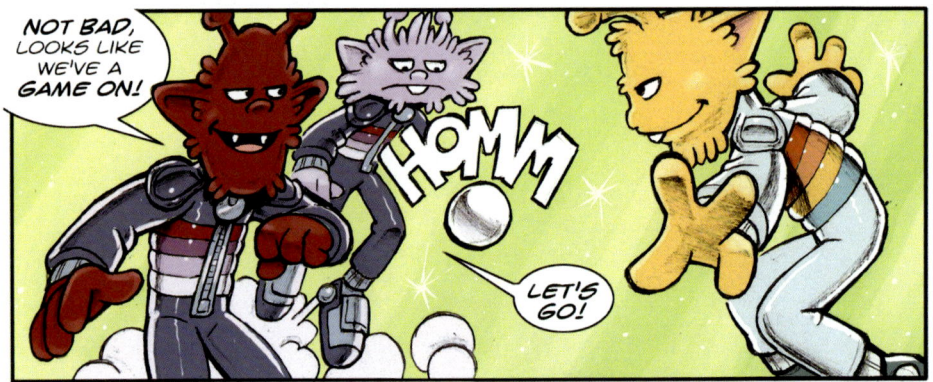

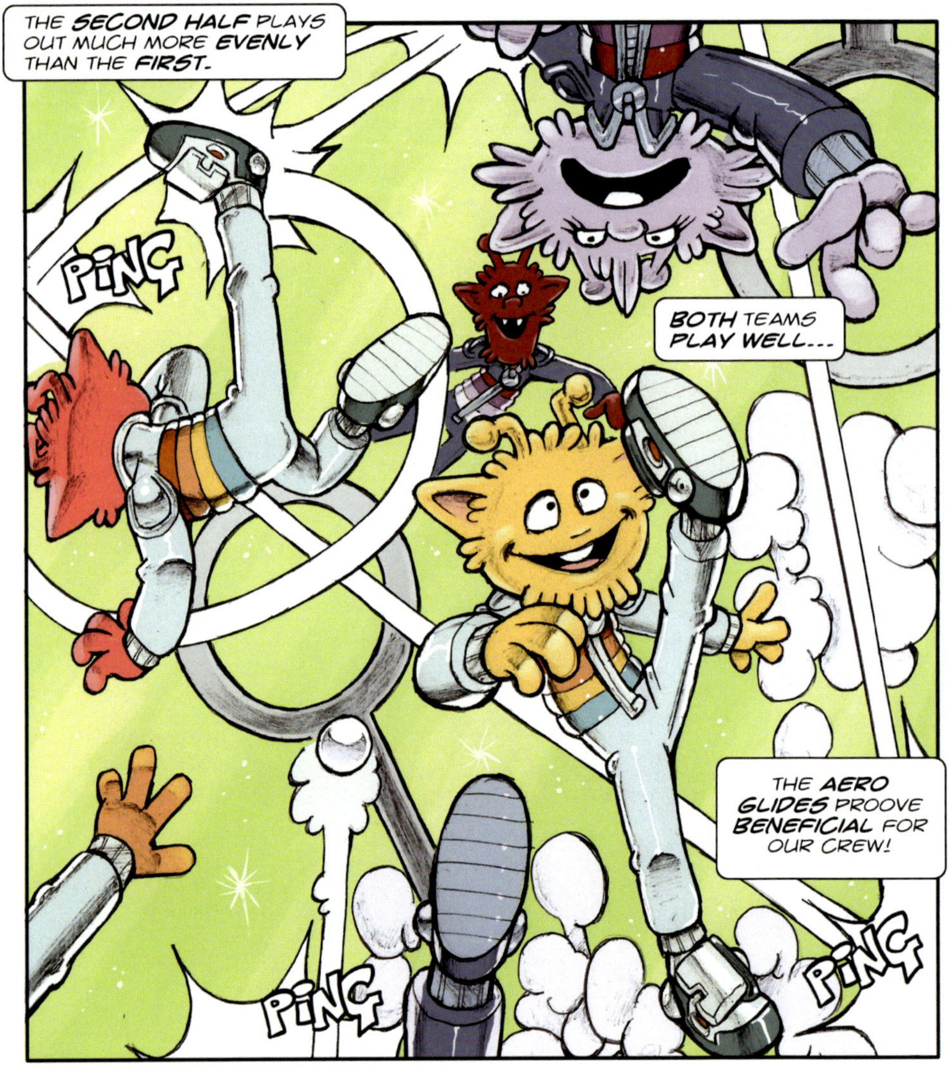

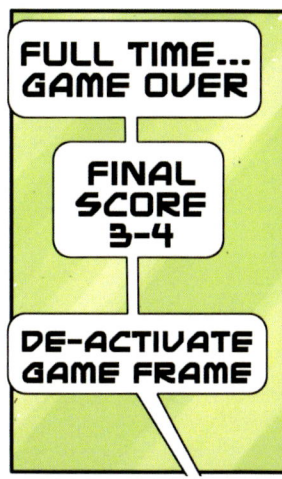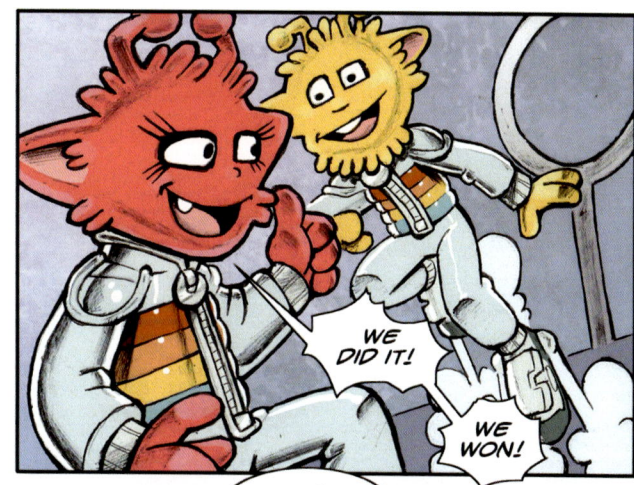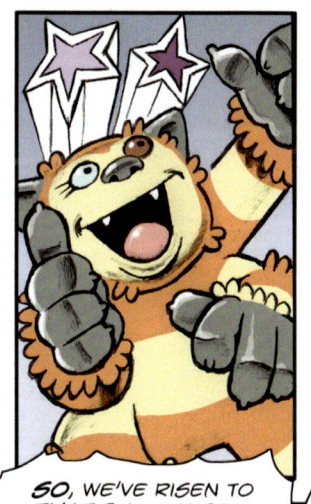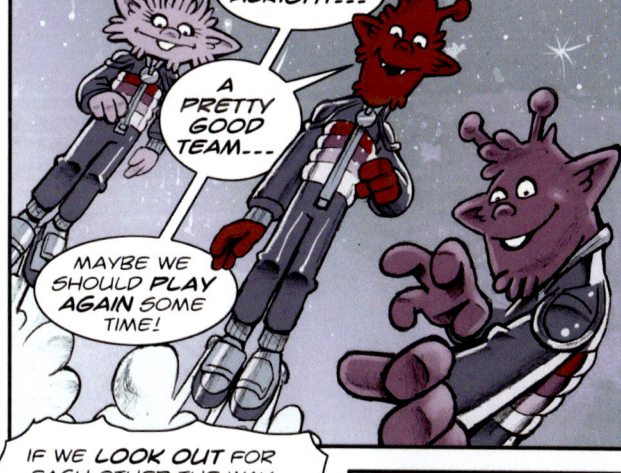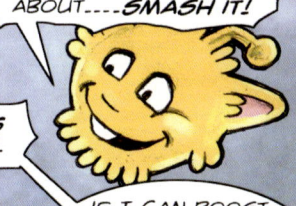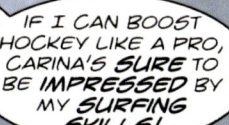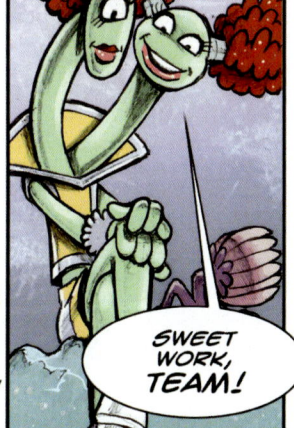

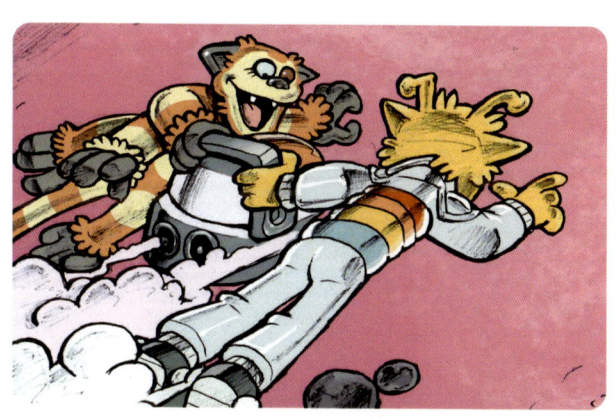

PART THREE

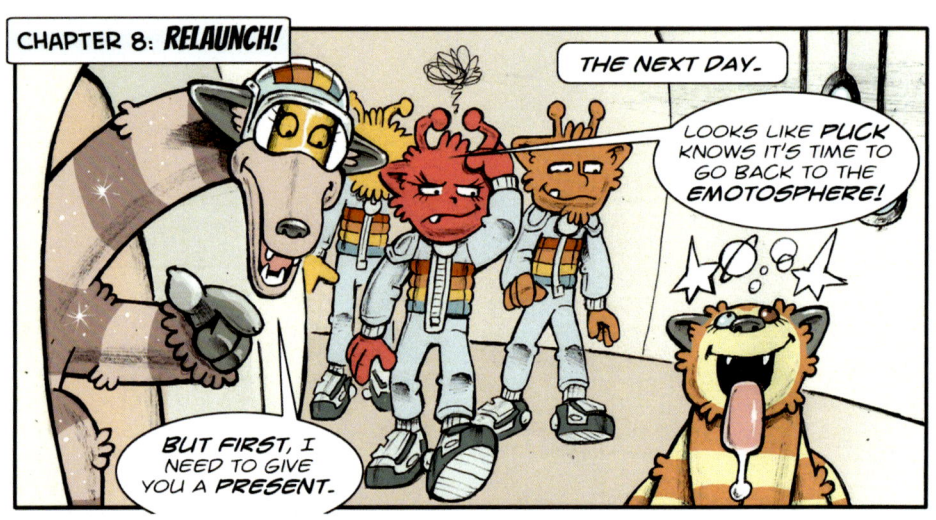
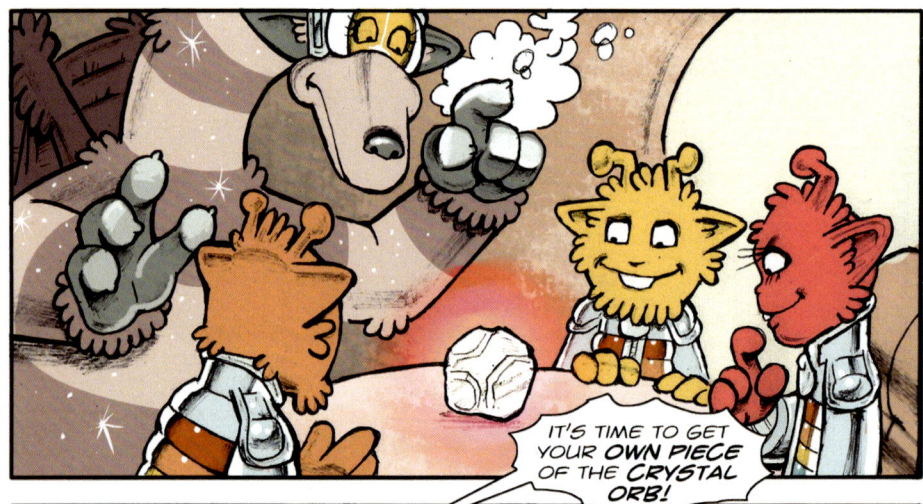
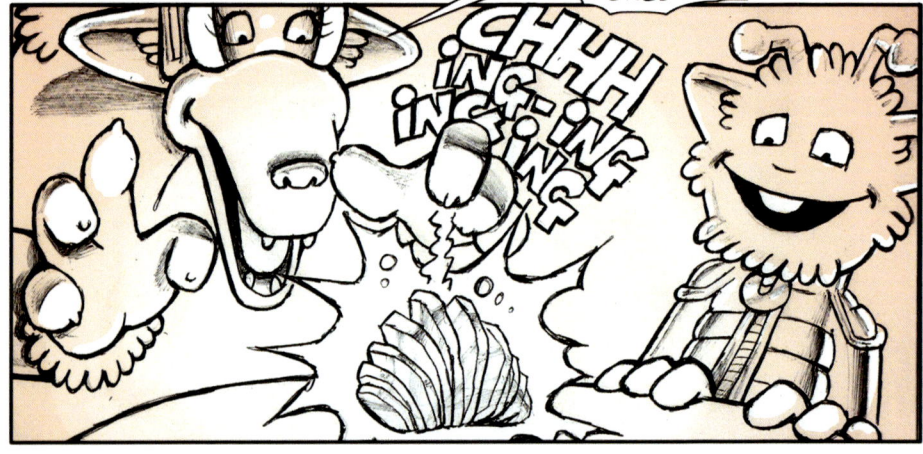

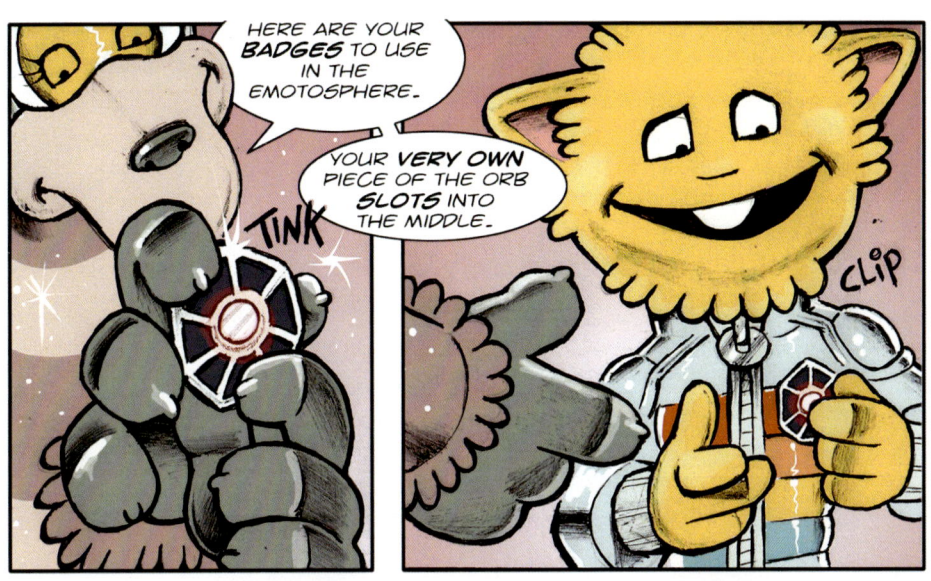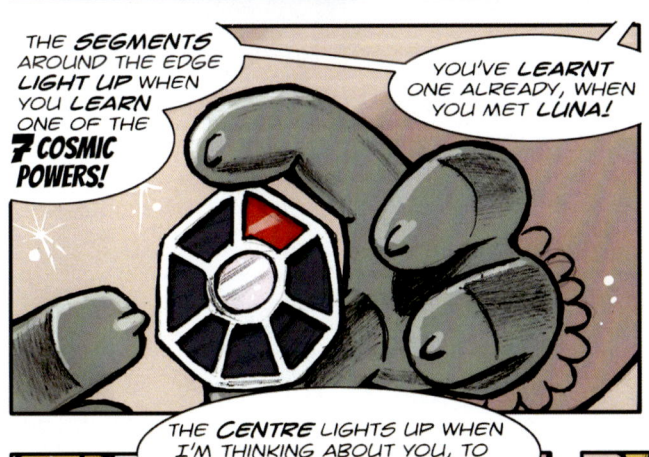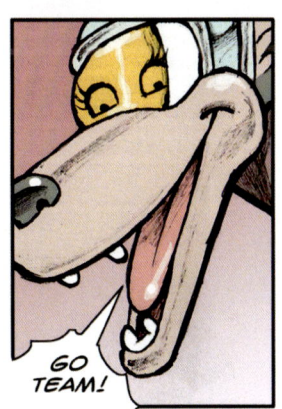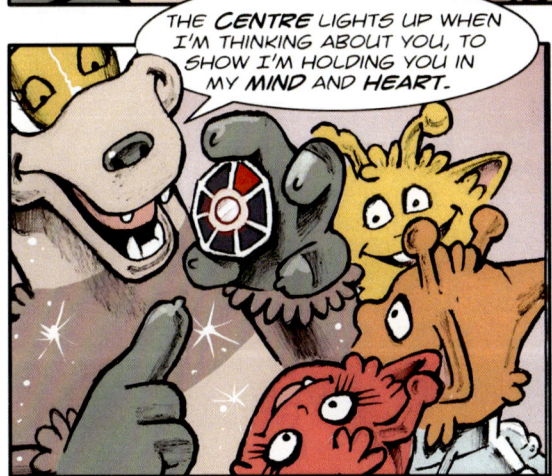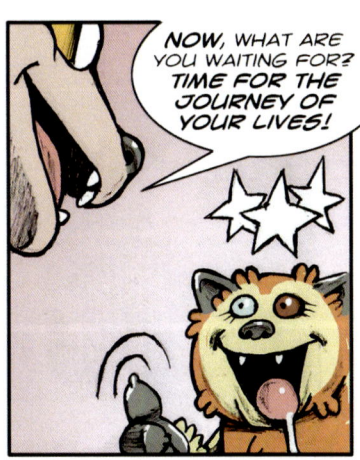

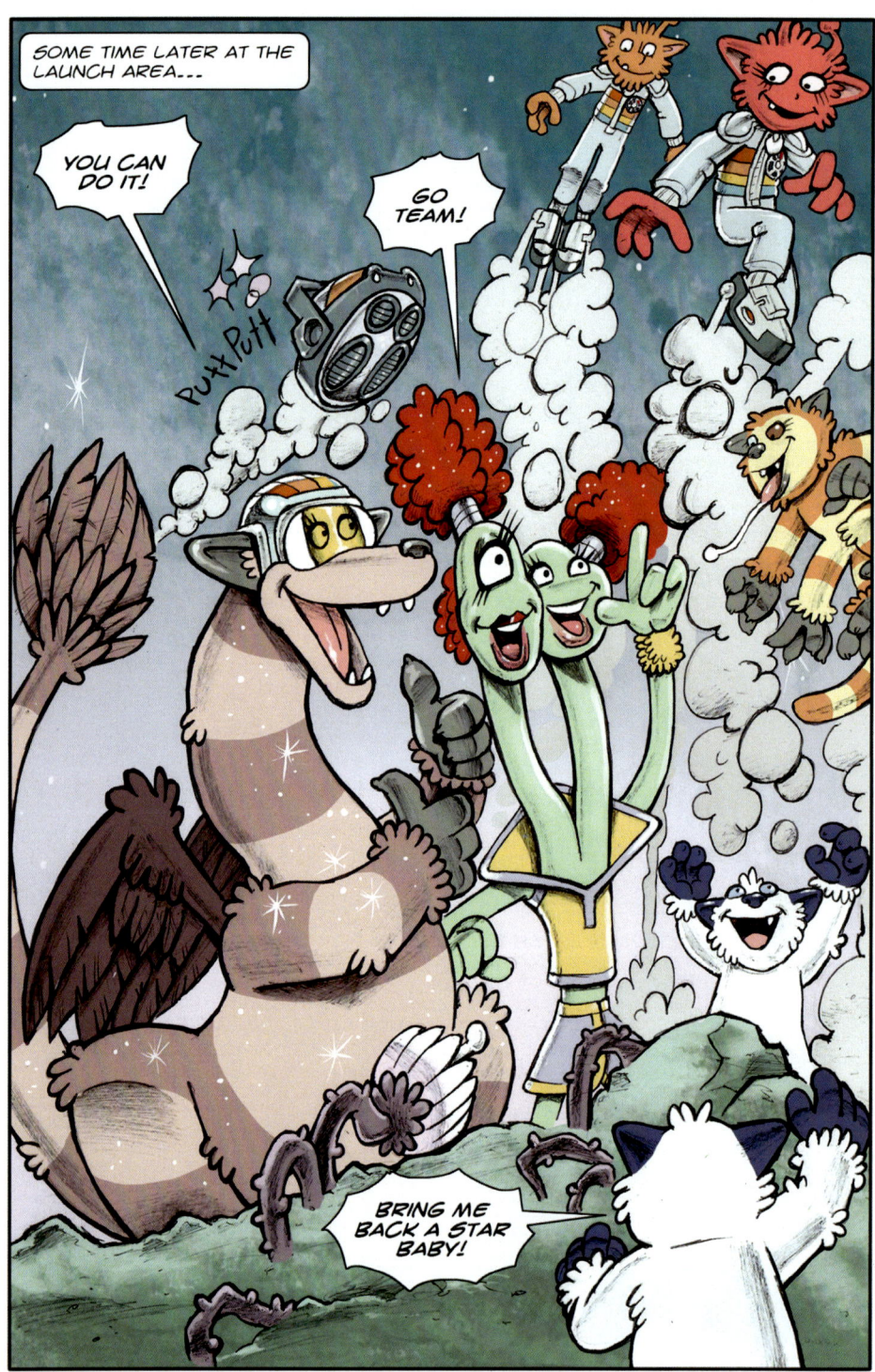

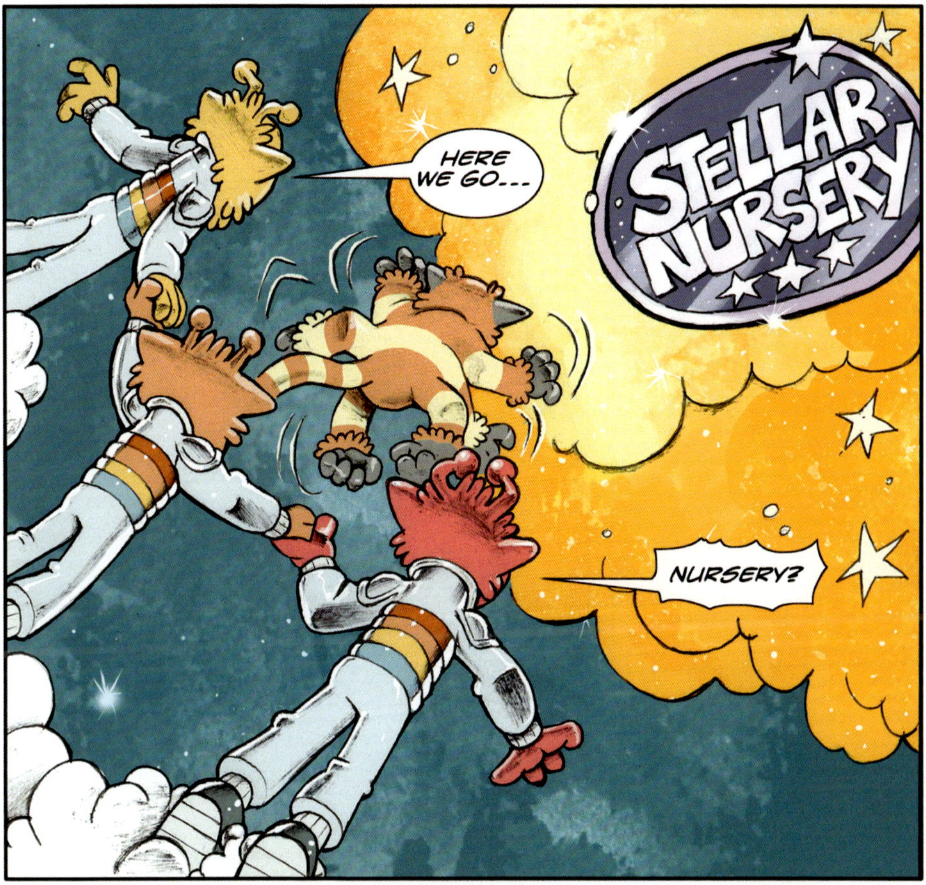

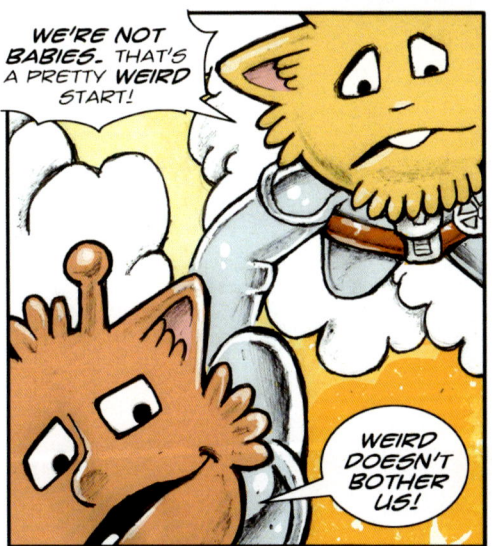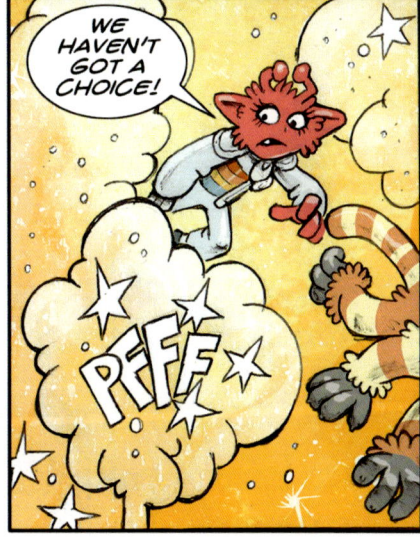

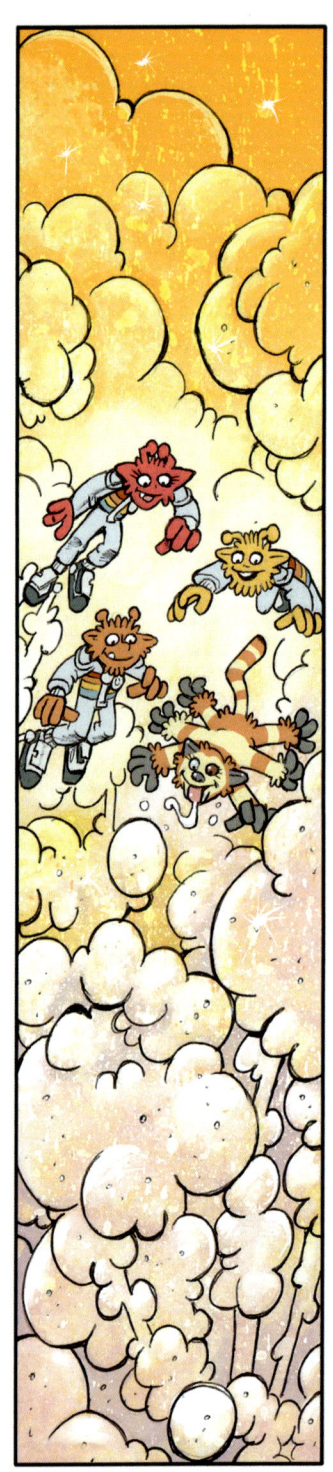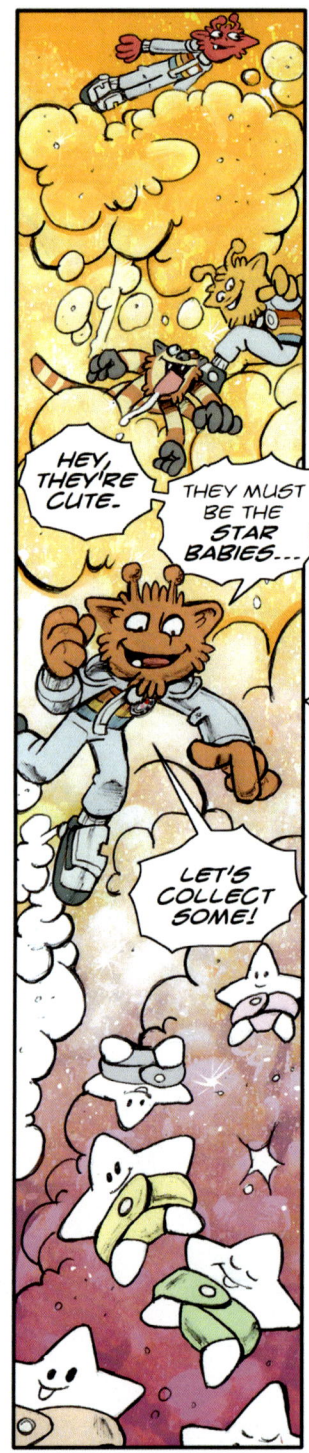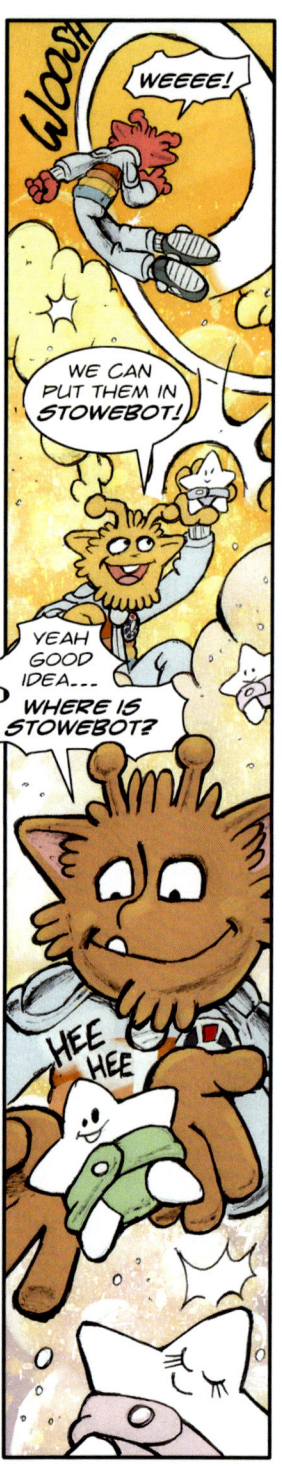

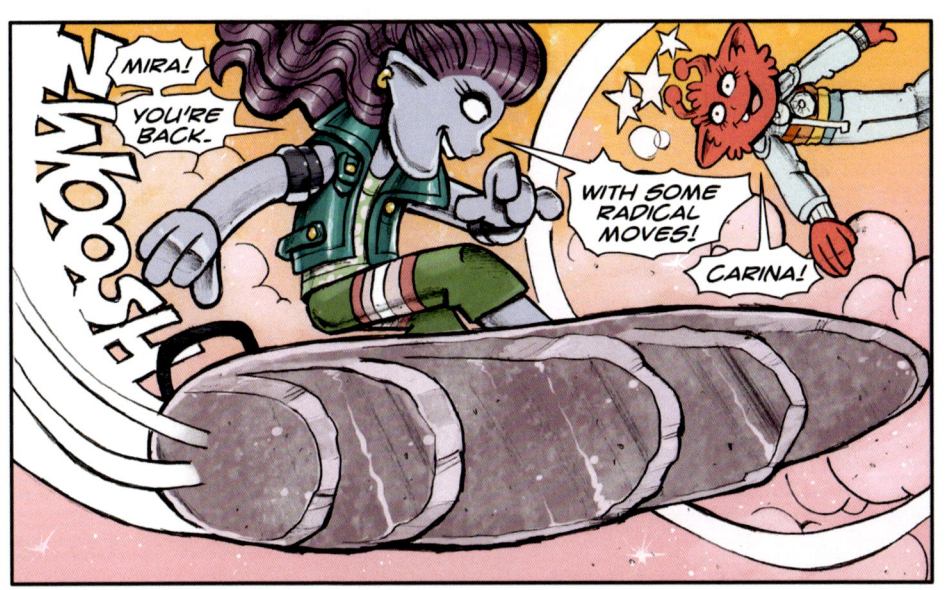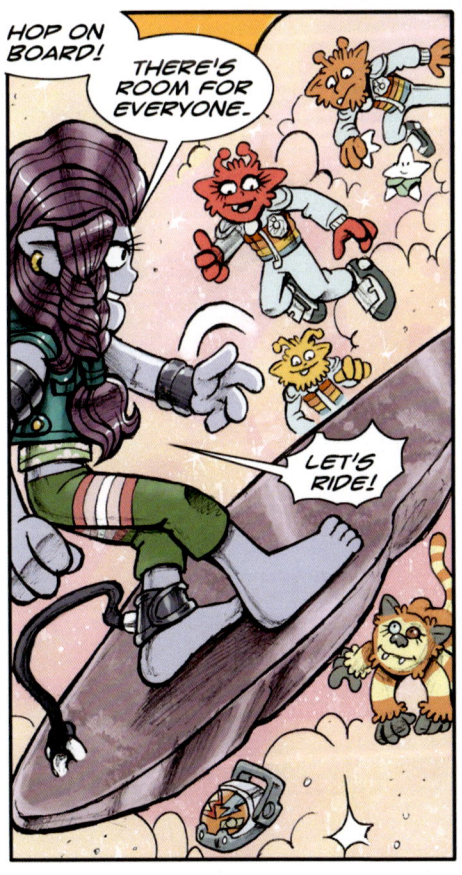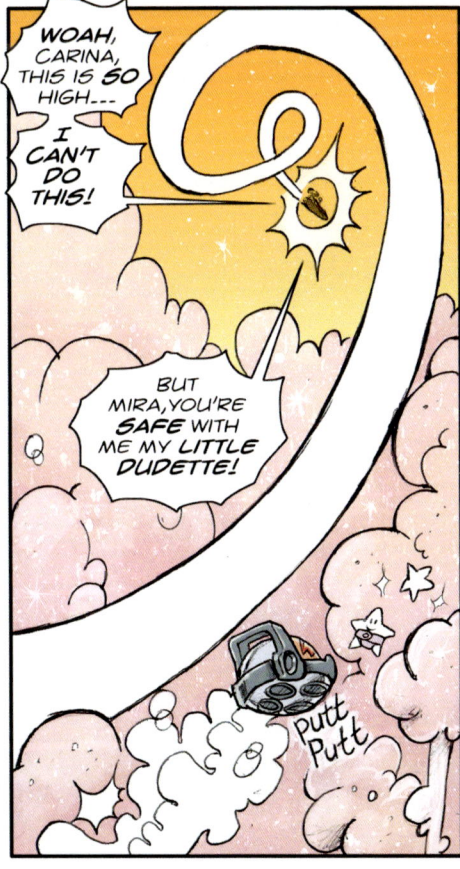

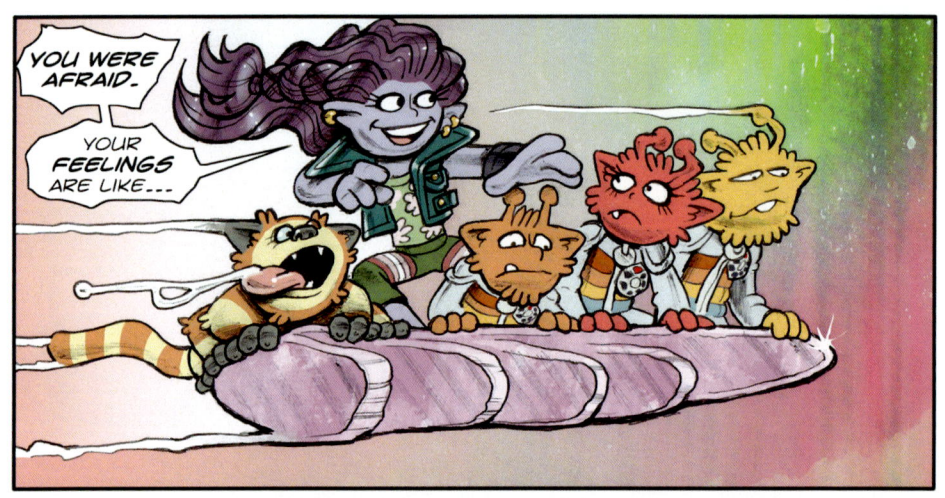

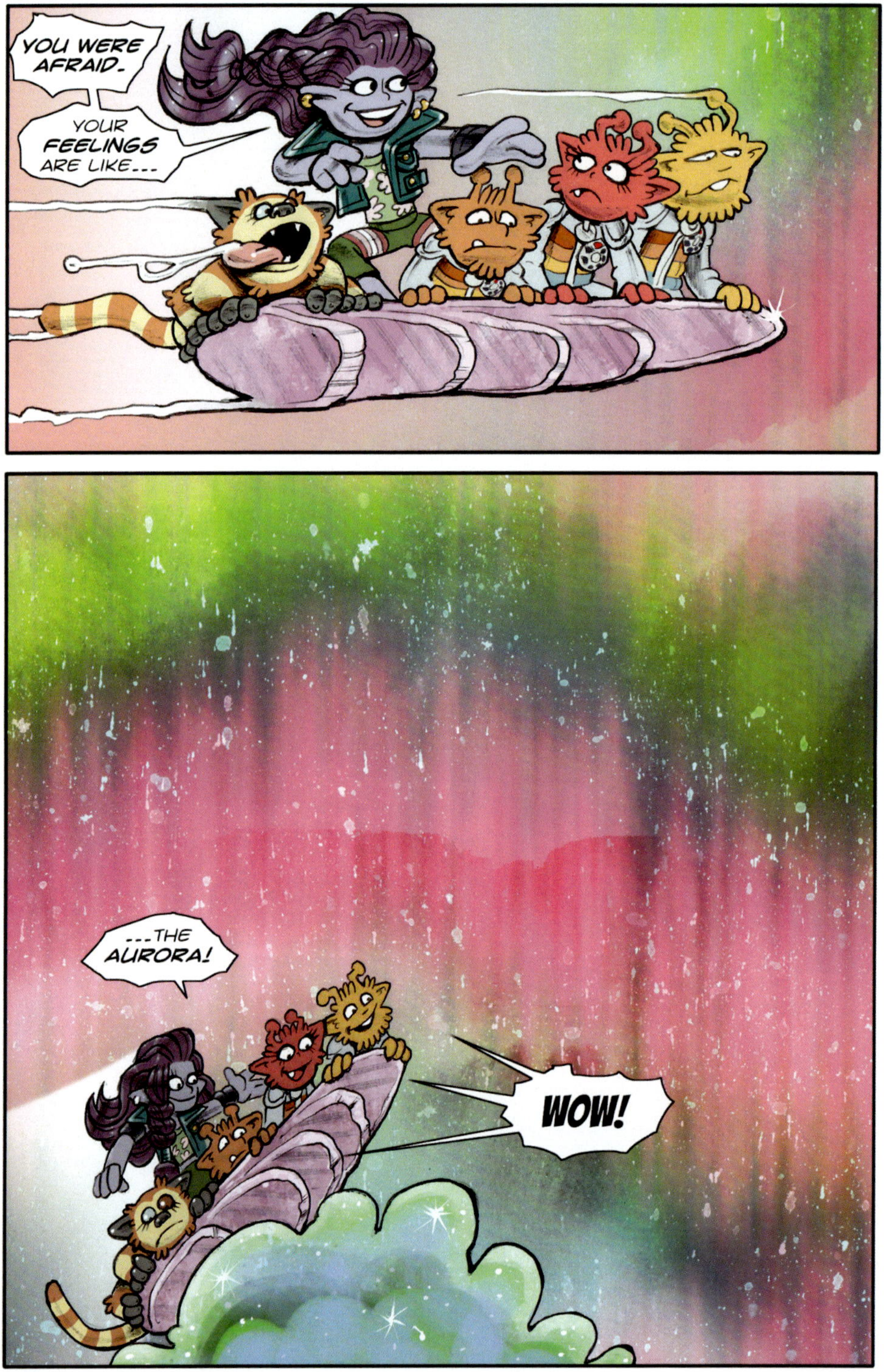

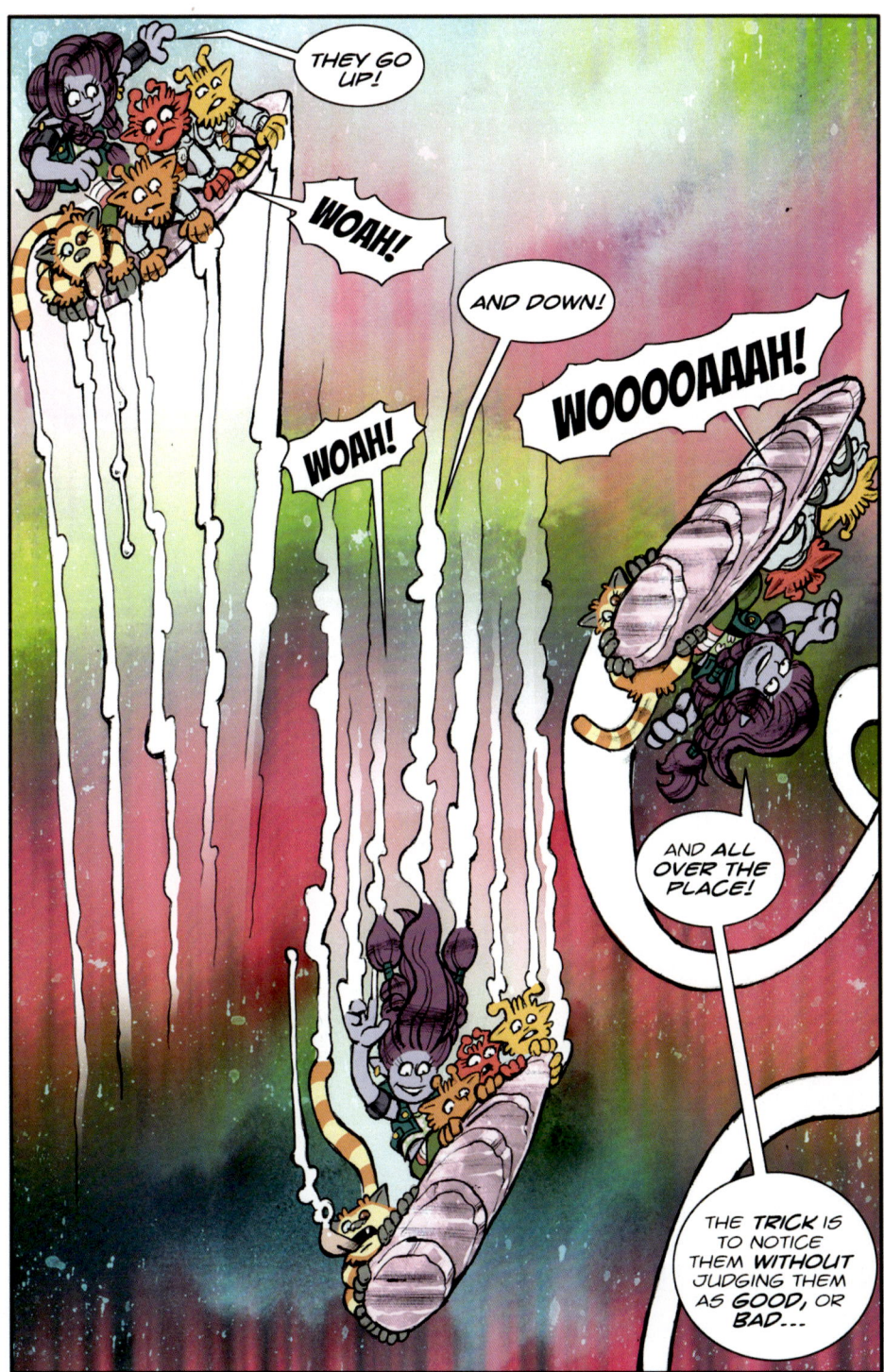

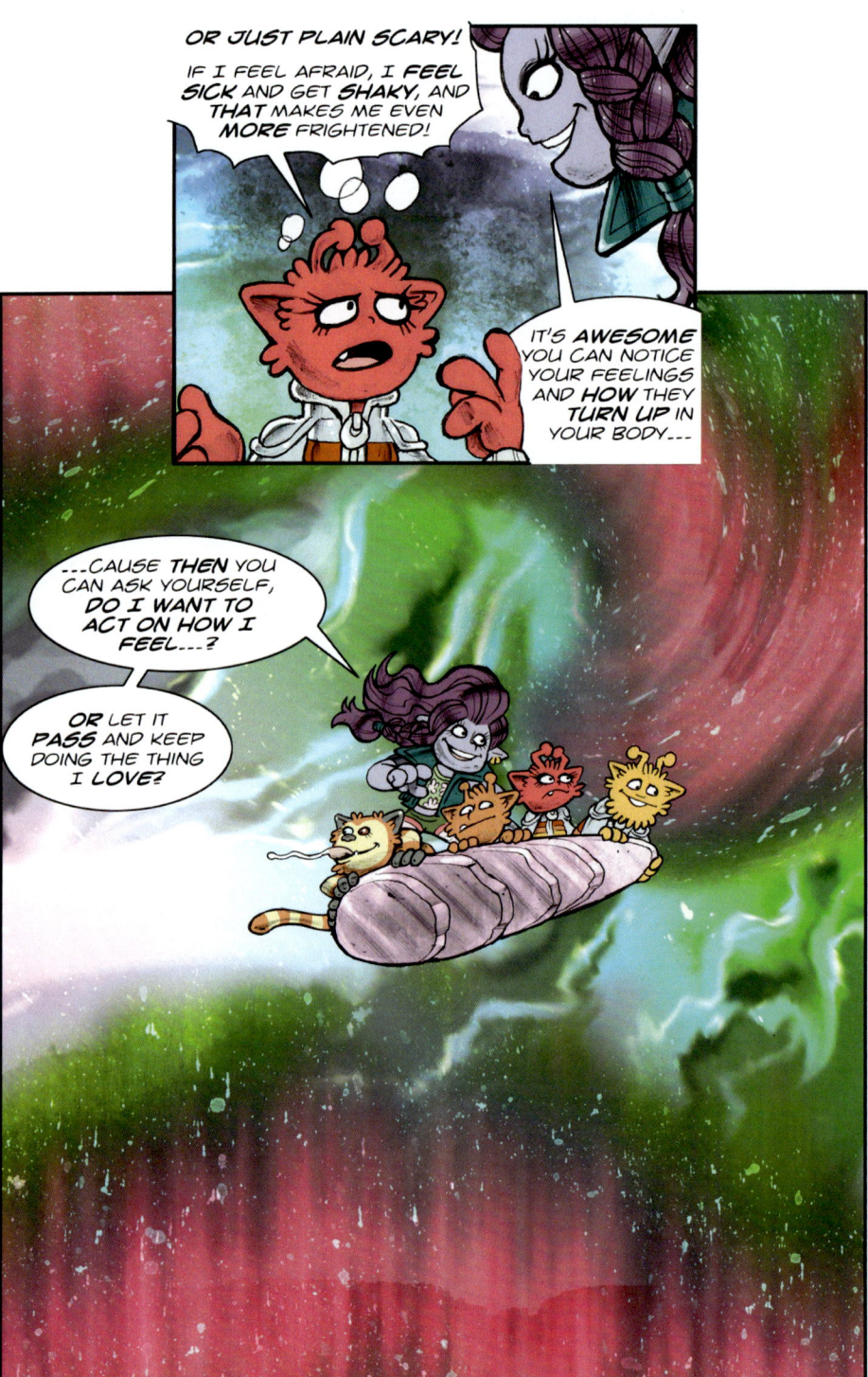

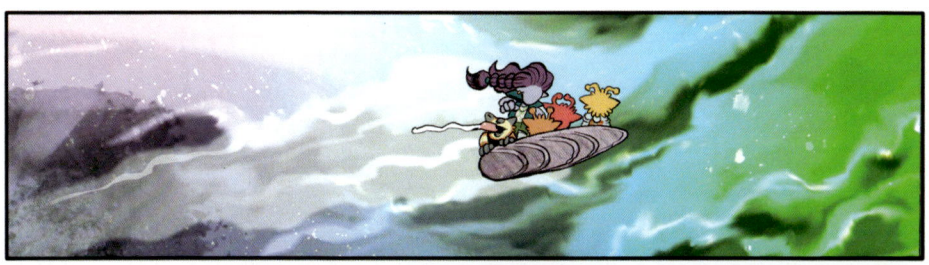

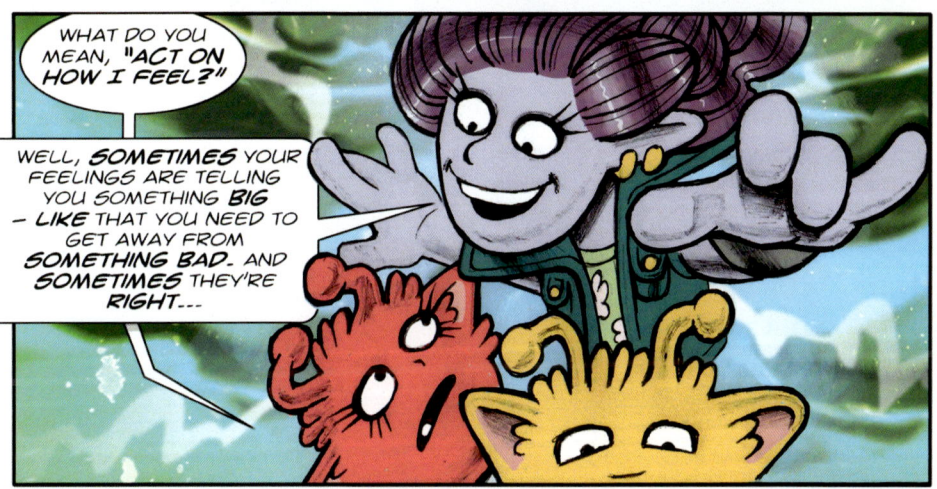

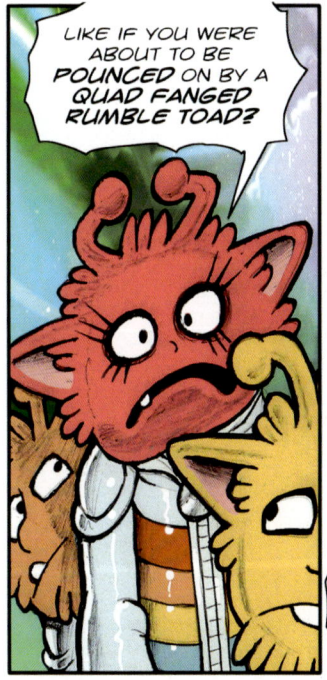

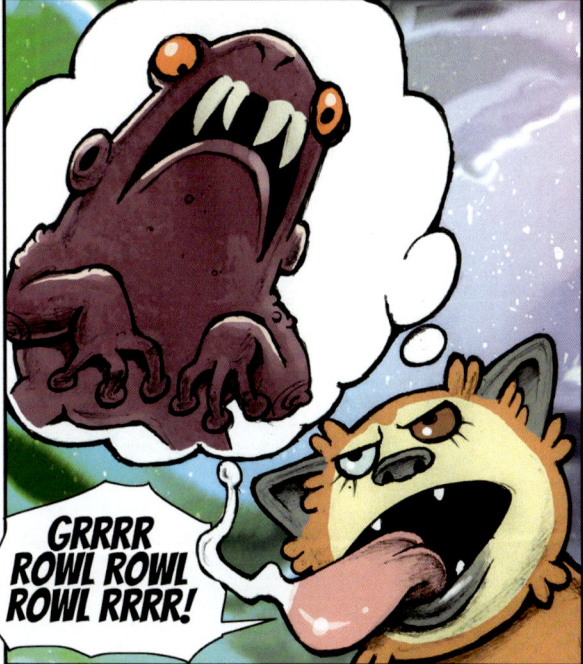

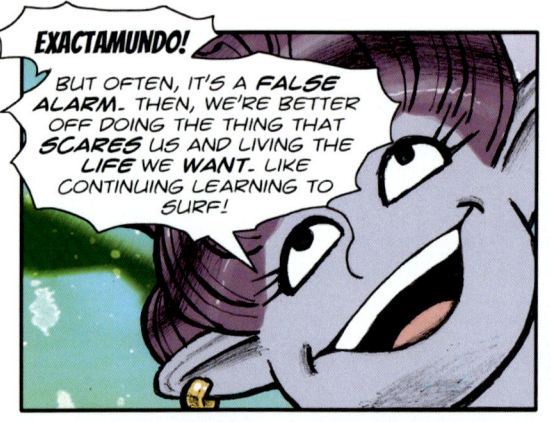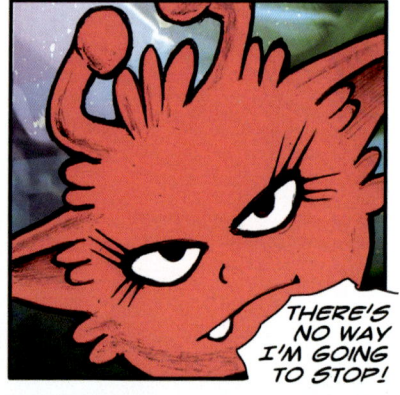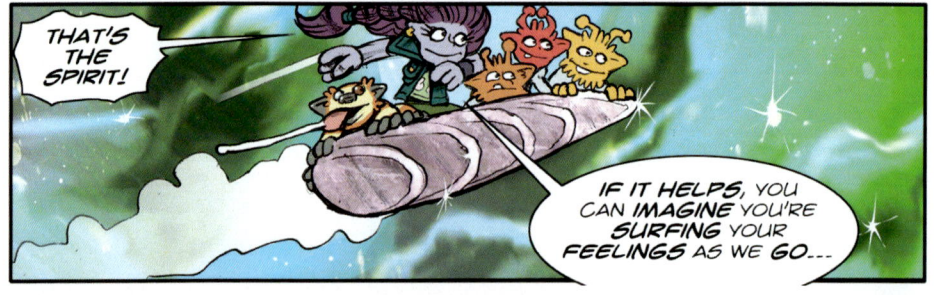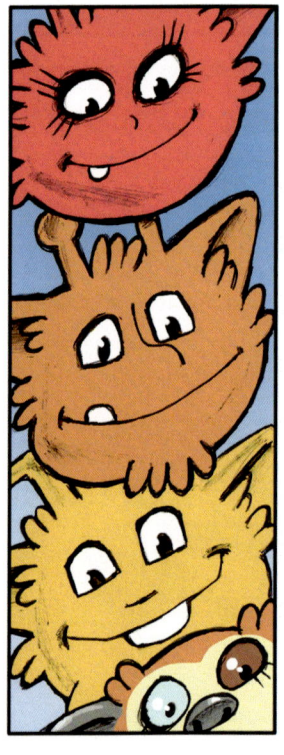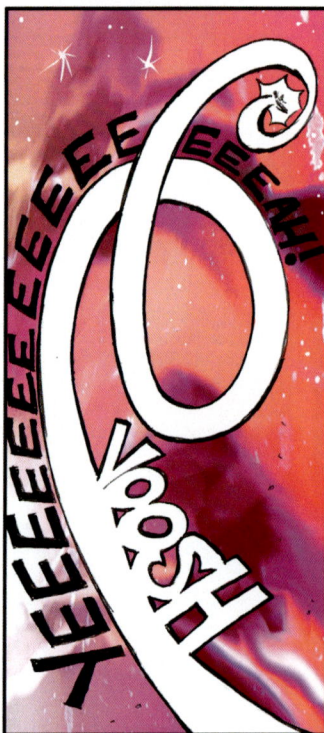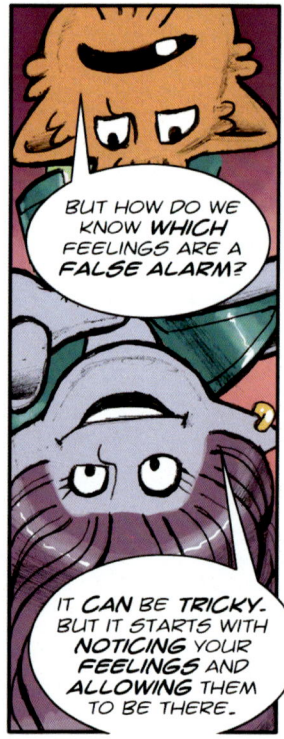

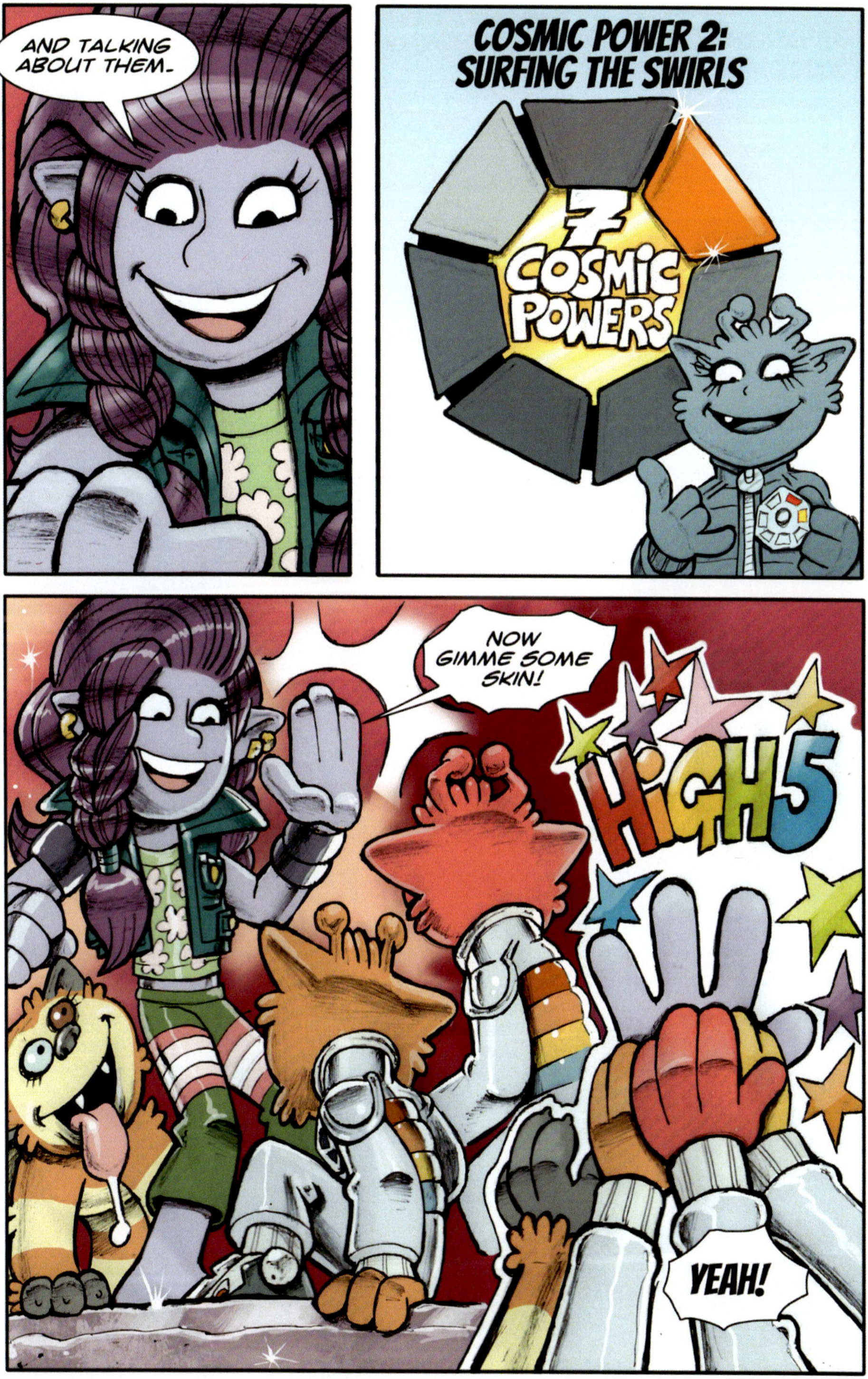

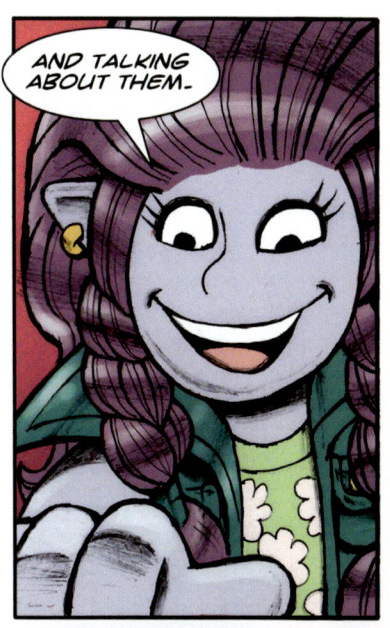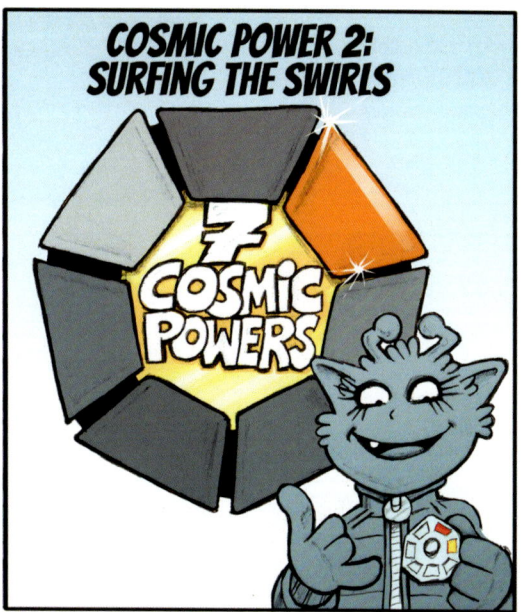

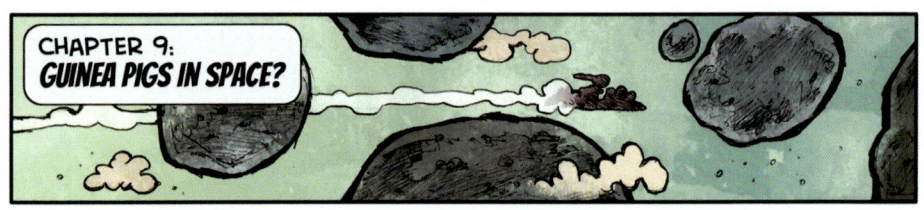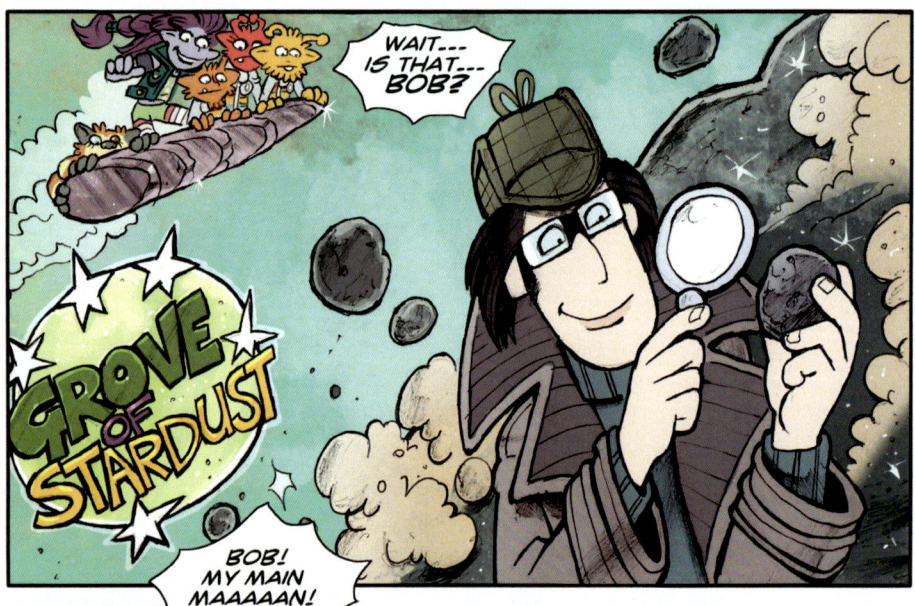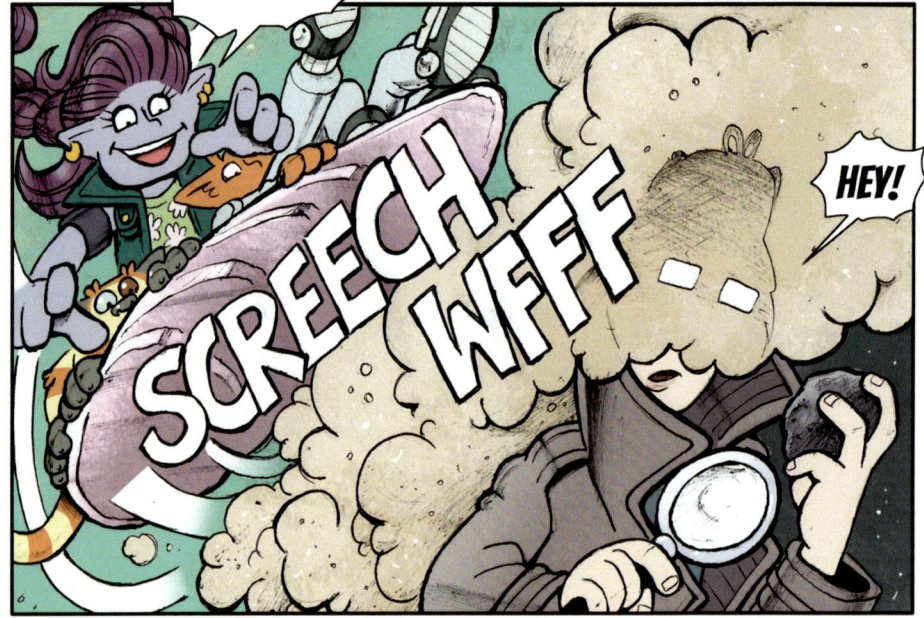

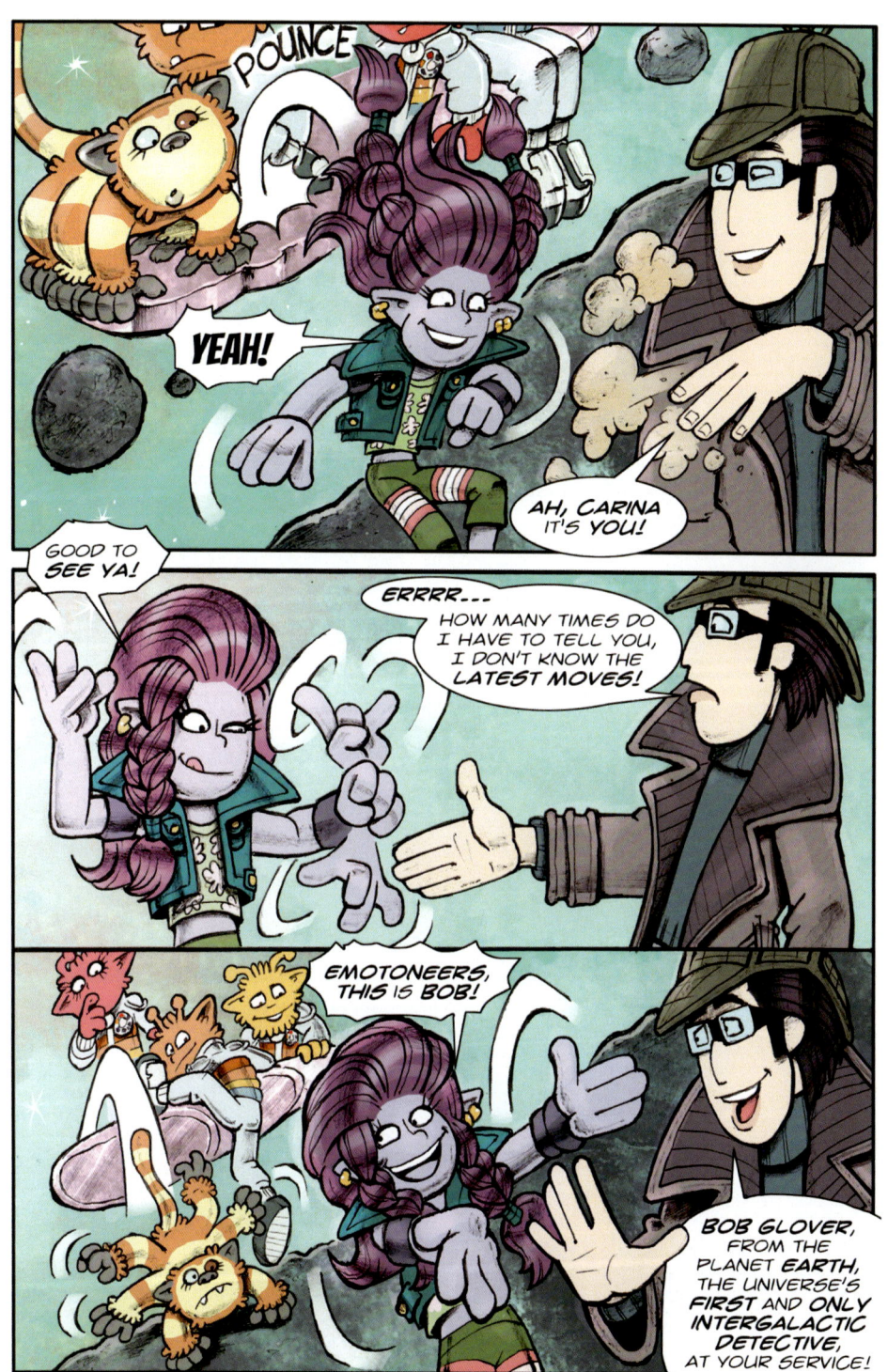

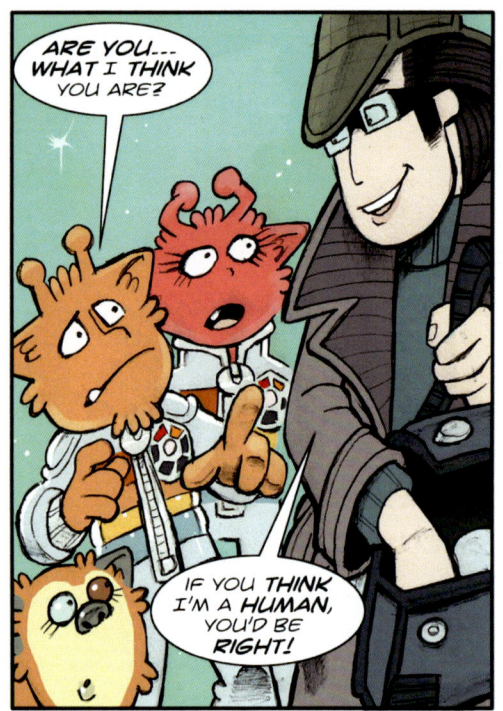
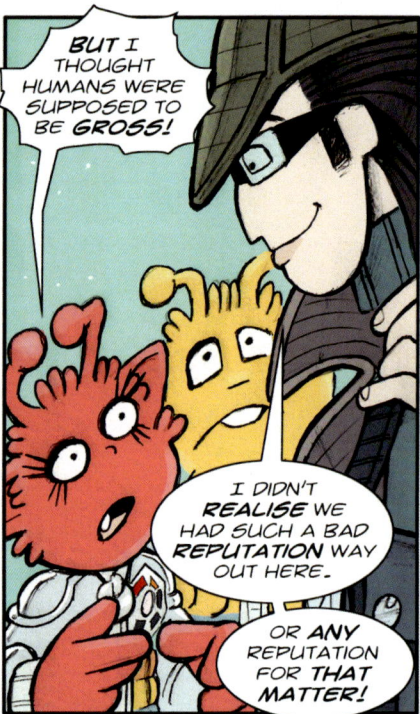
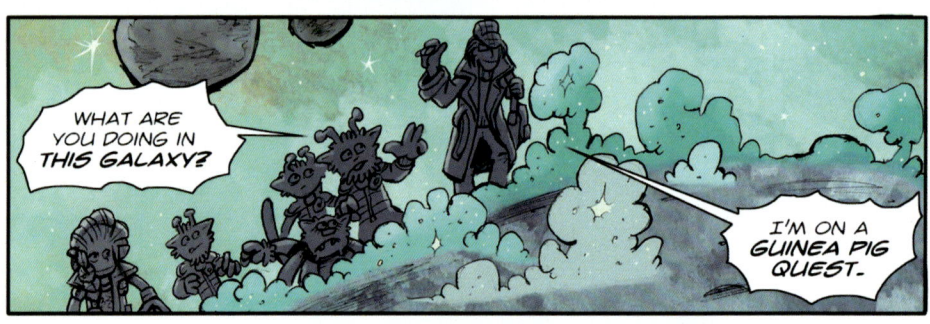
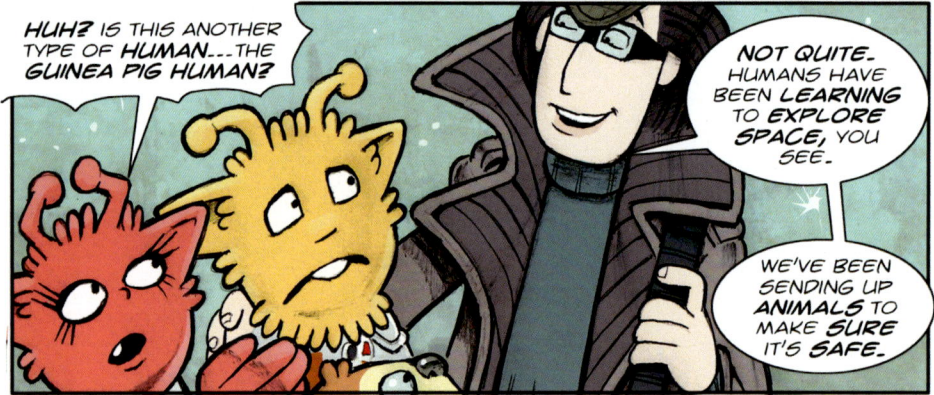

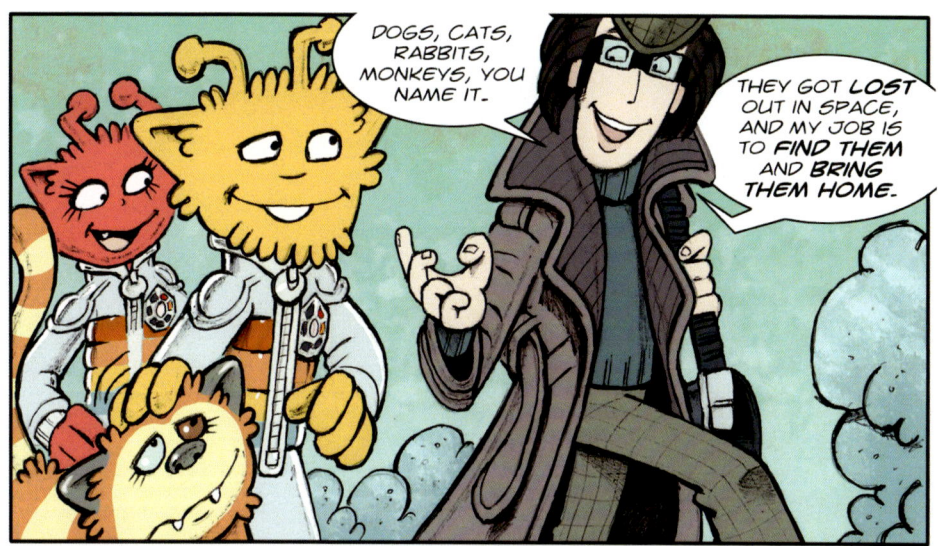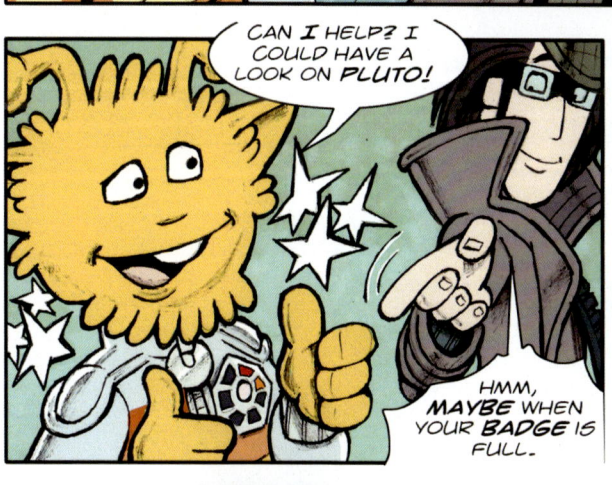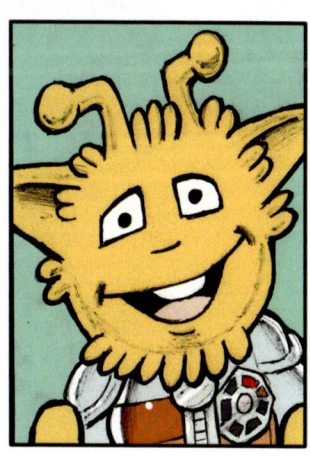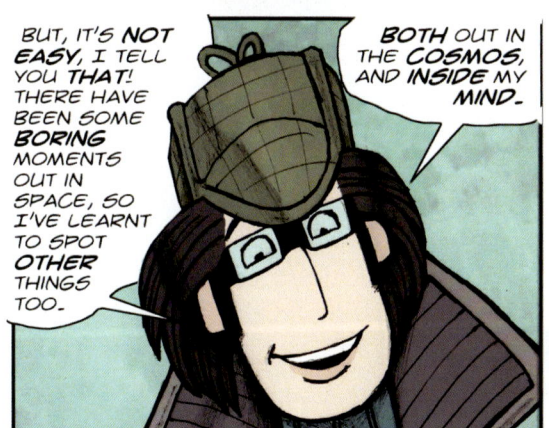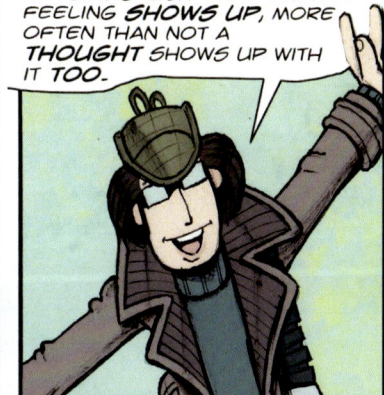

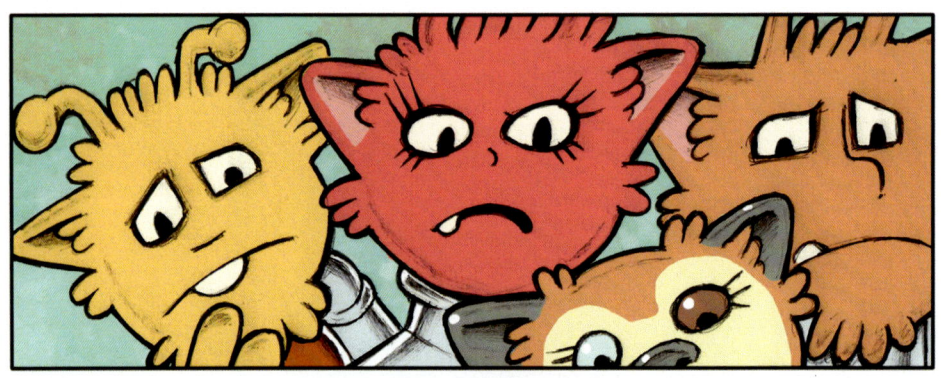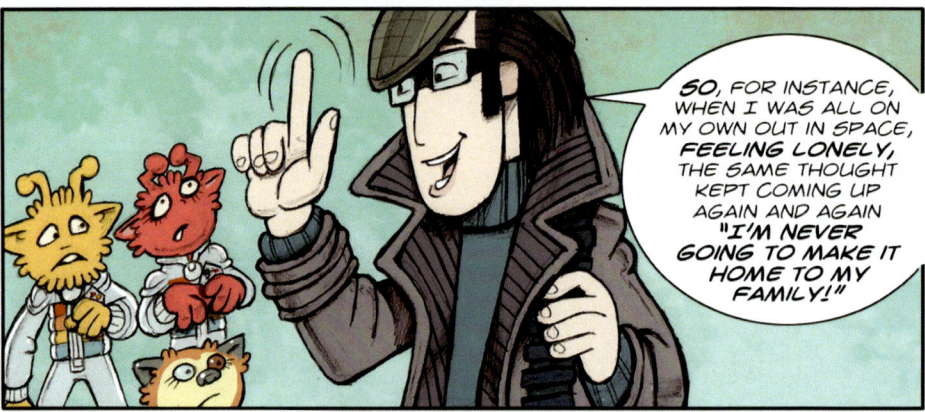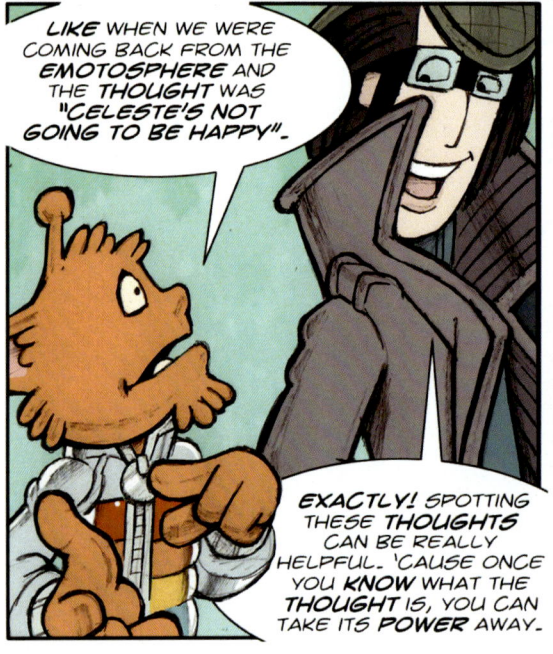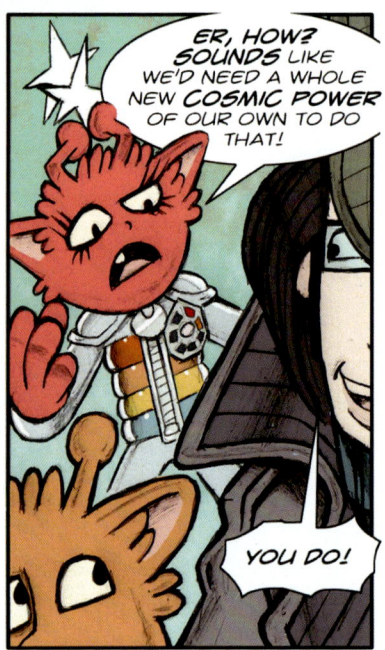

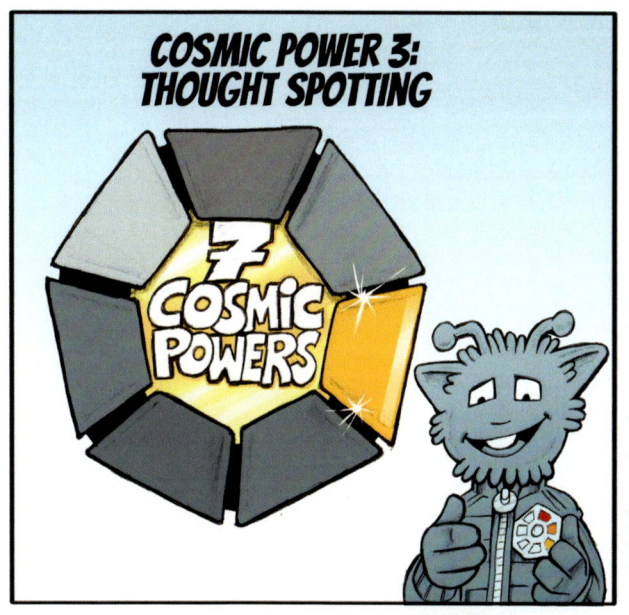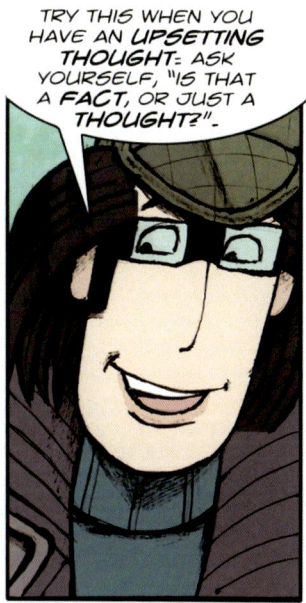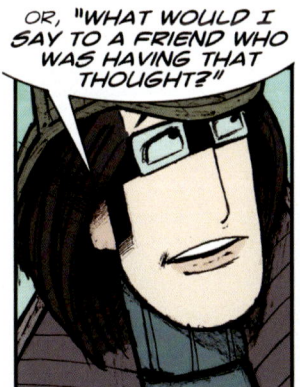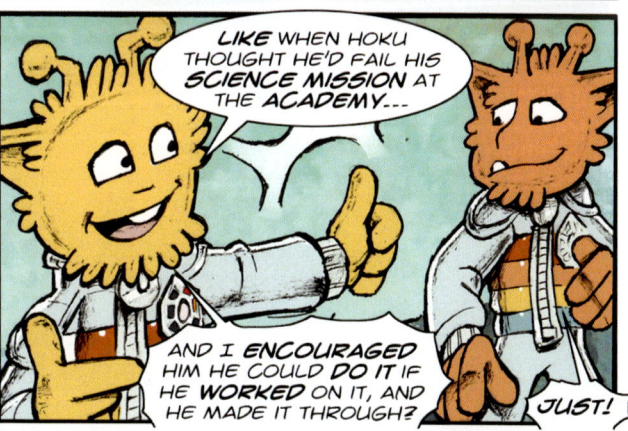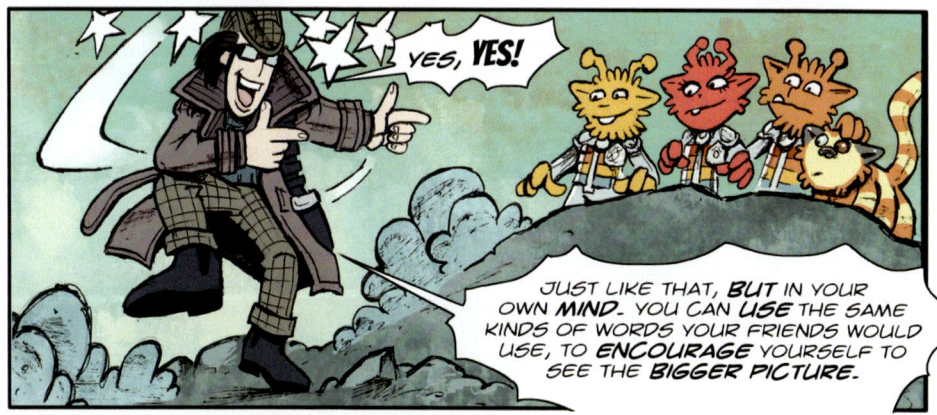

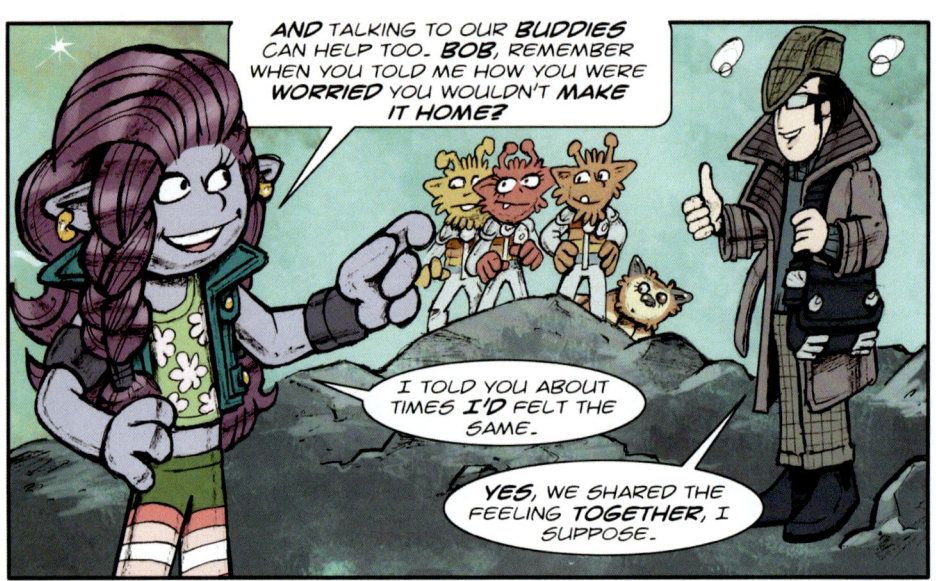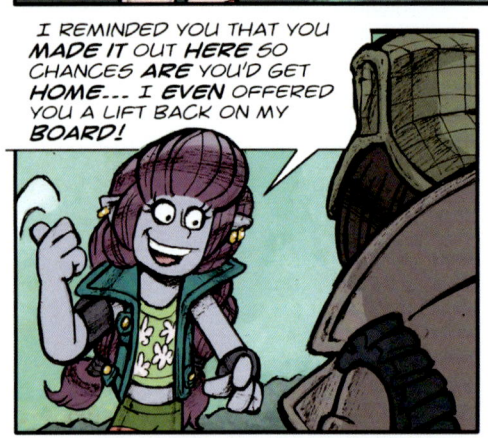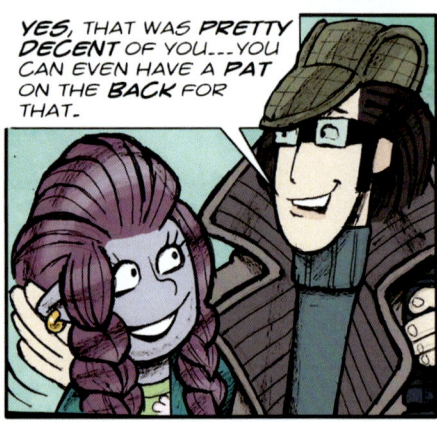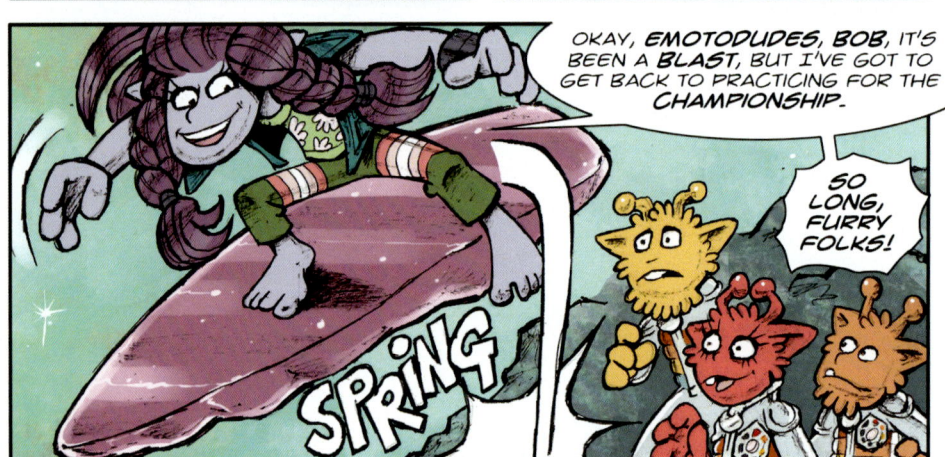

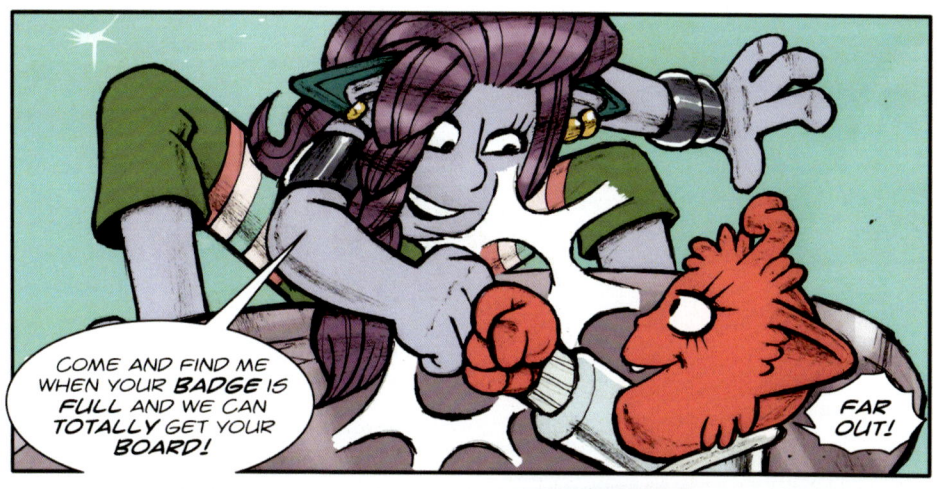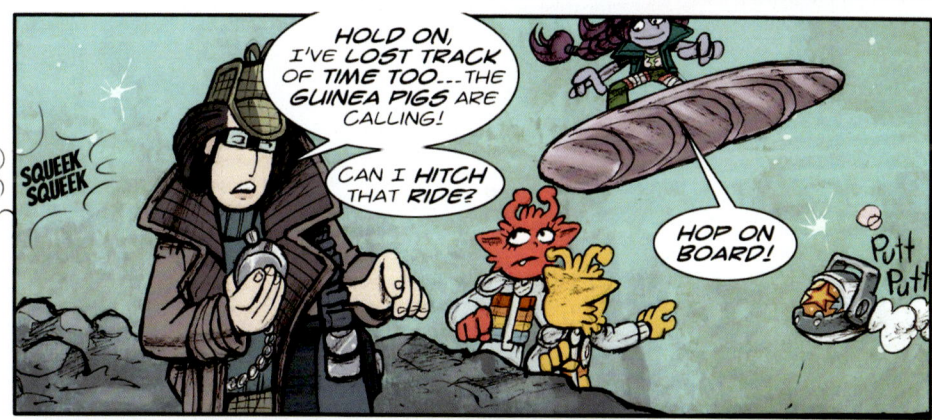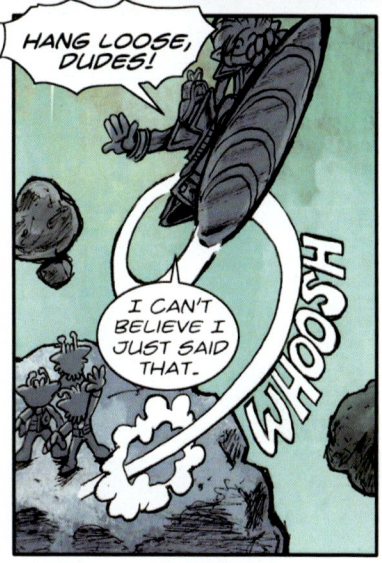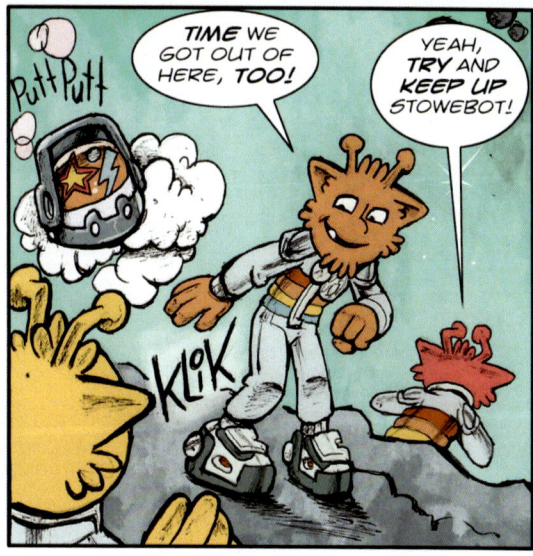

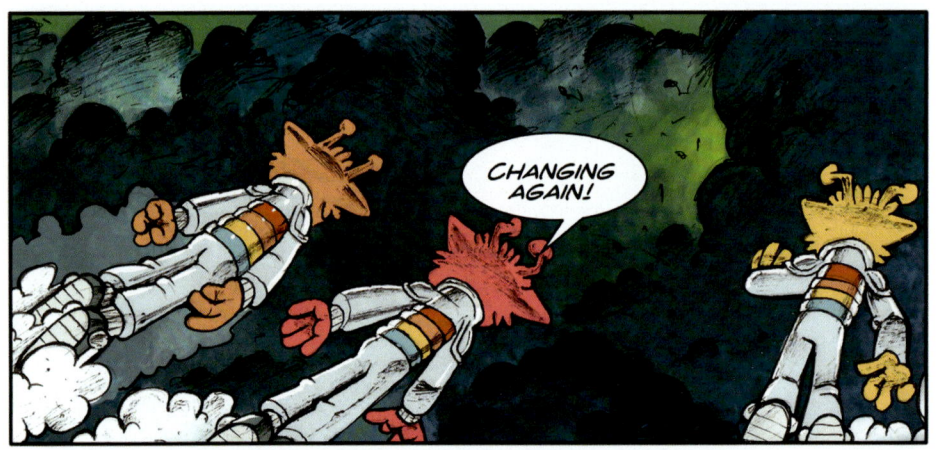
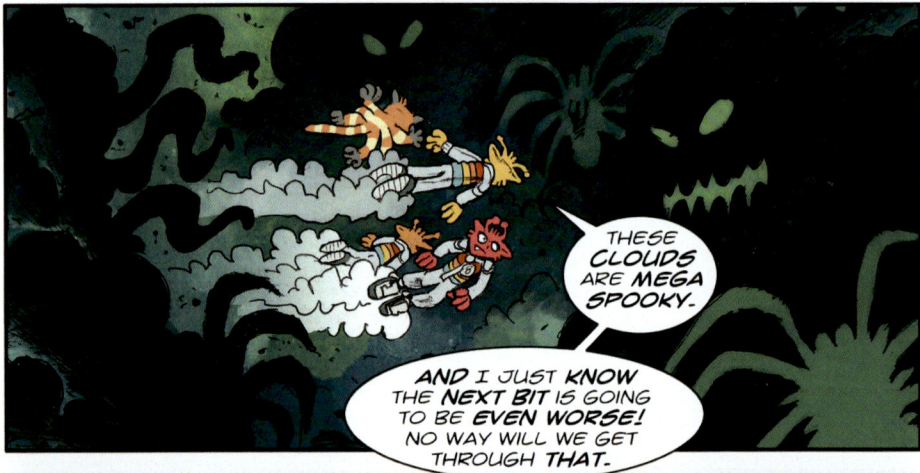
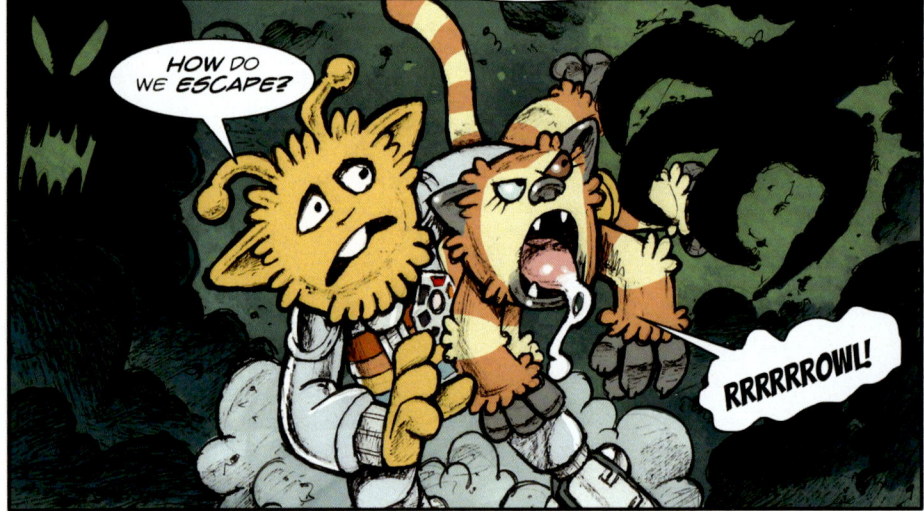

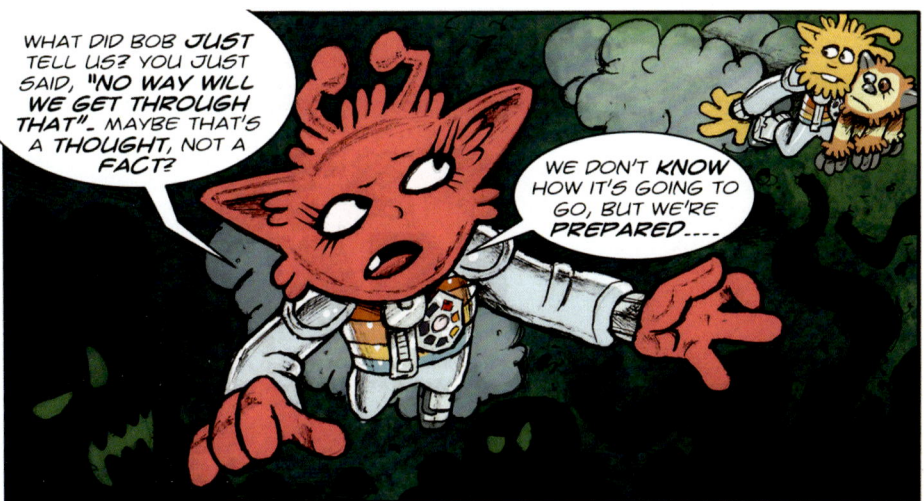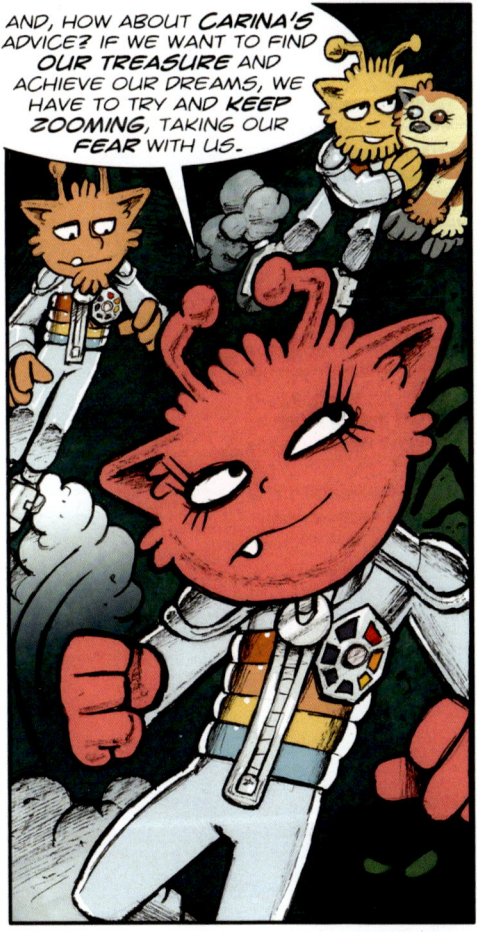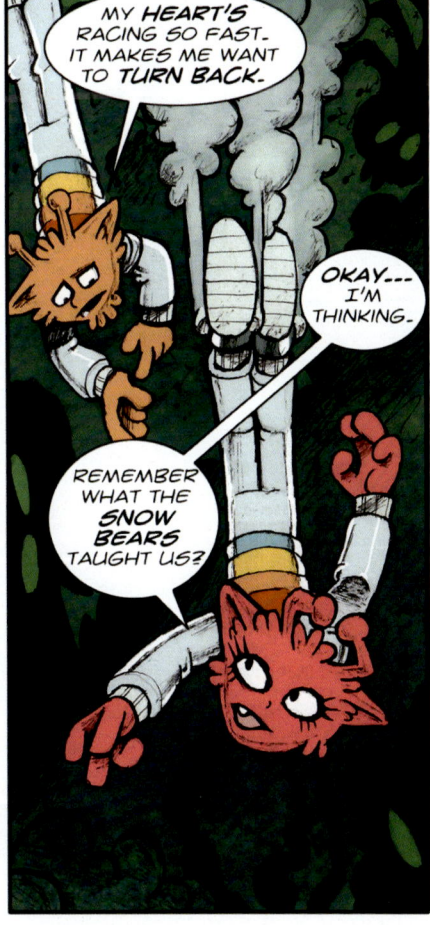

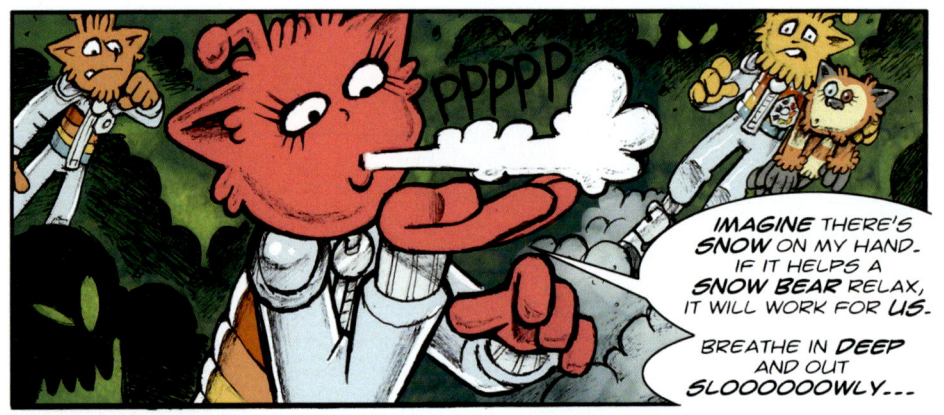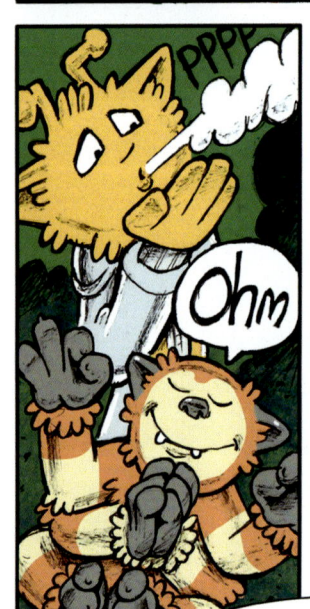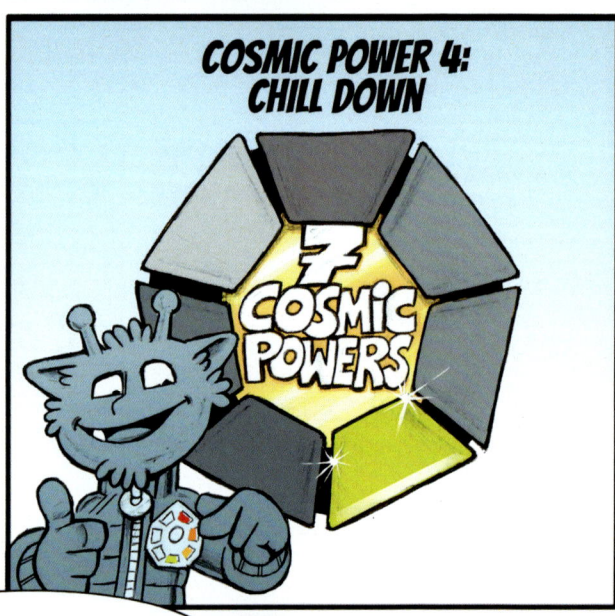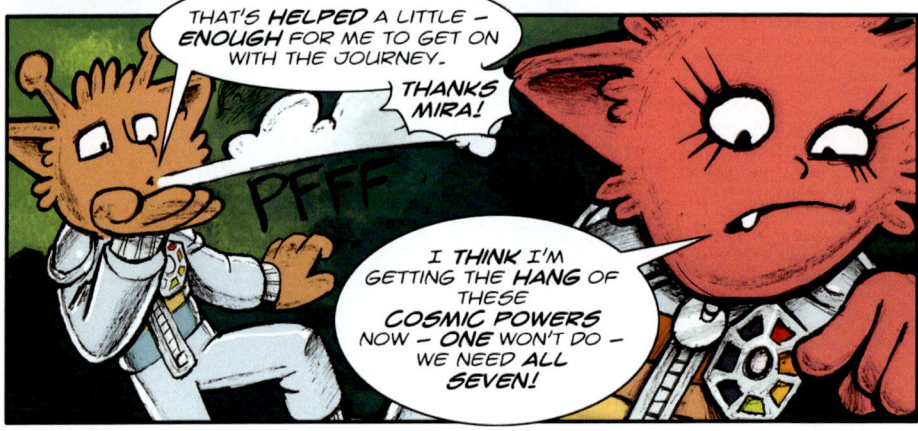

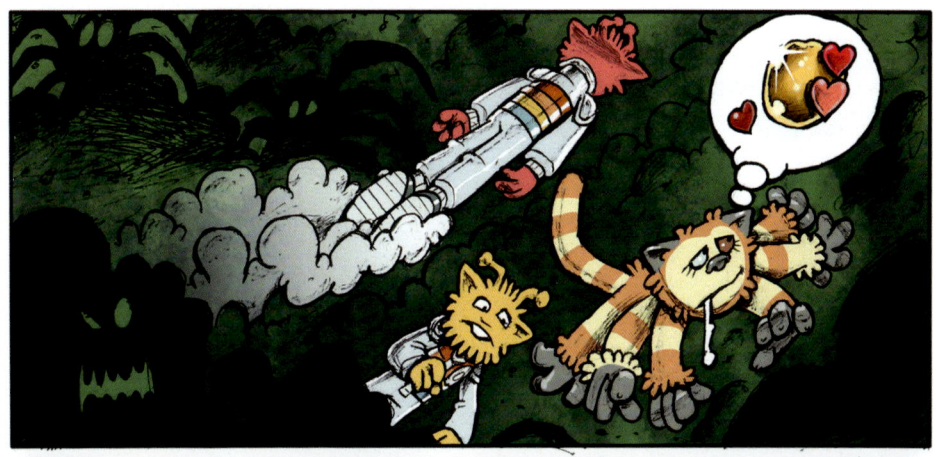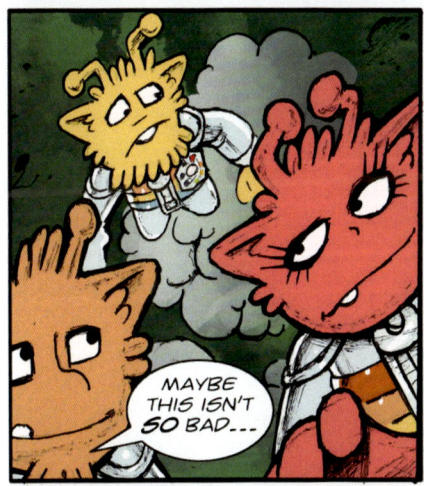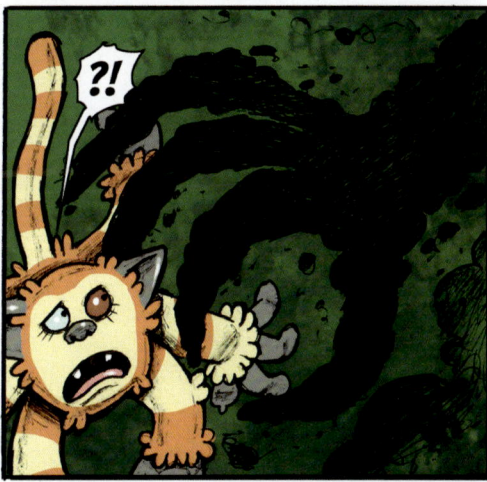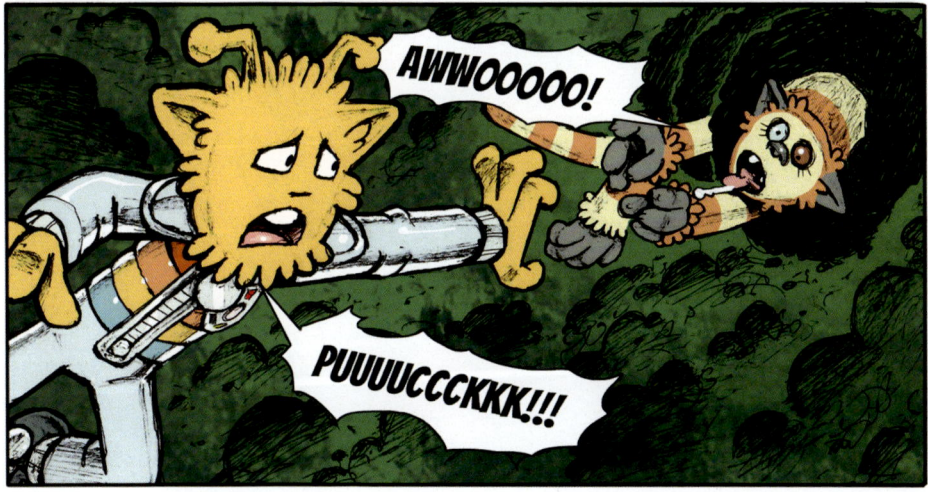

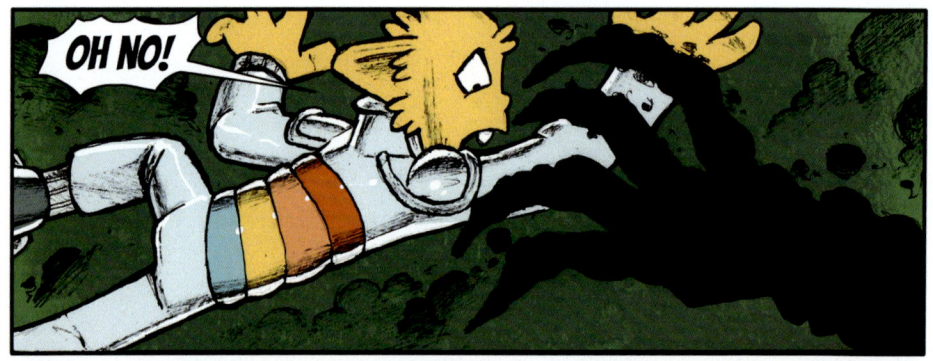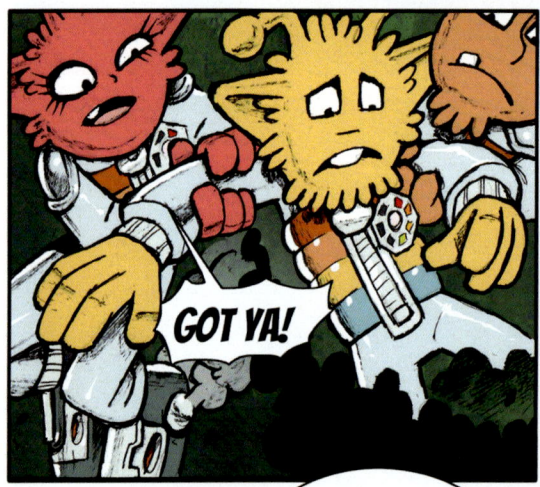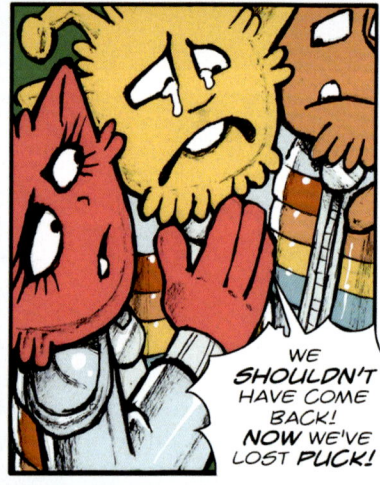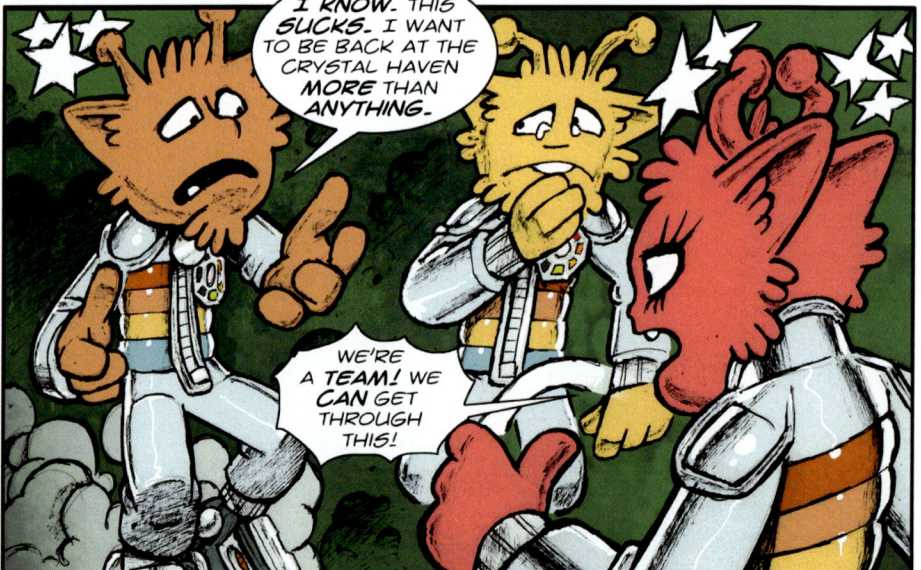

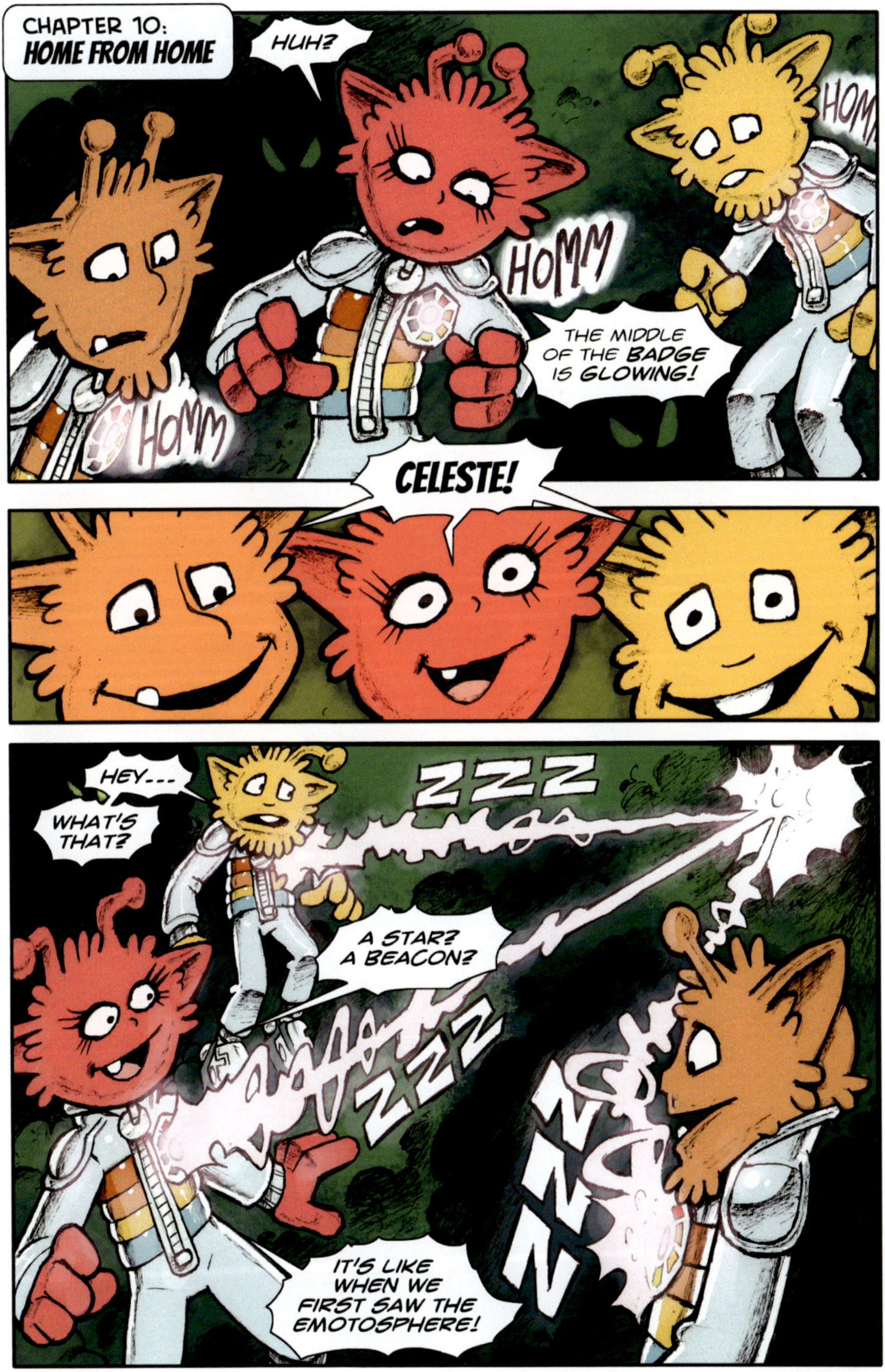

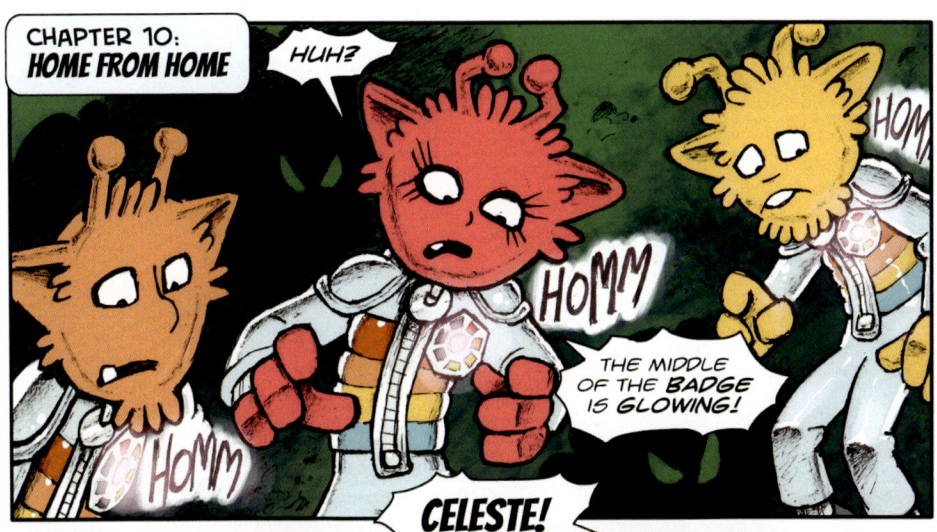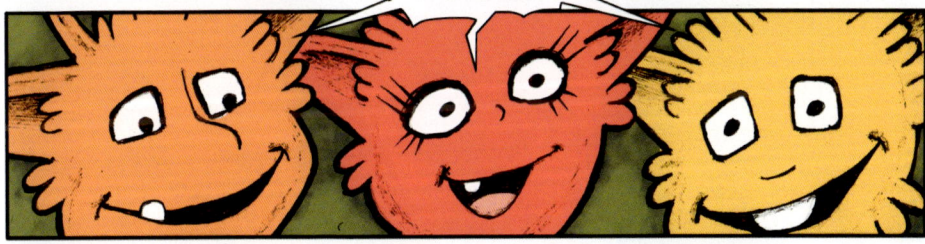

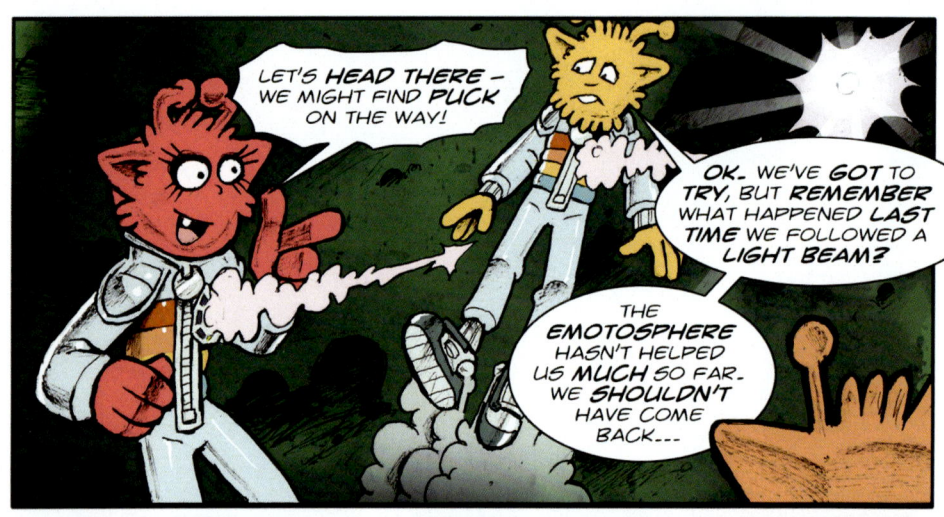

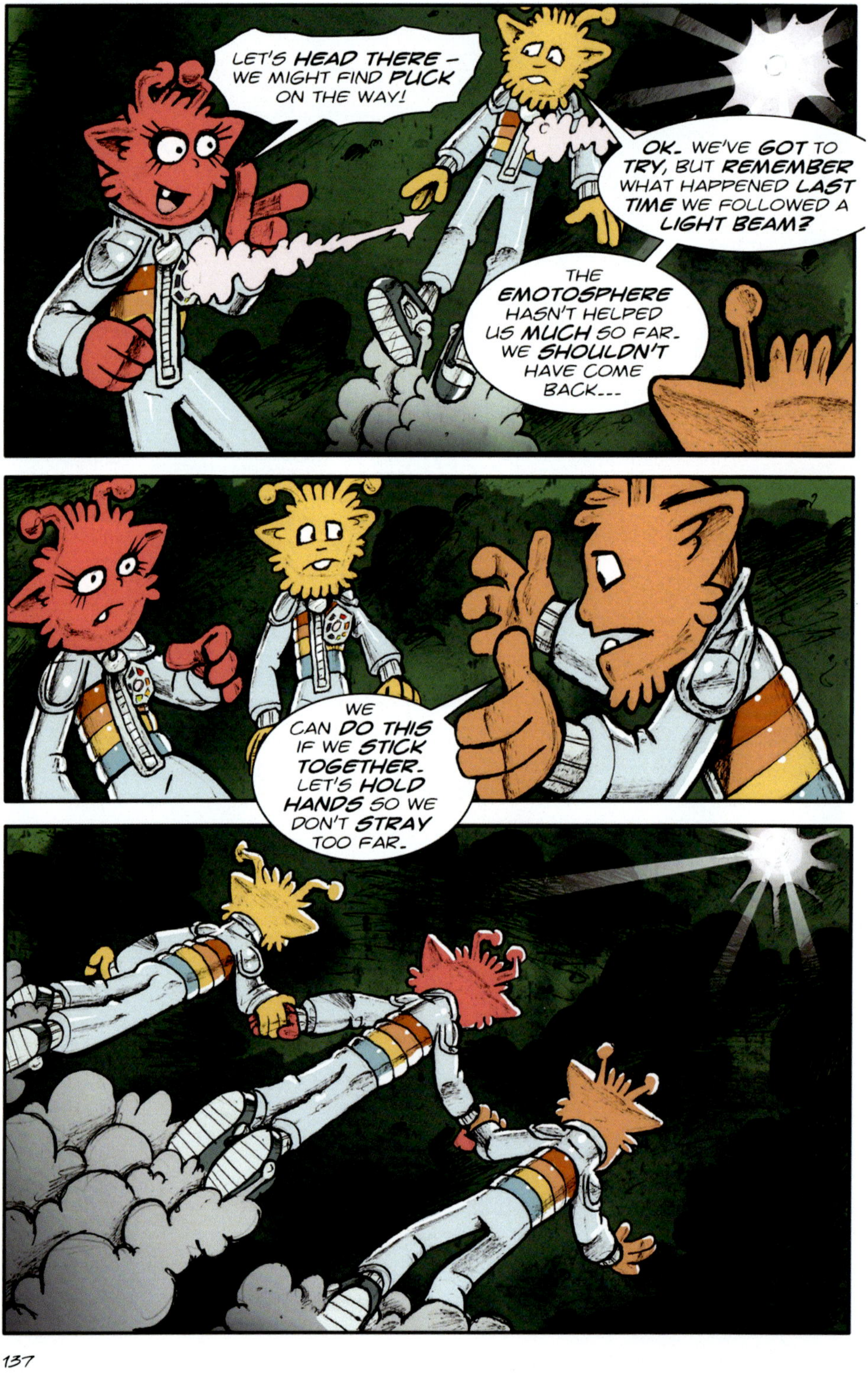

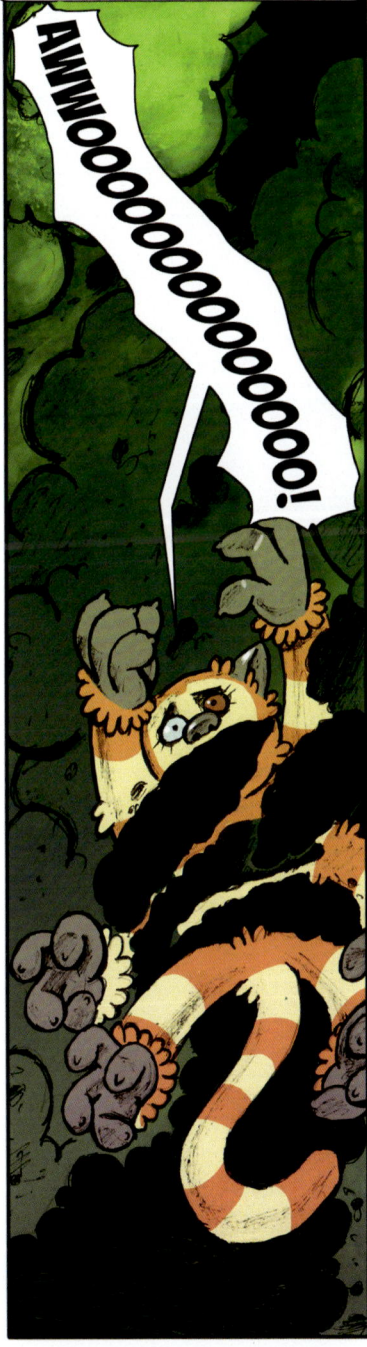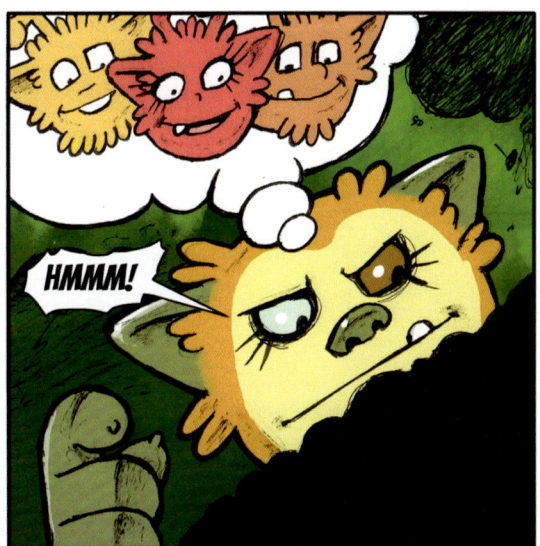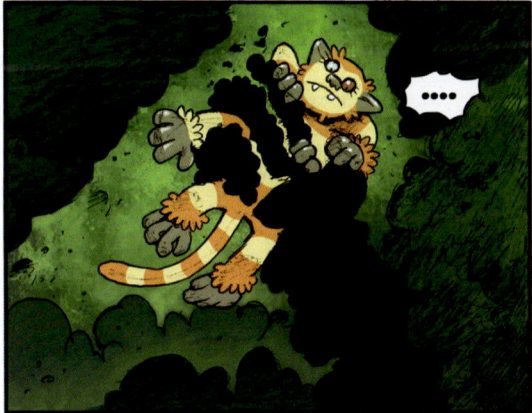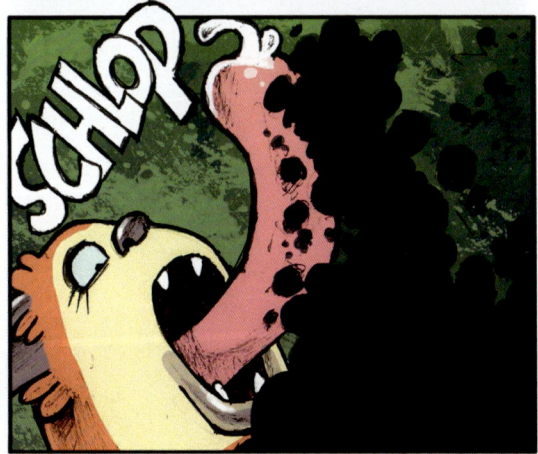

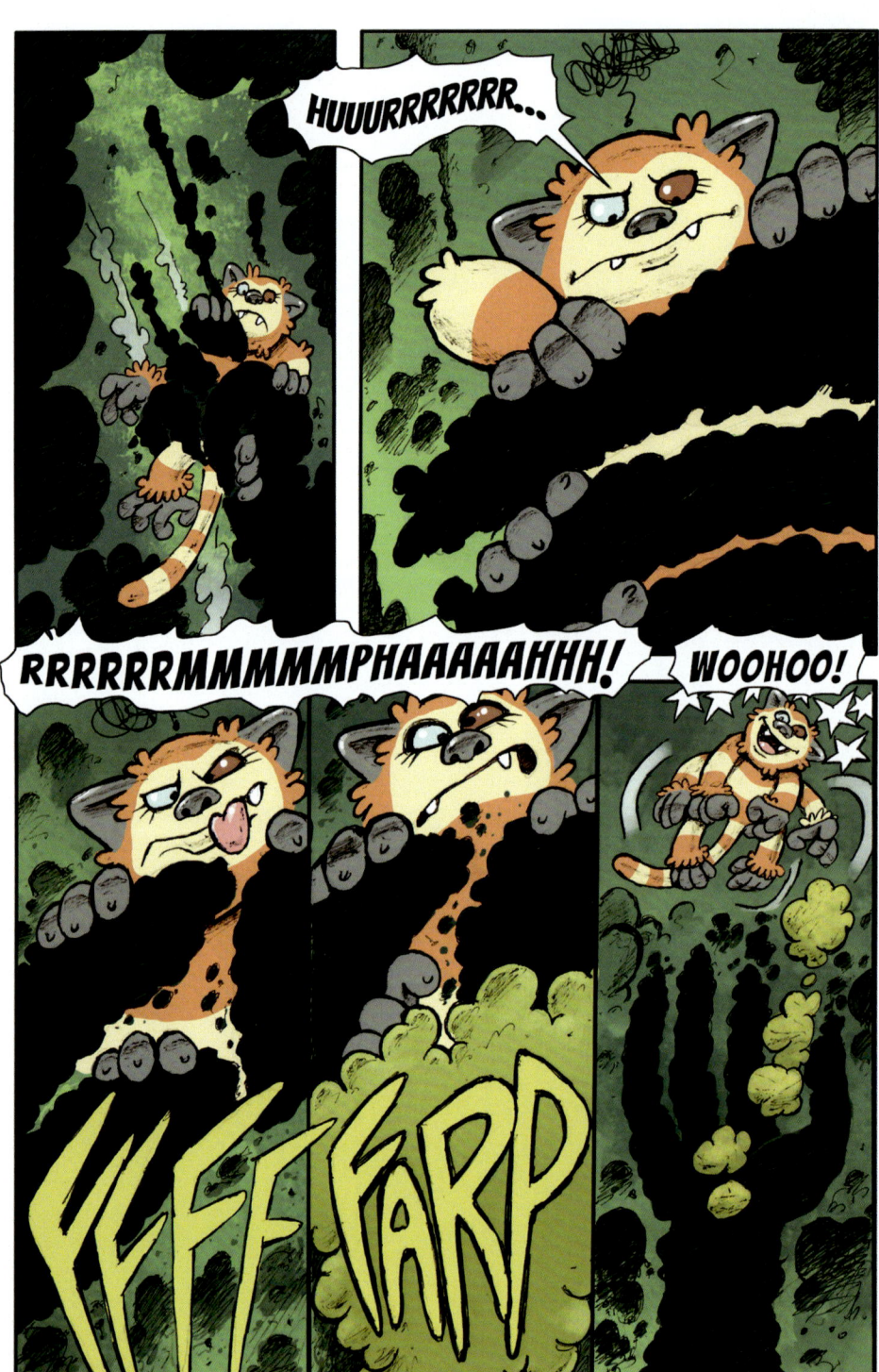

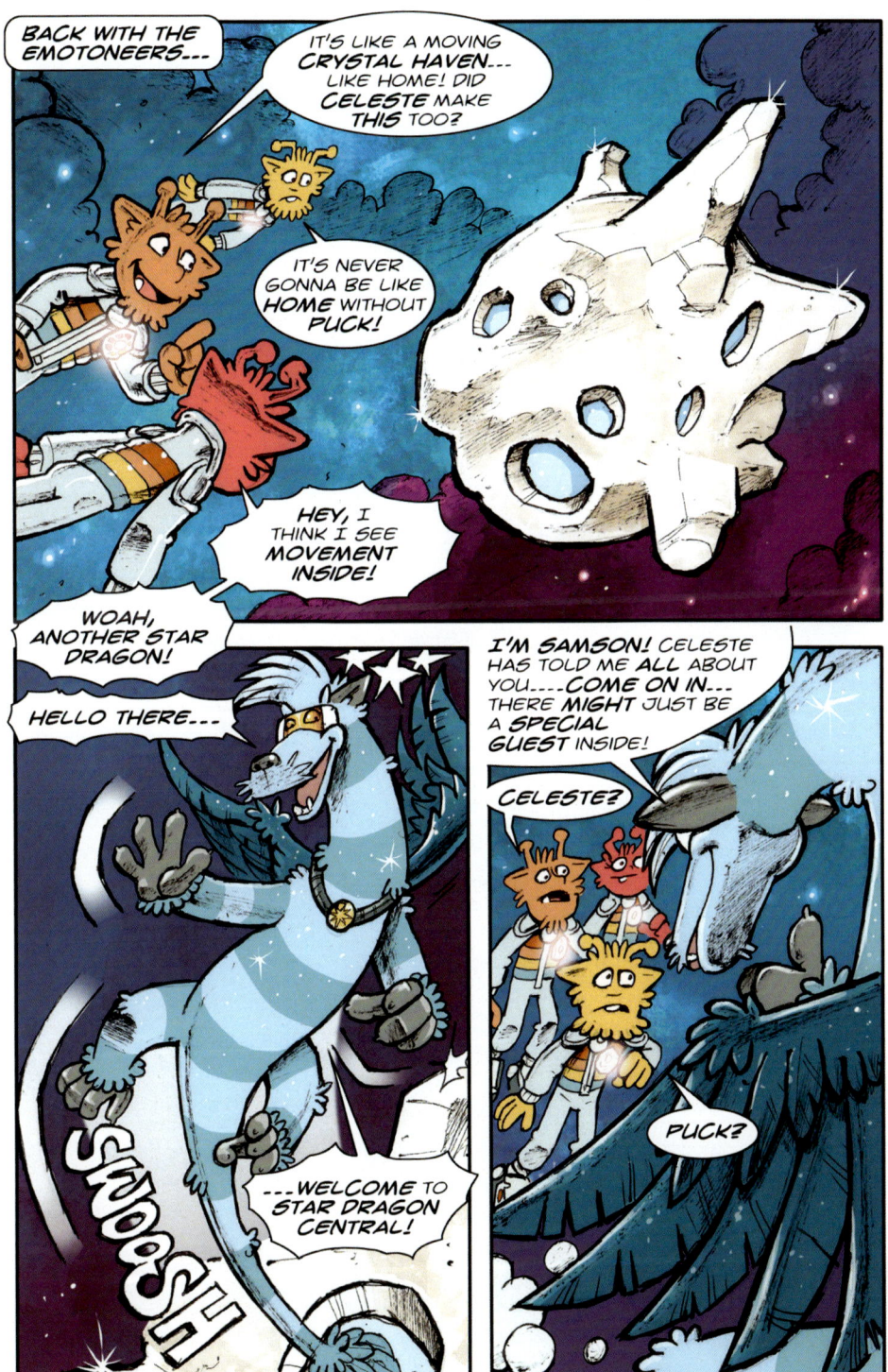

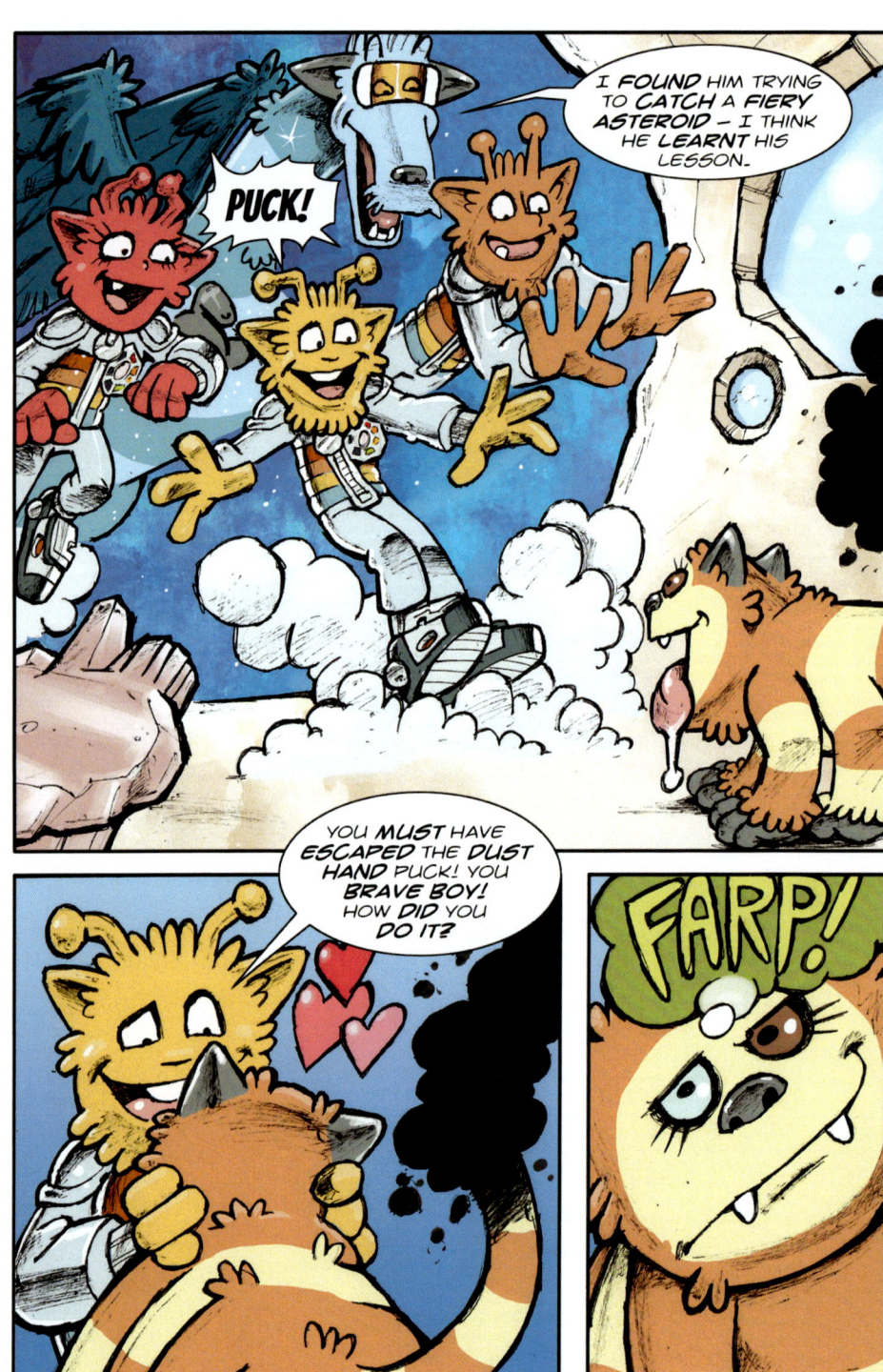

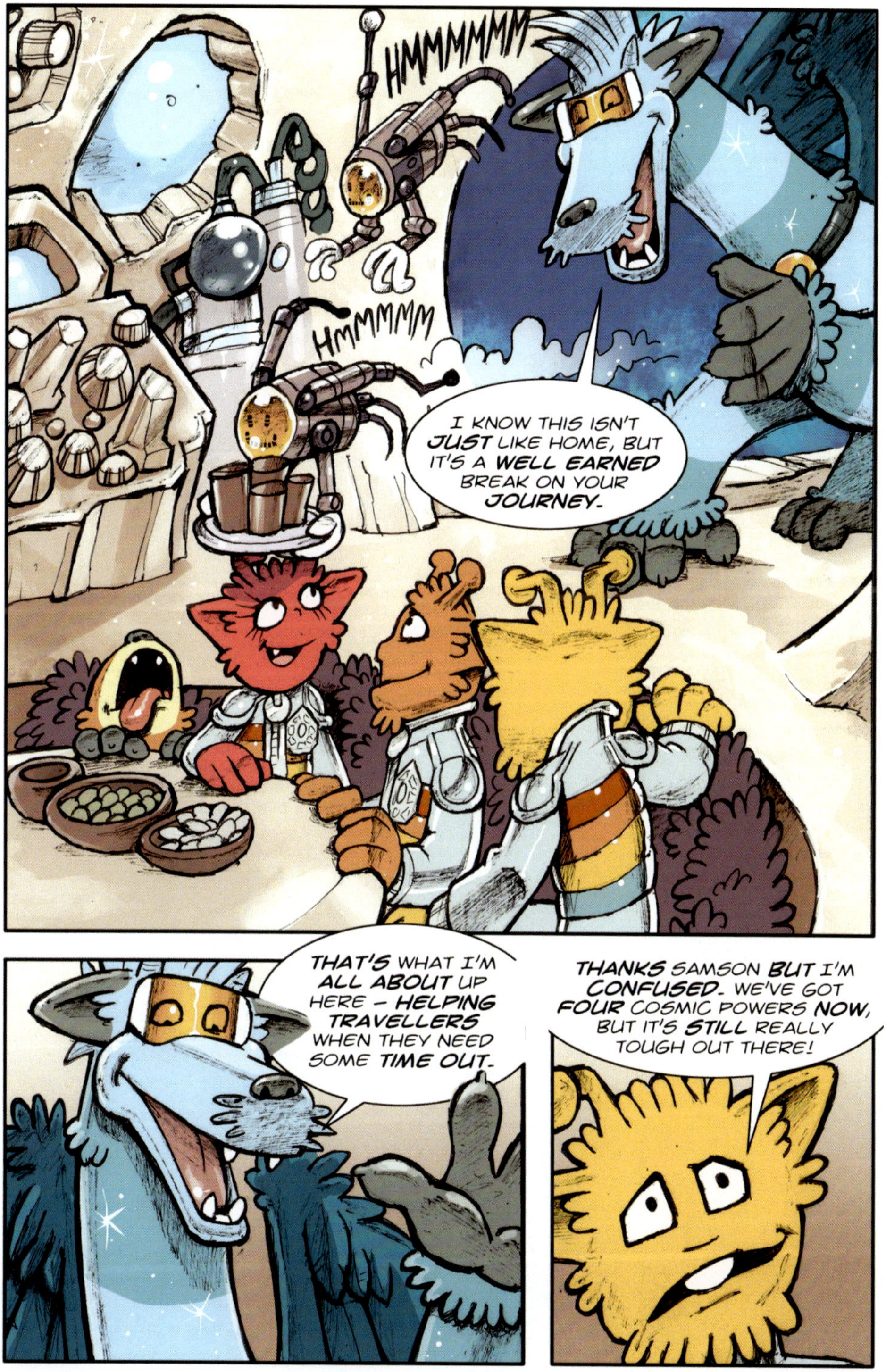

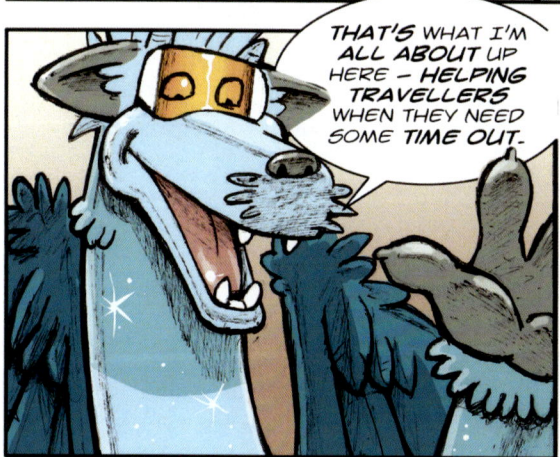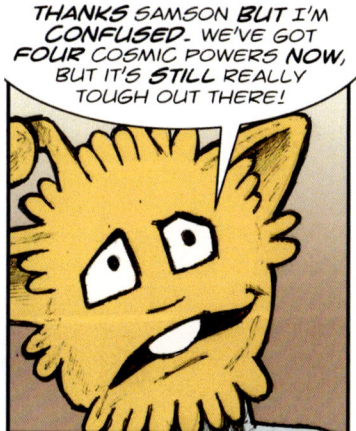

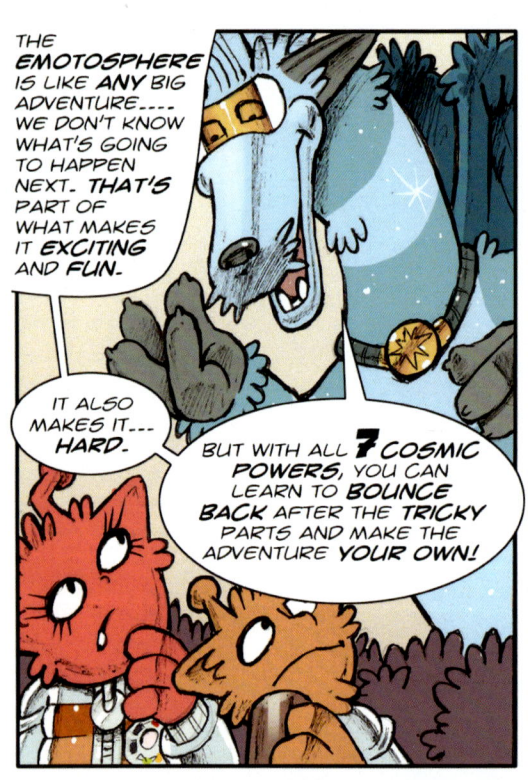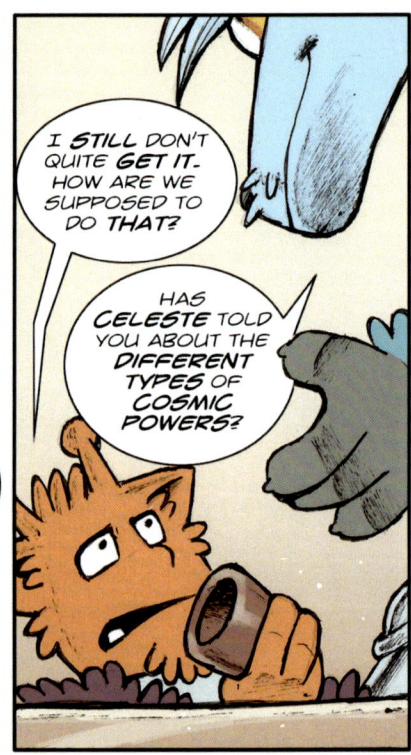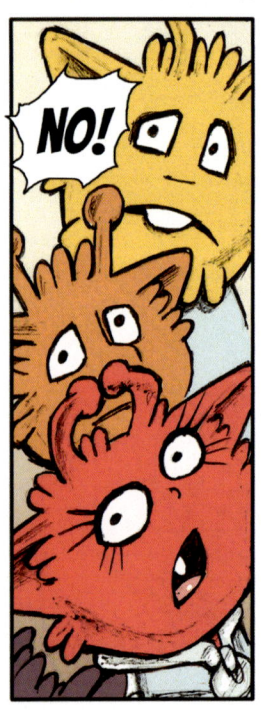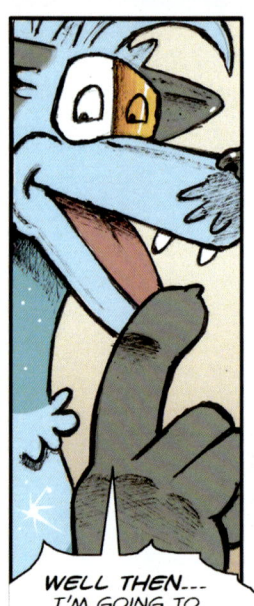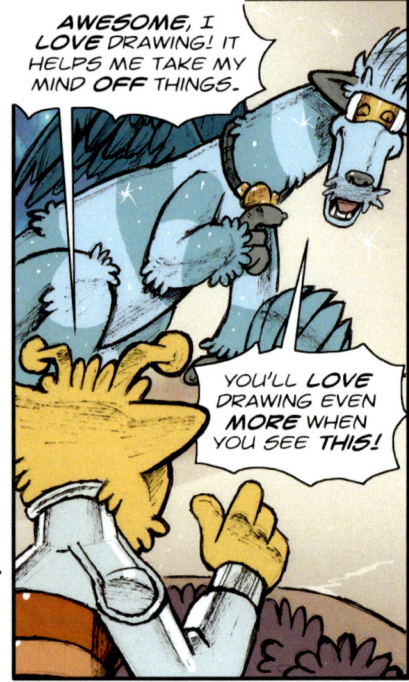

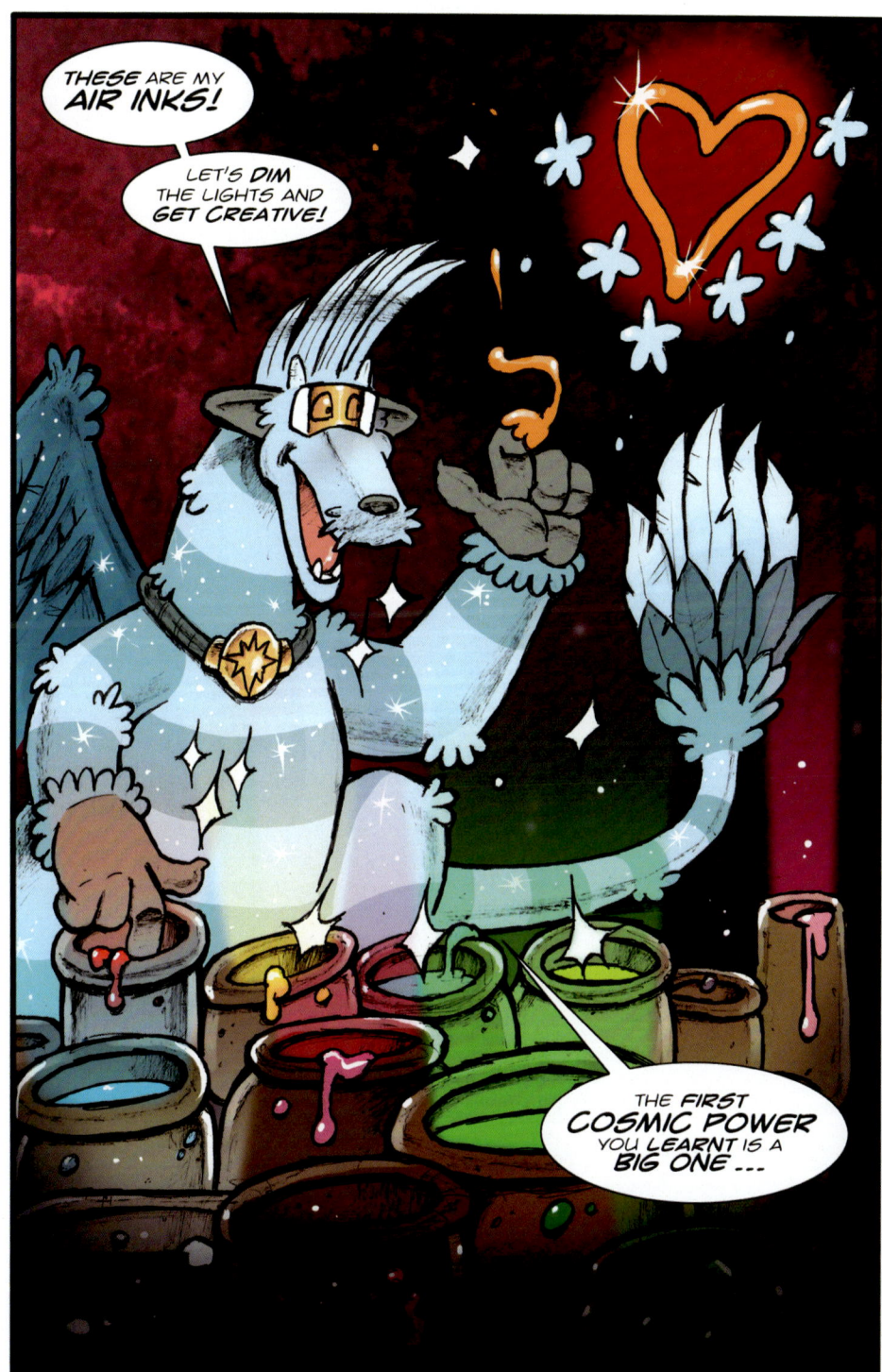

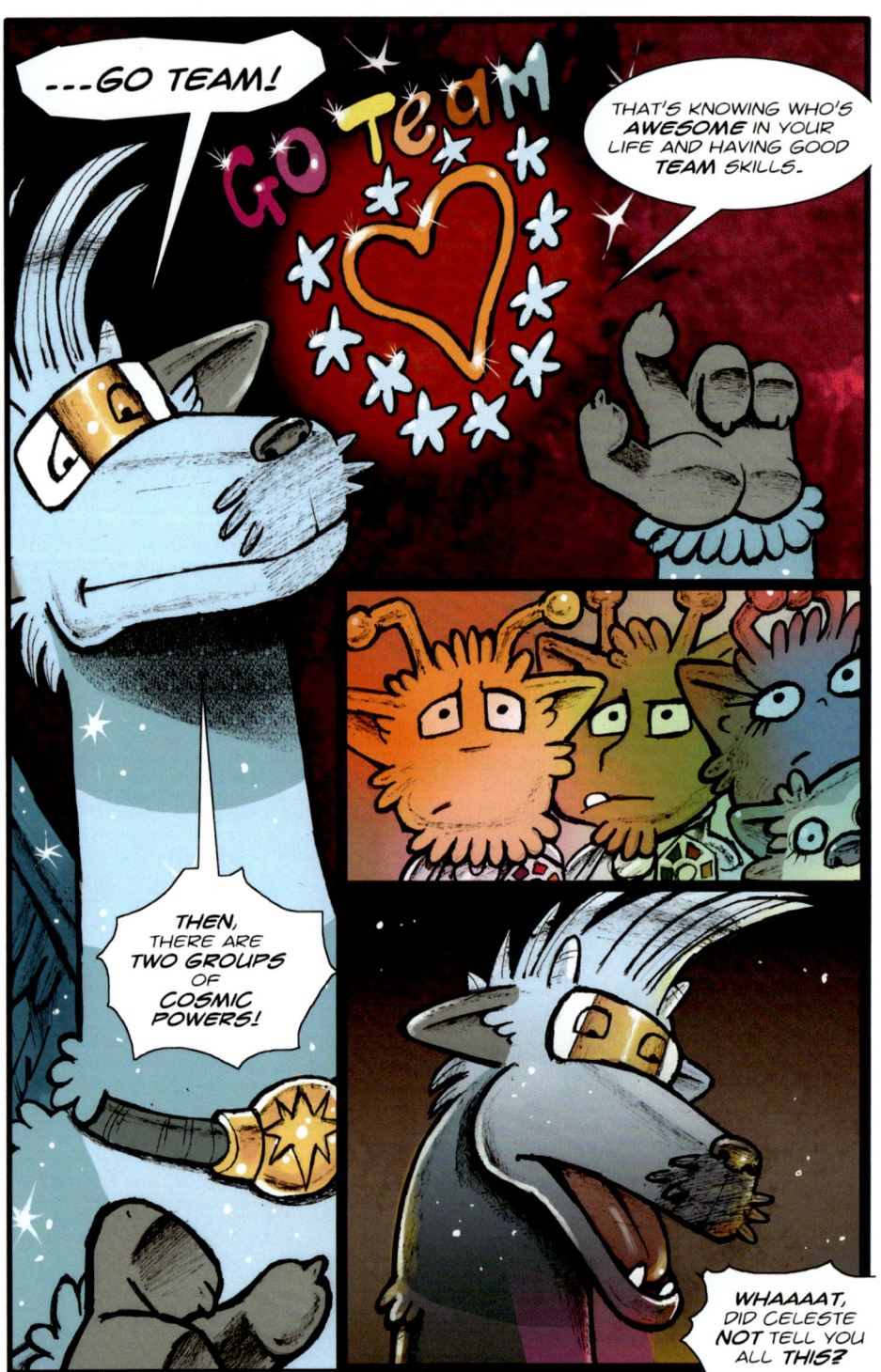

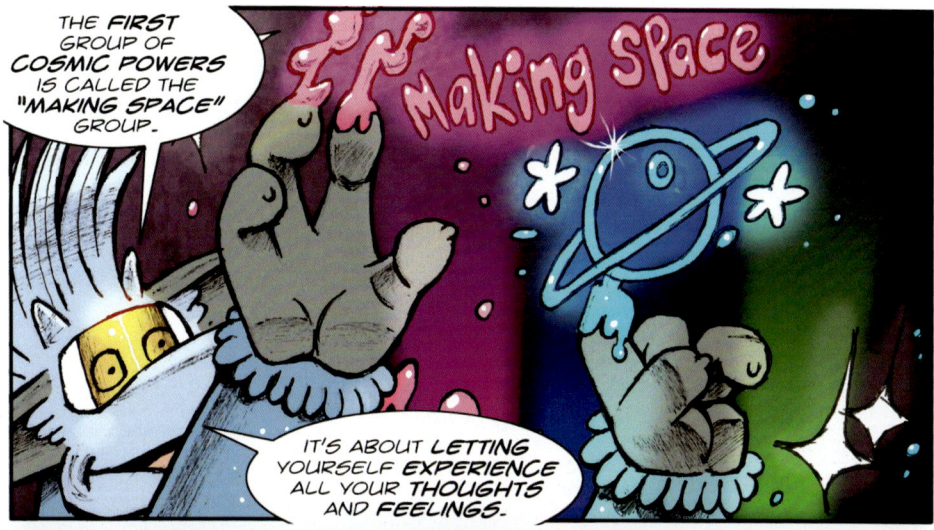
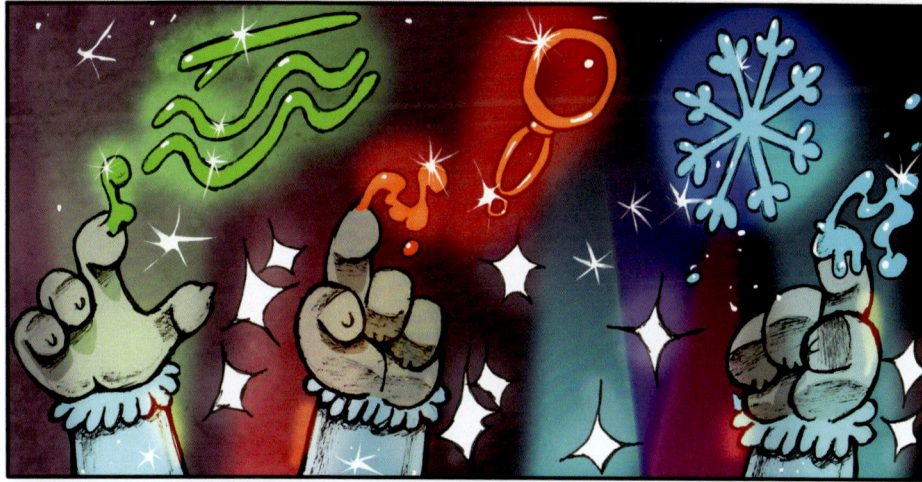
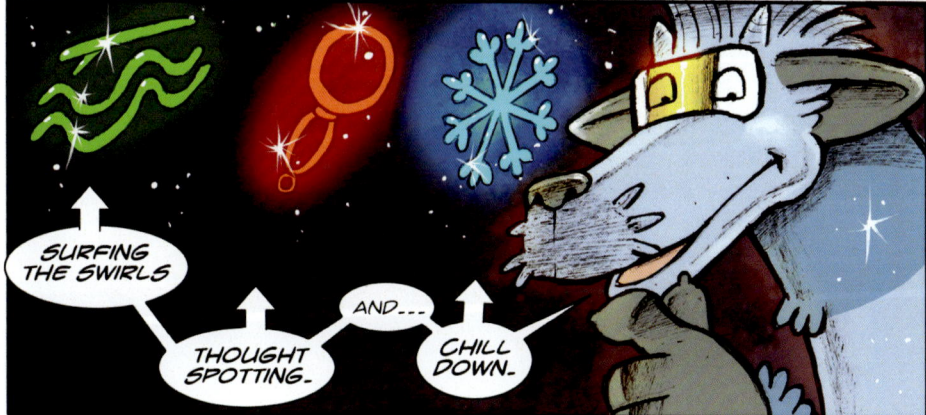

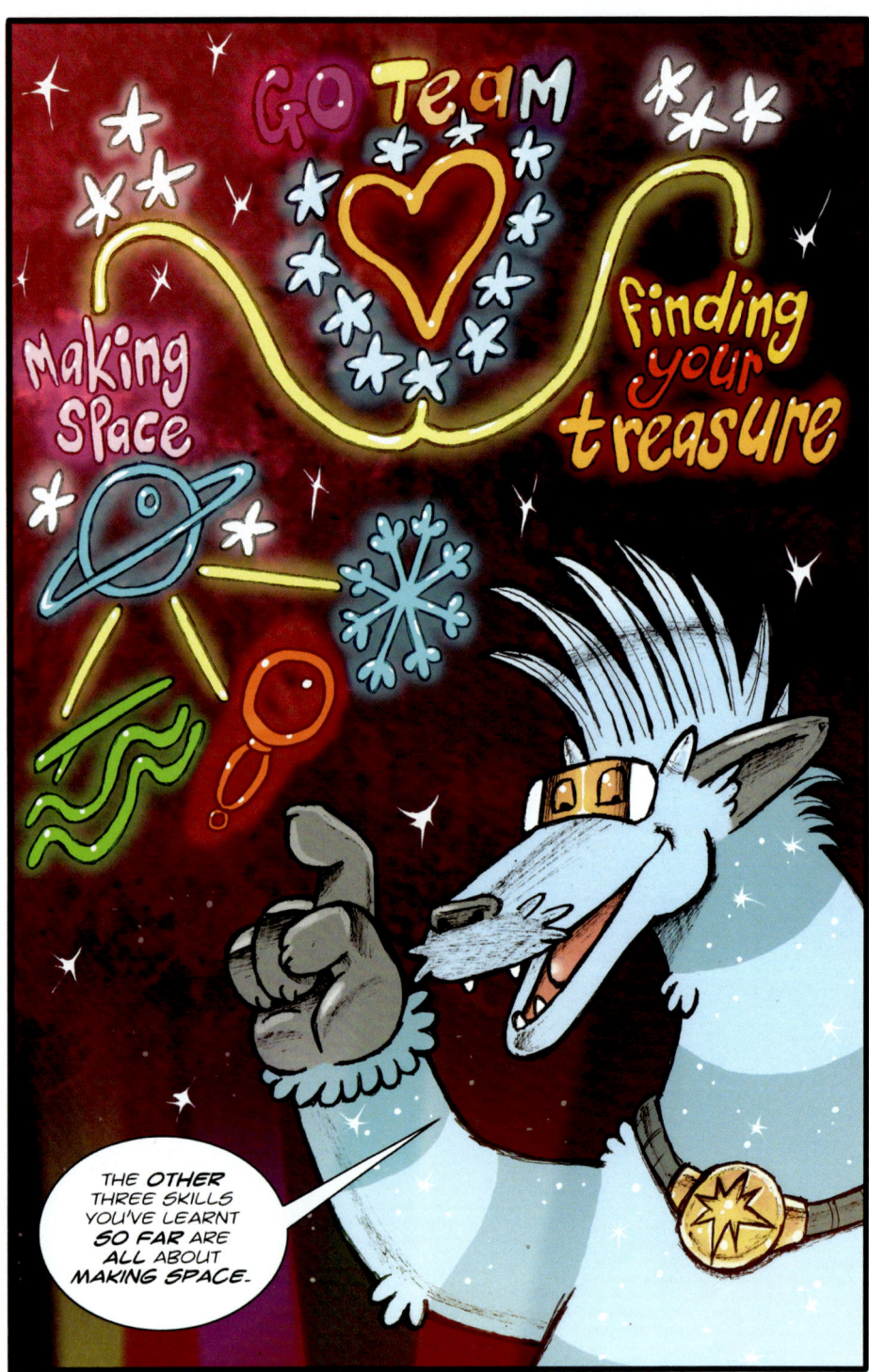

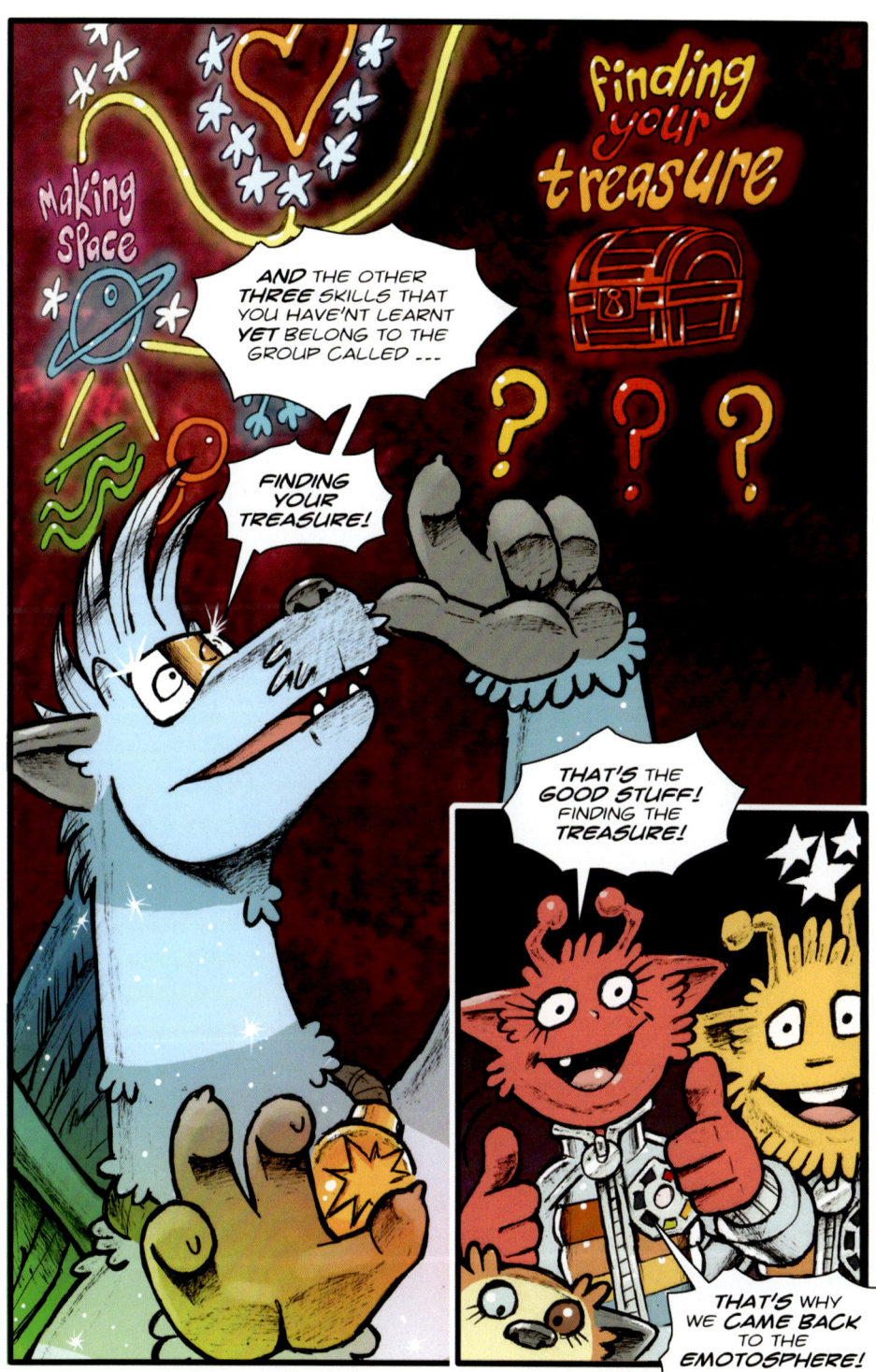

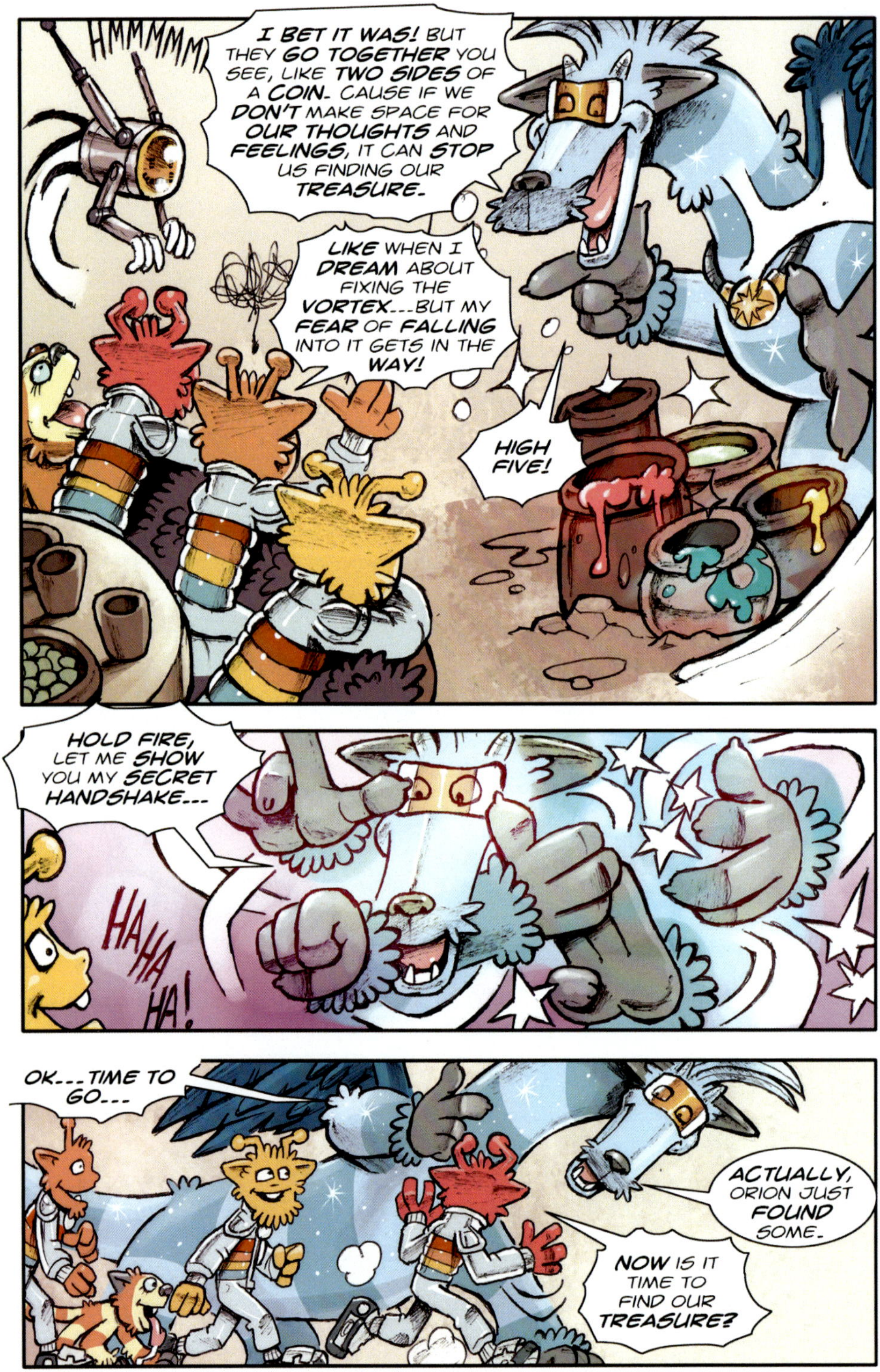

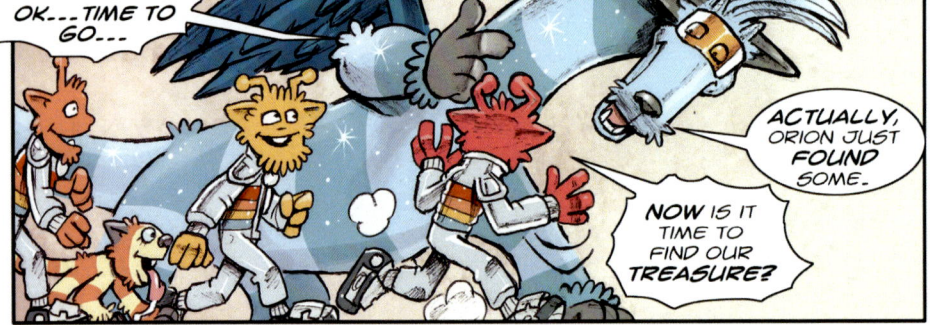

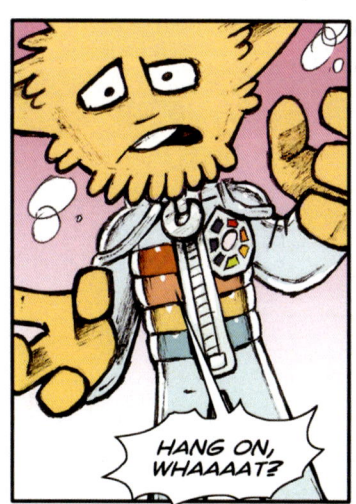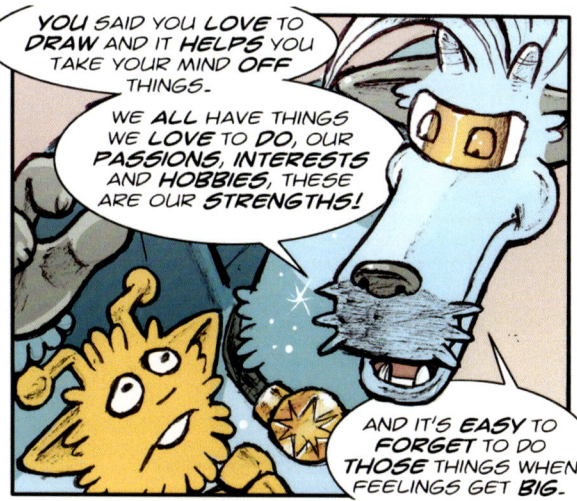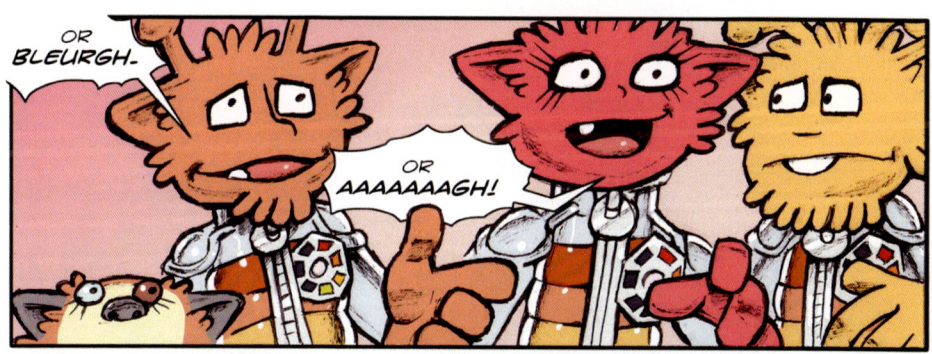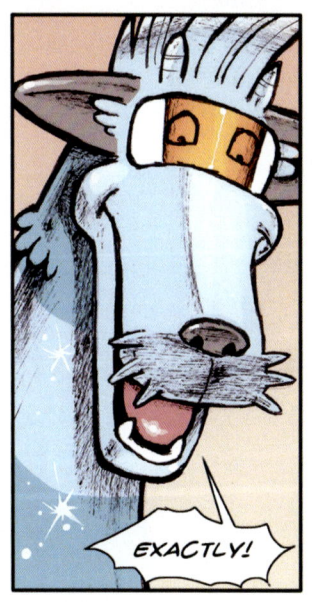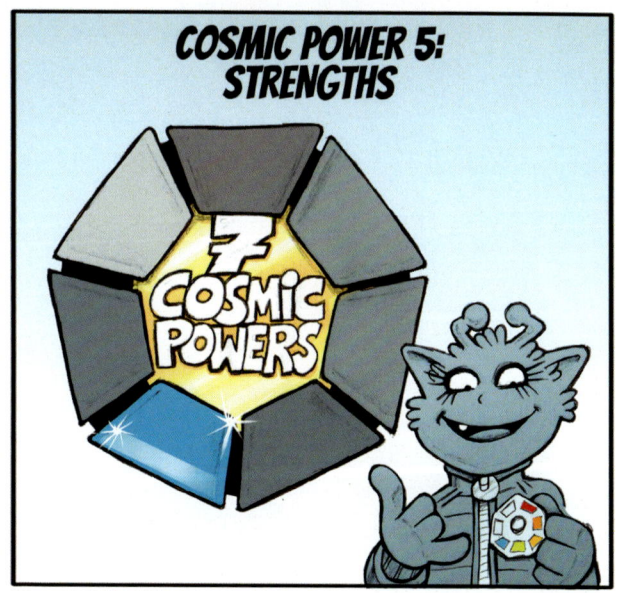

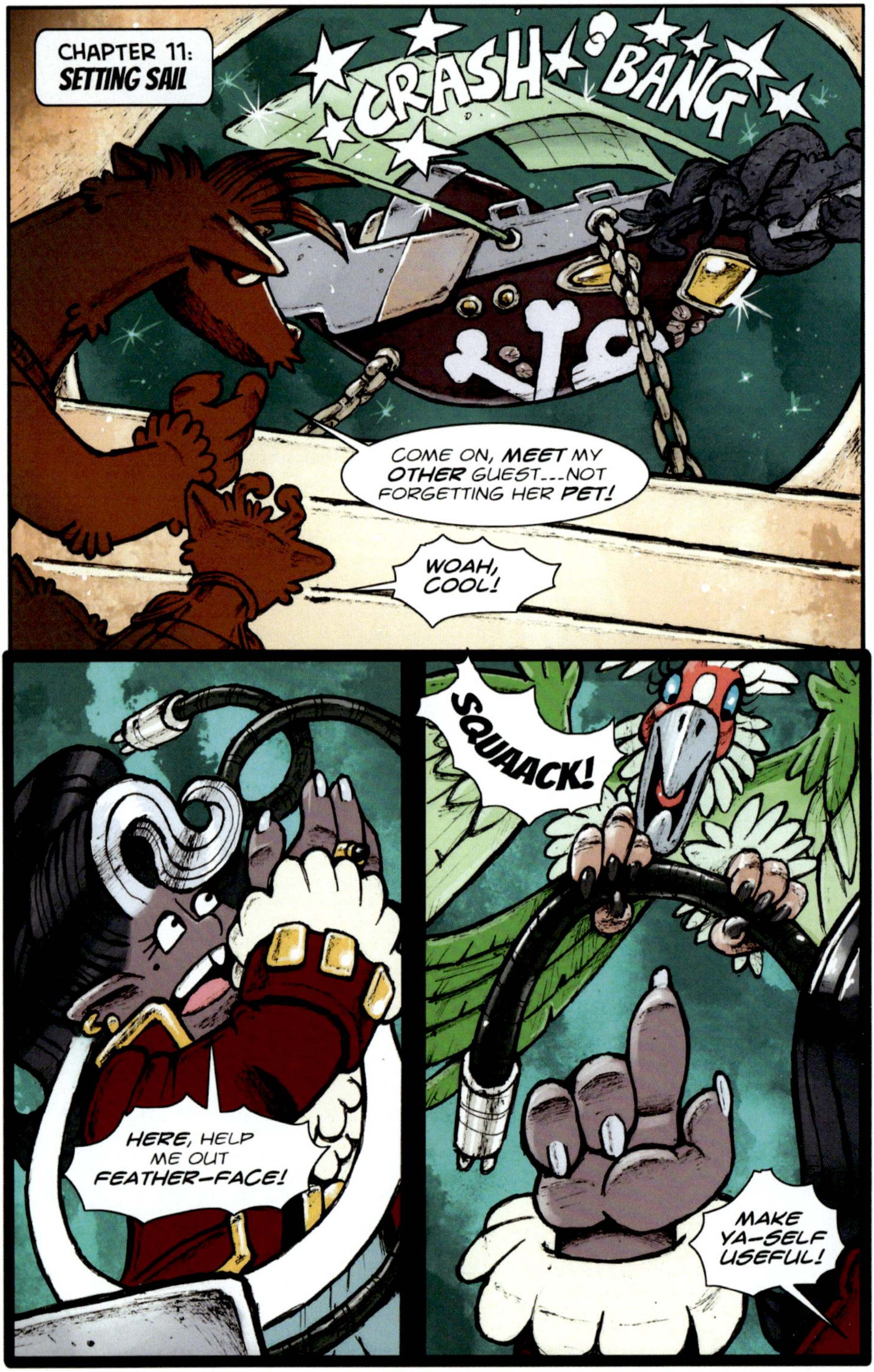

CHAPTER 11:
SETTING SAIL

CRASH BANG

"Come on, *meet* my *other* guest... not forgetting her *pet*!"

"Woah, cool!"

SQUAACK!

"Here, help me out feather-face!"

"Make ya-self useful!"

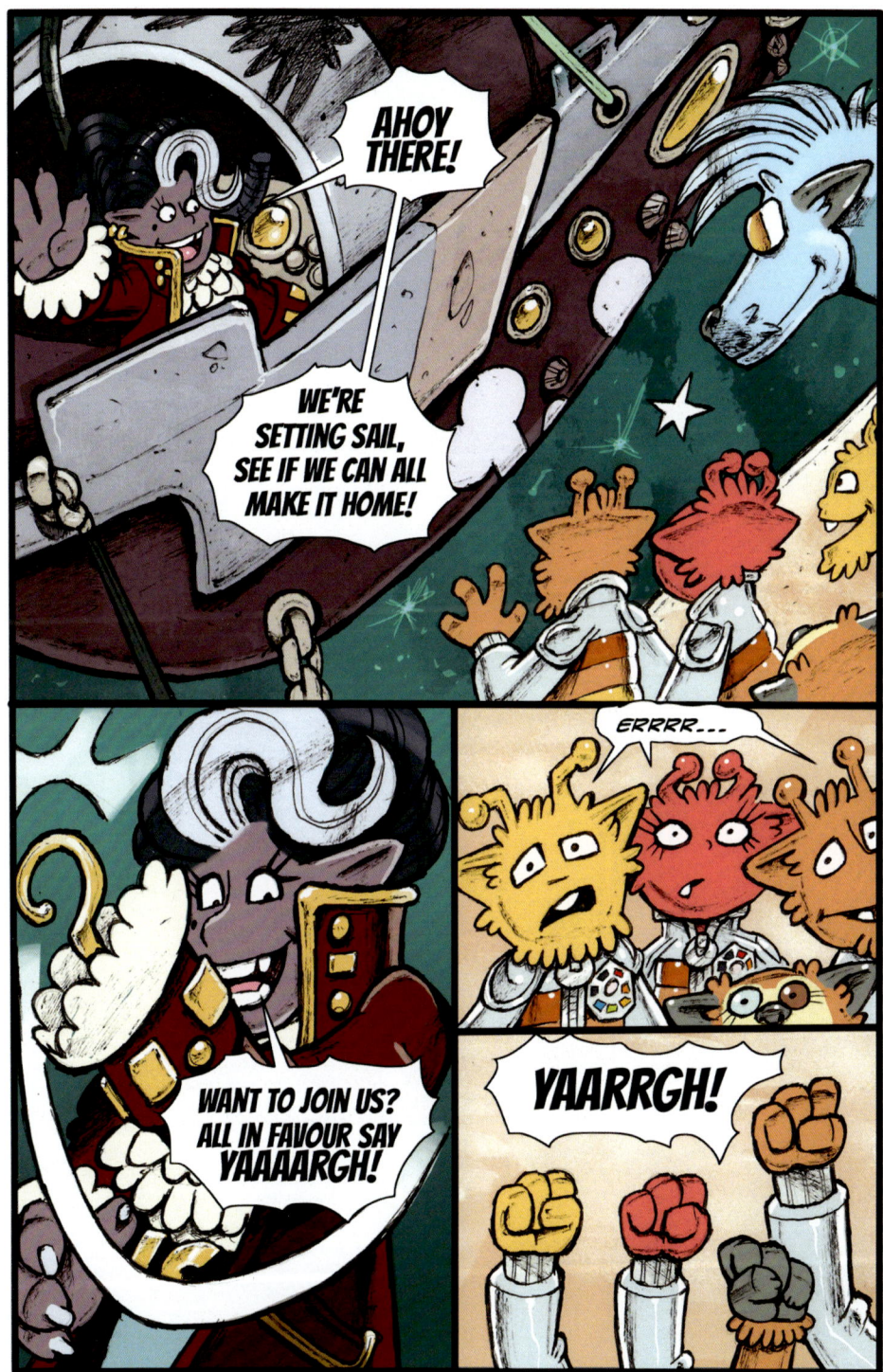

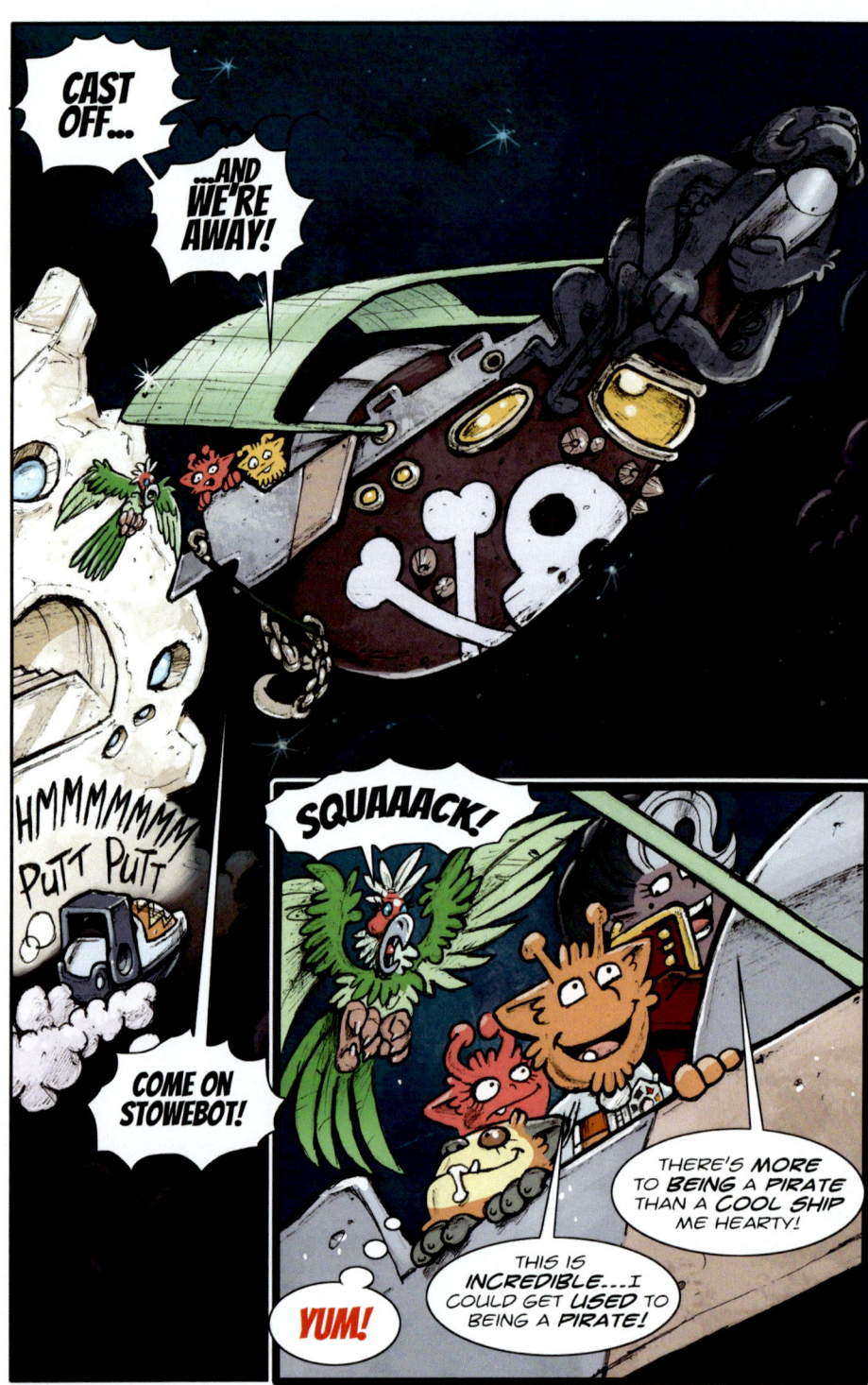

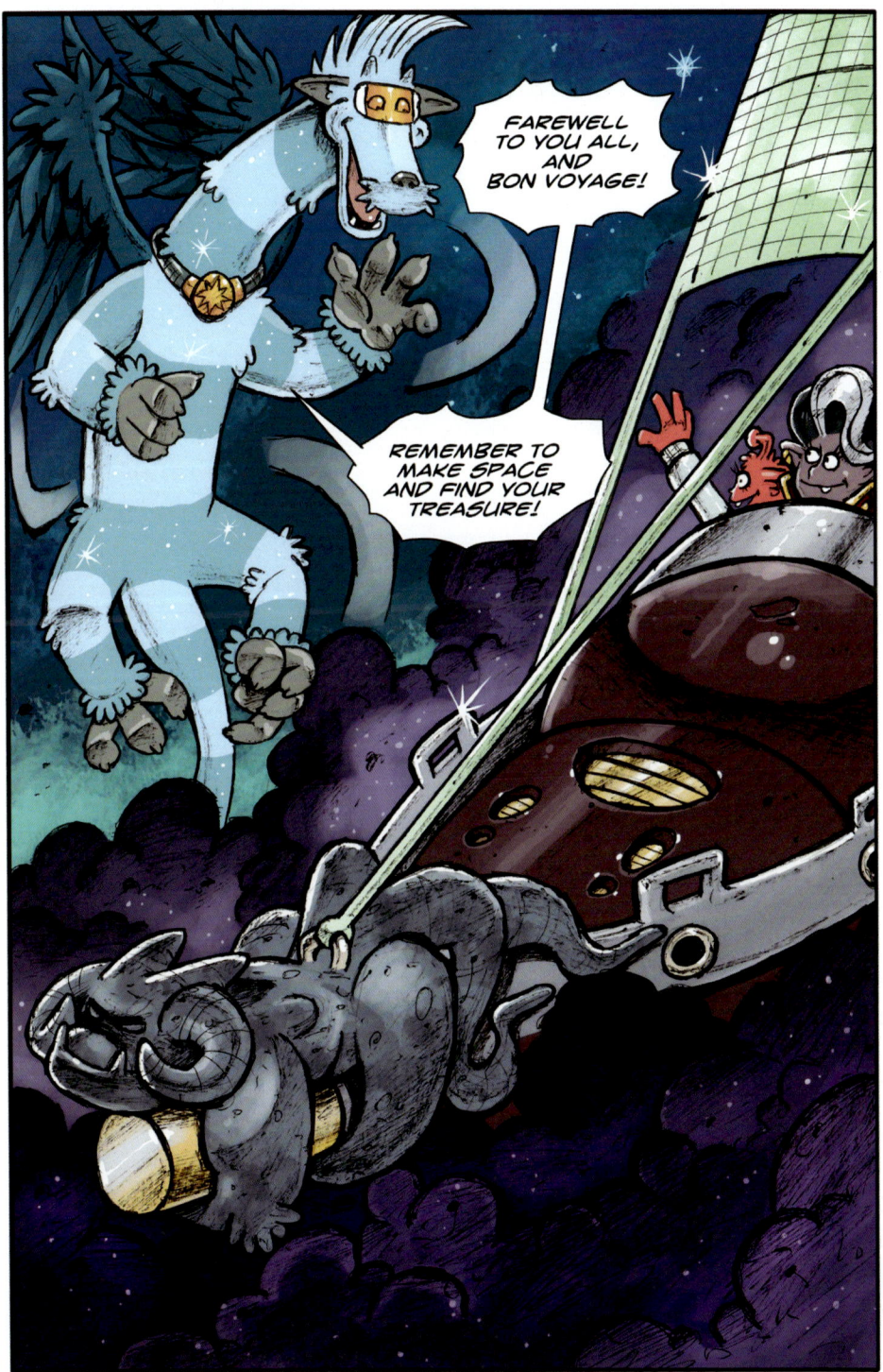

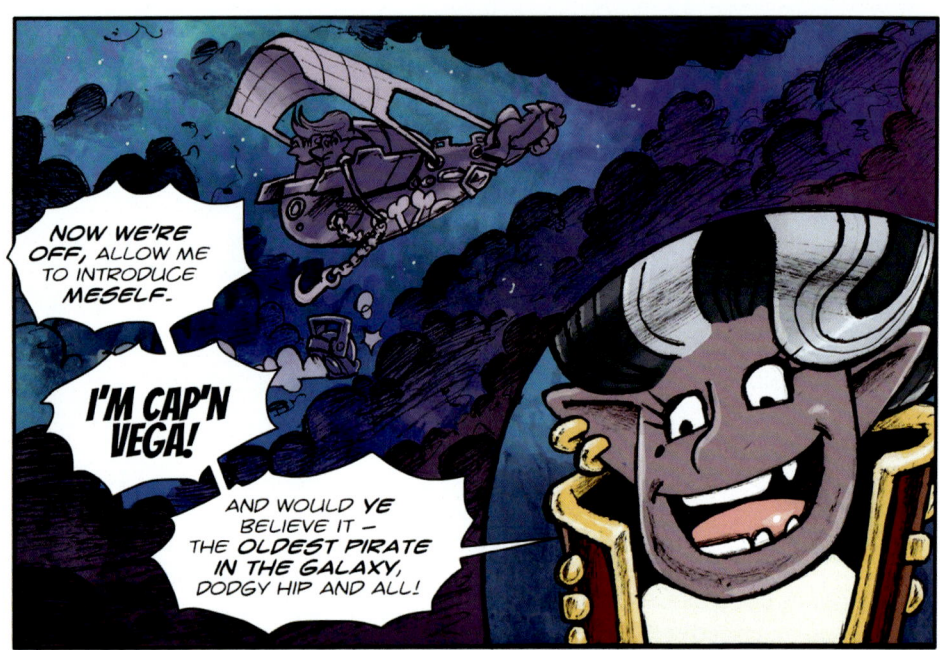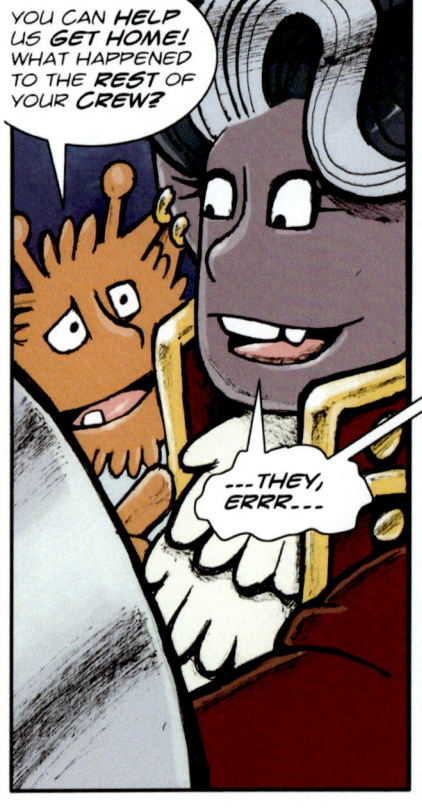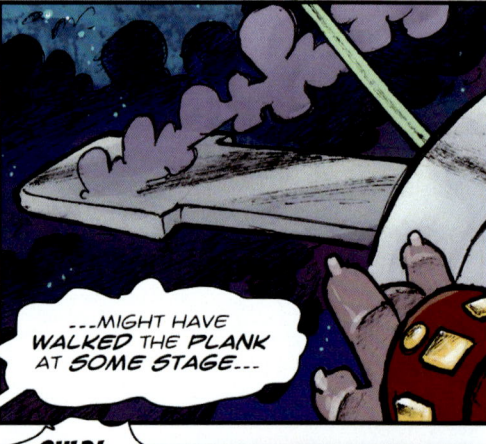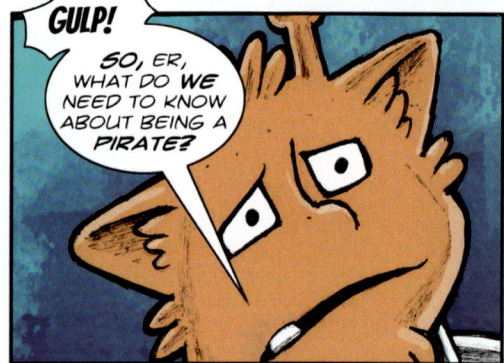

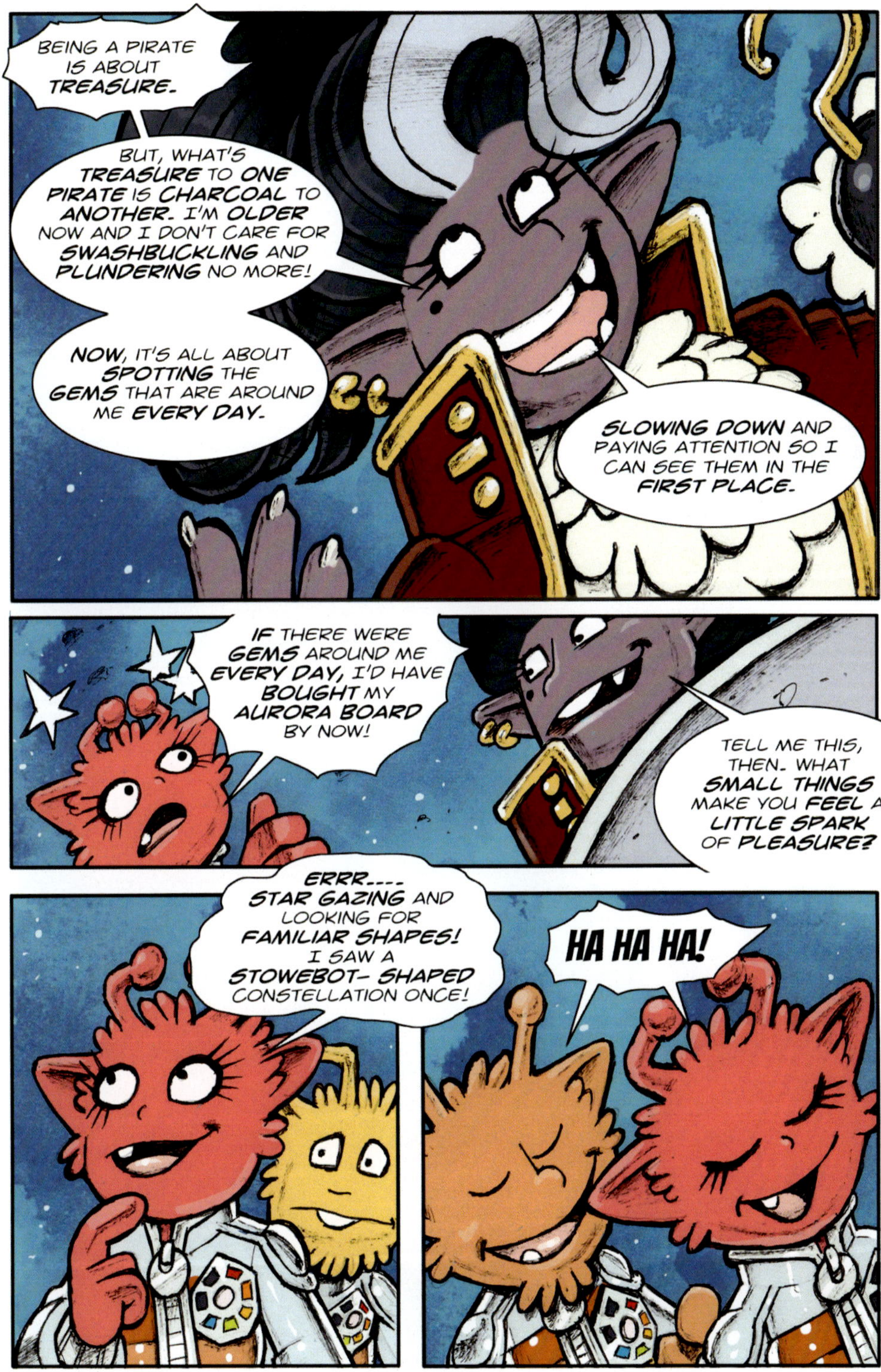

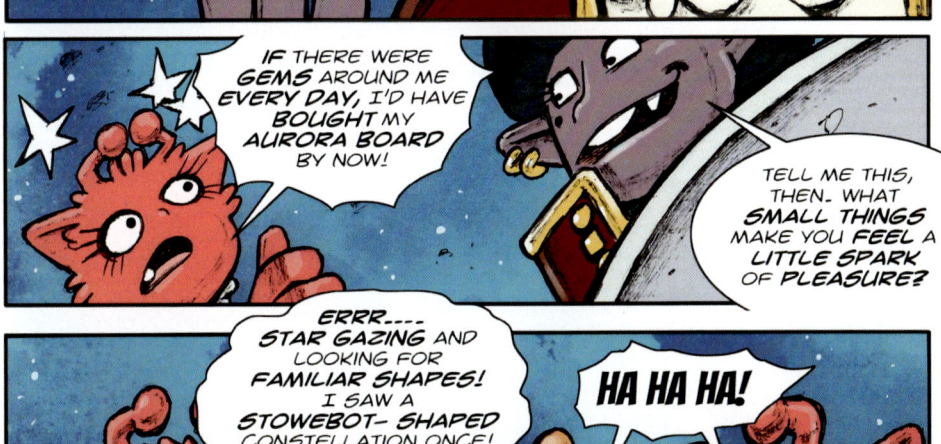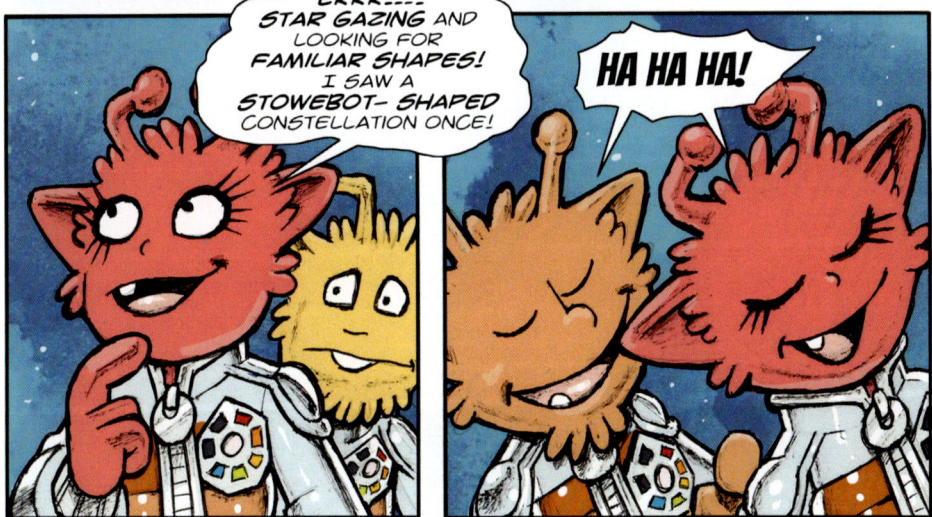

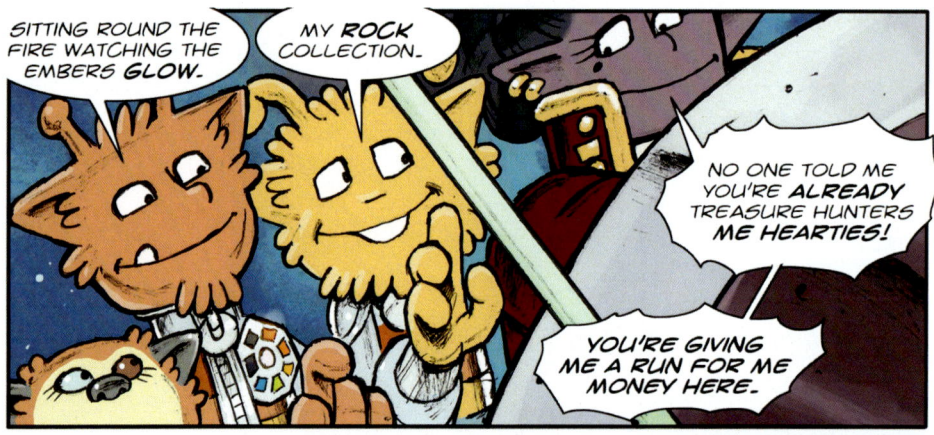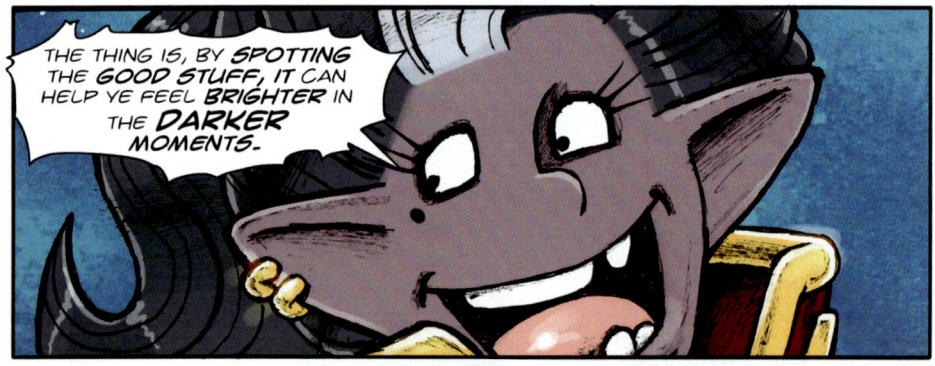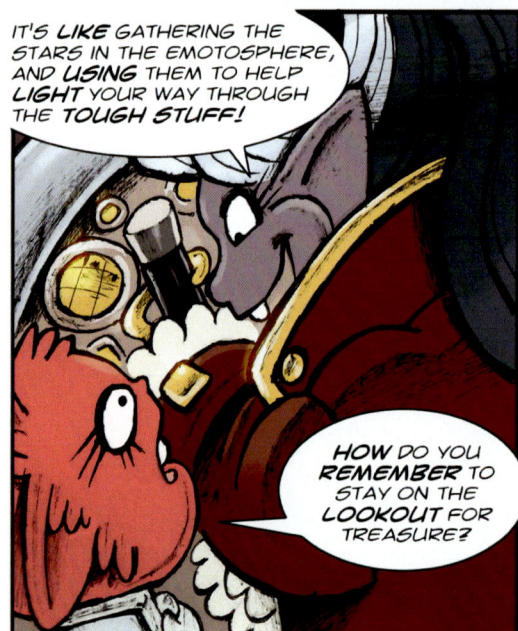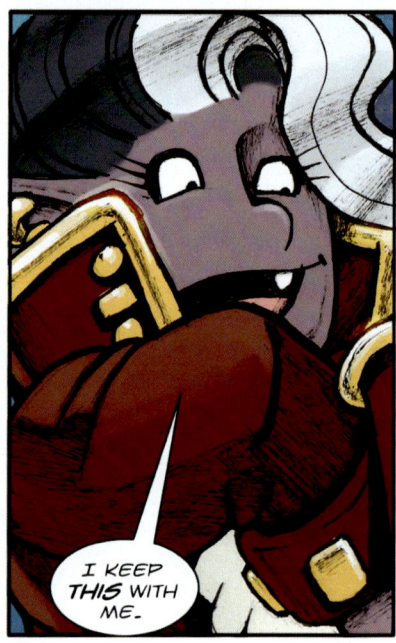

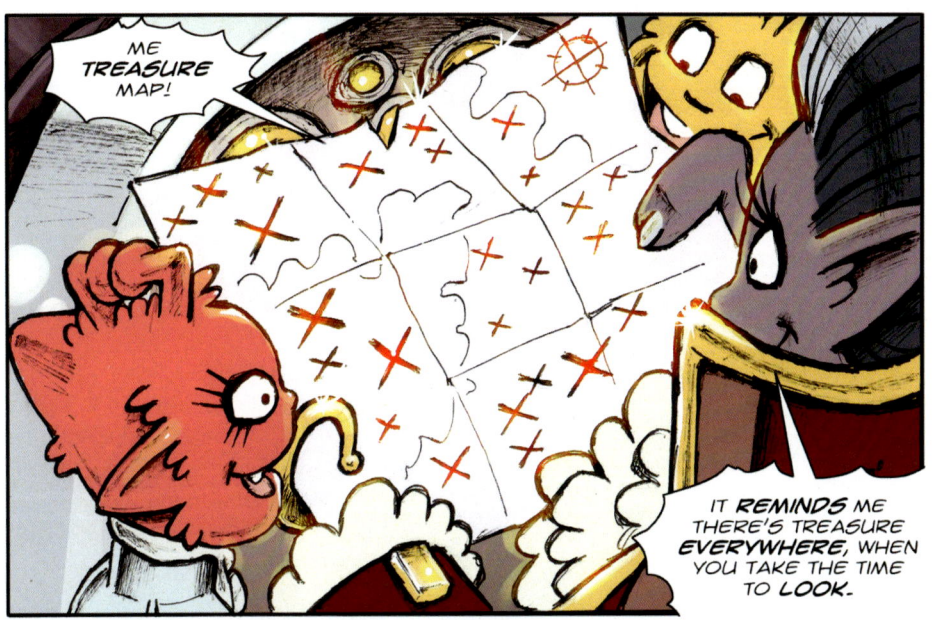

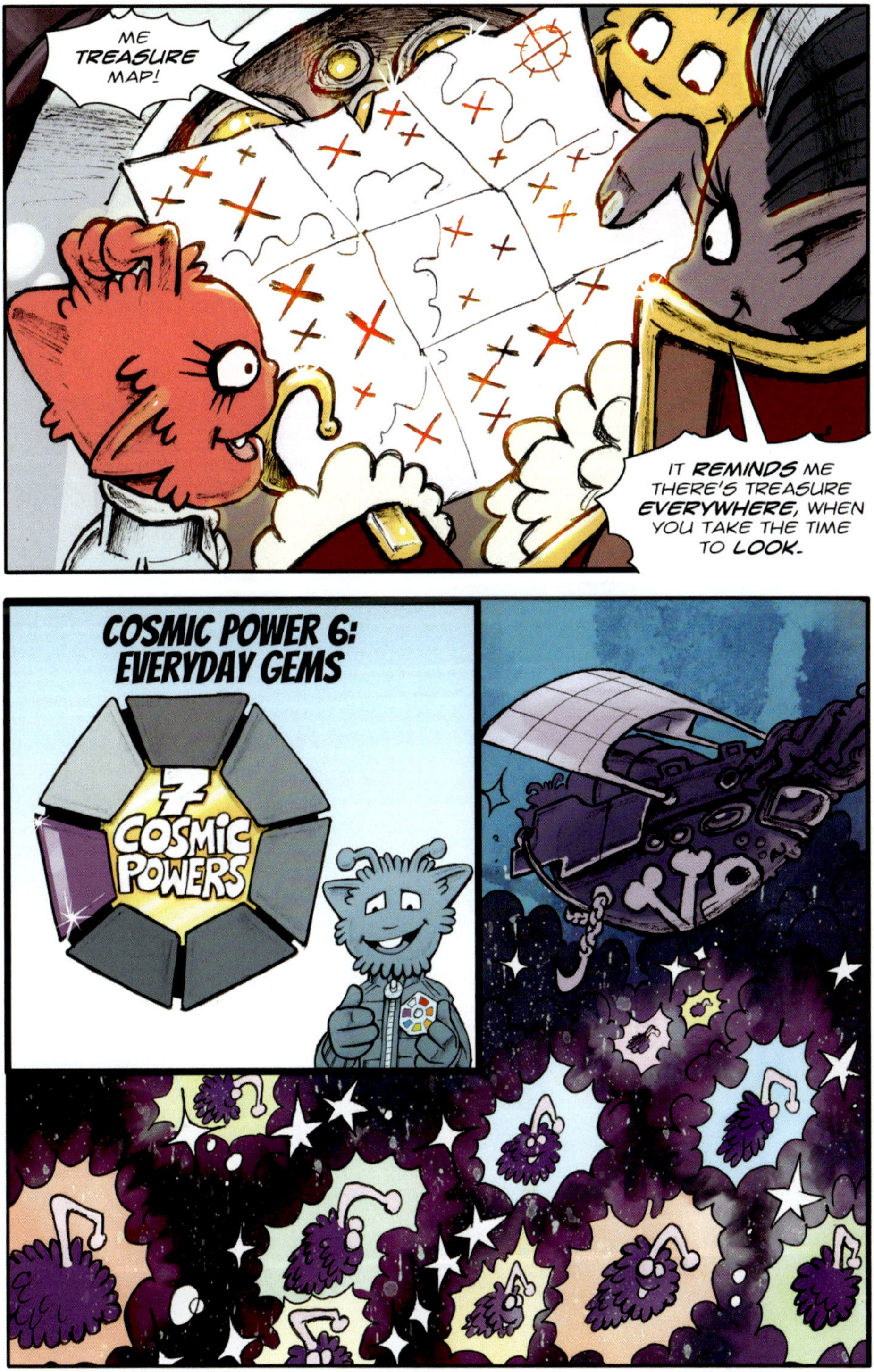

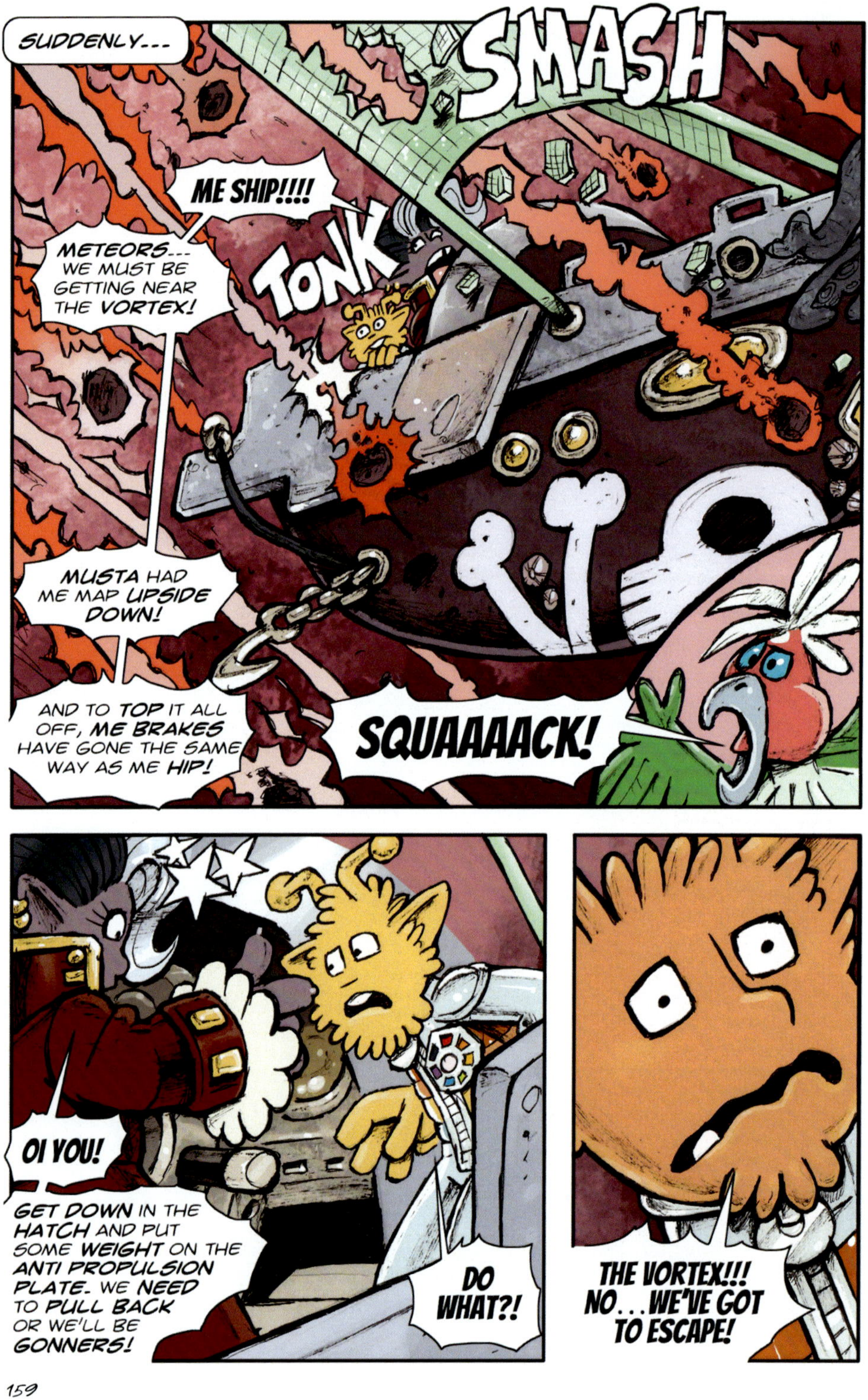

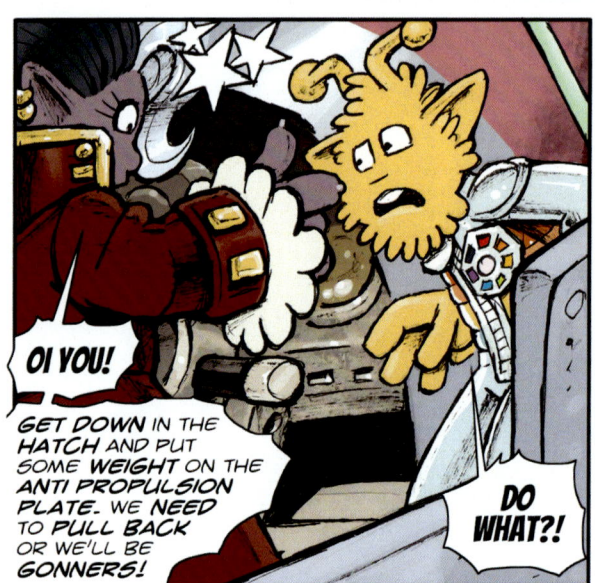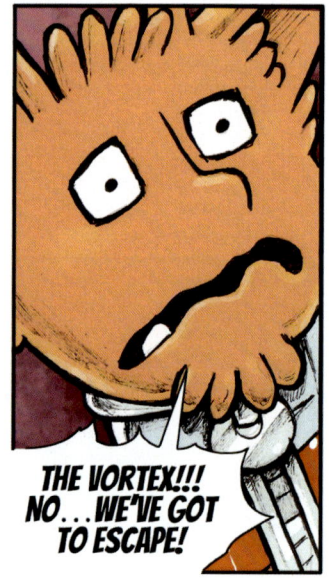

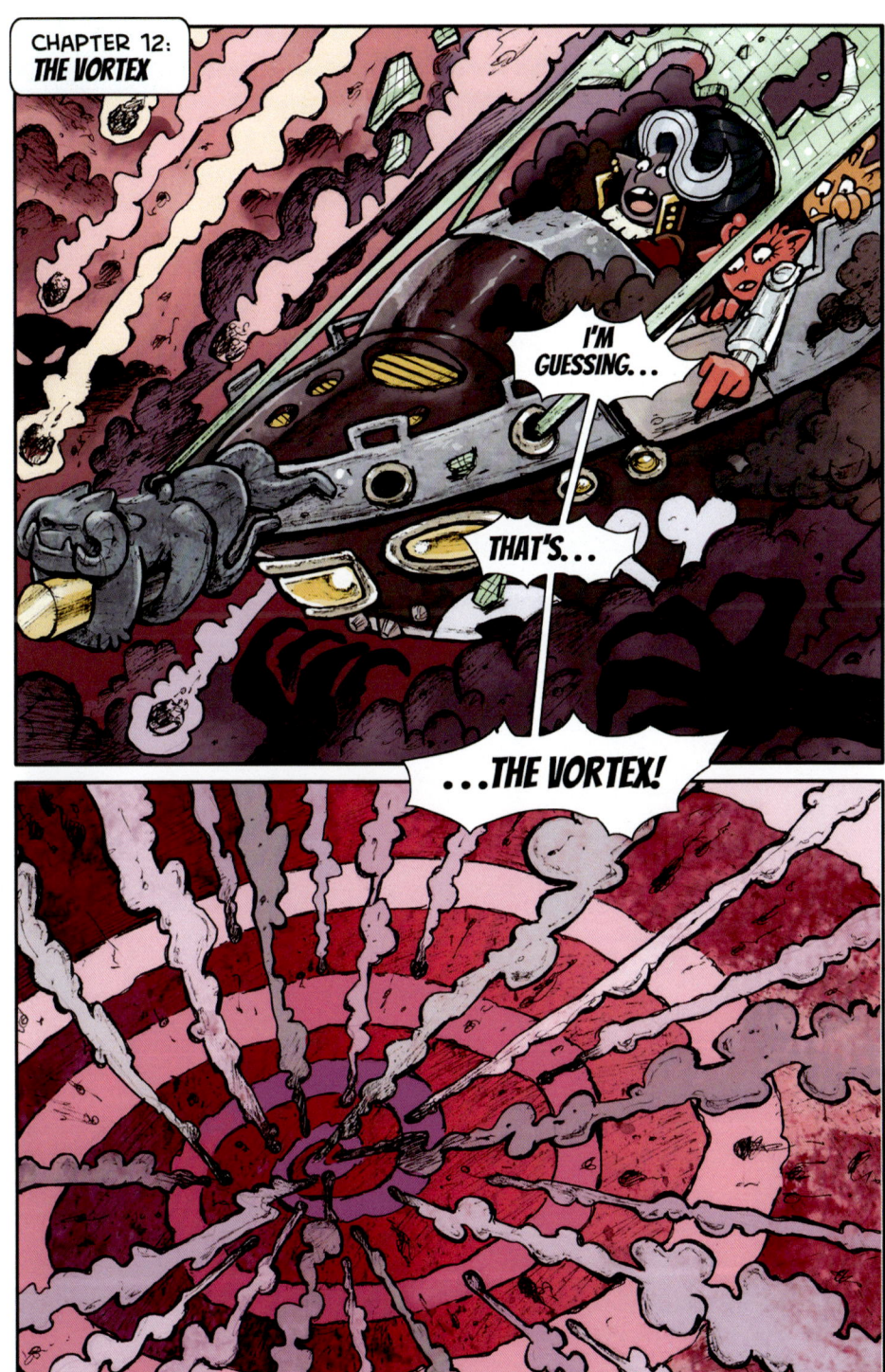

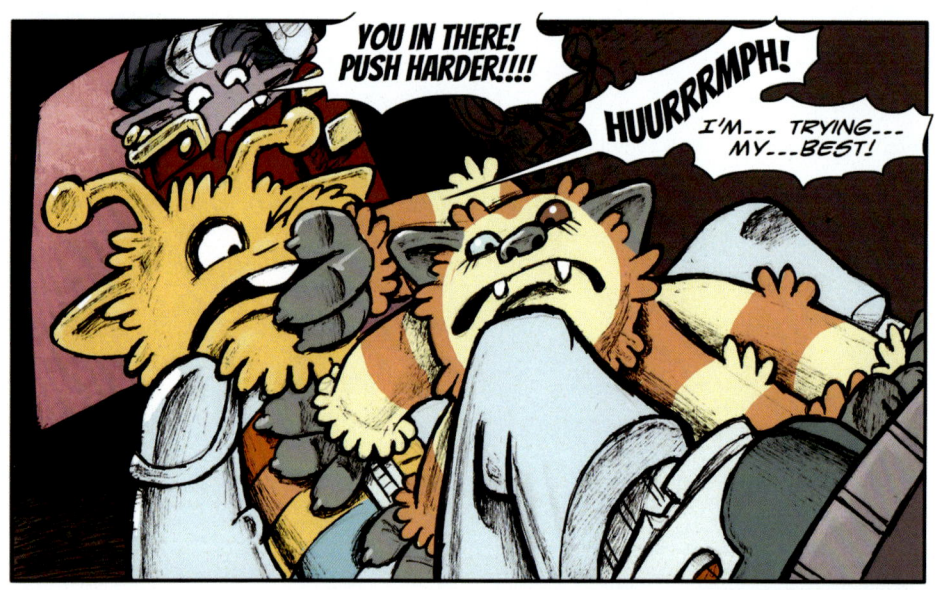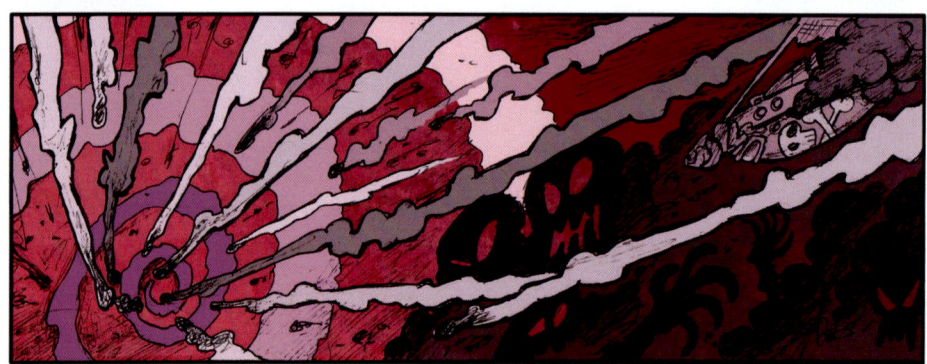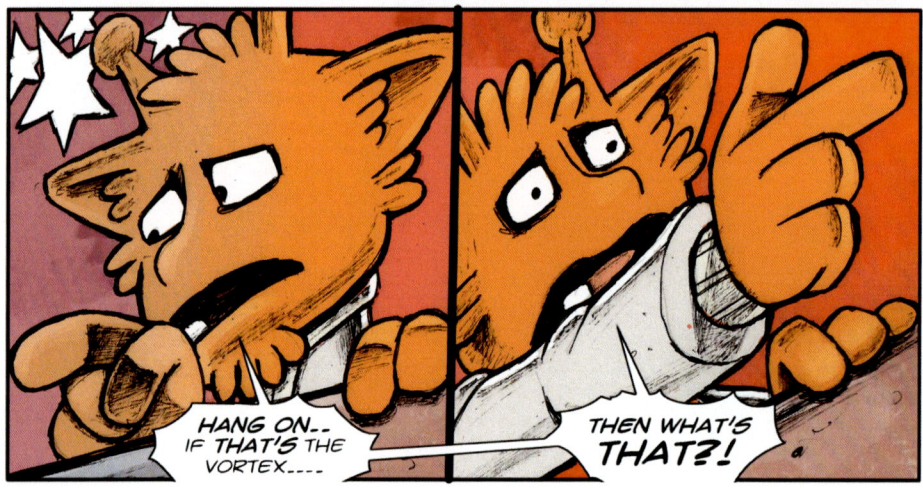

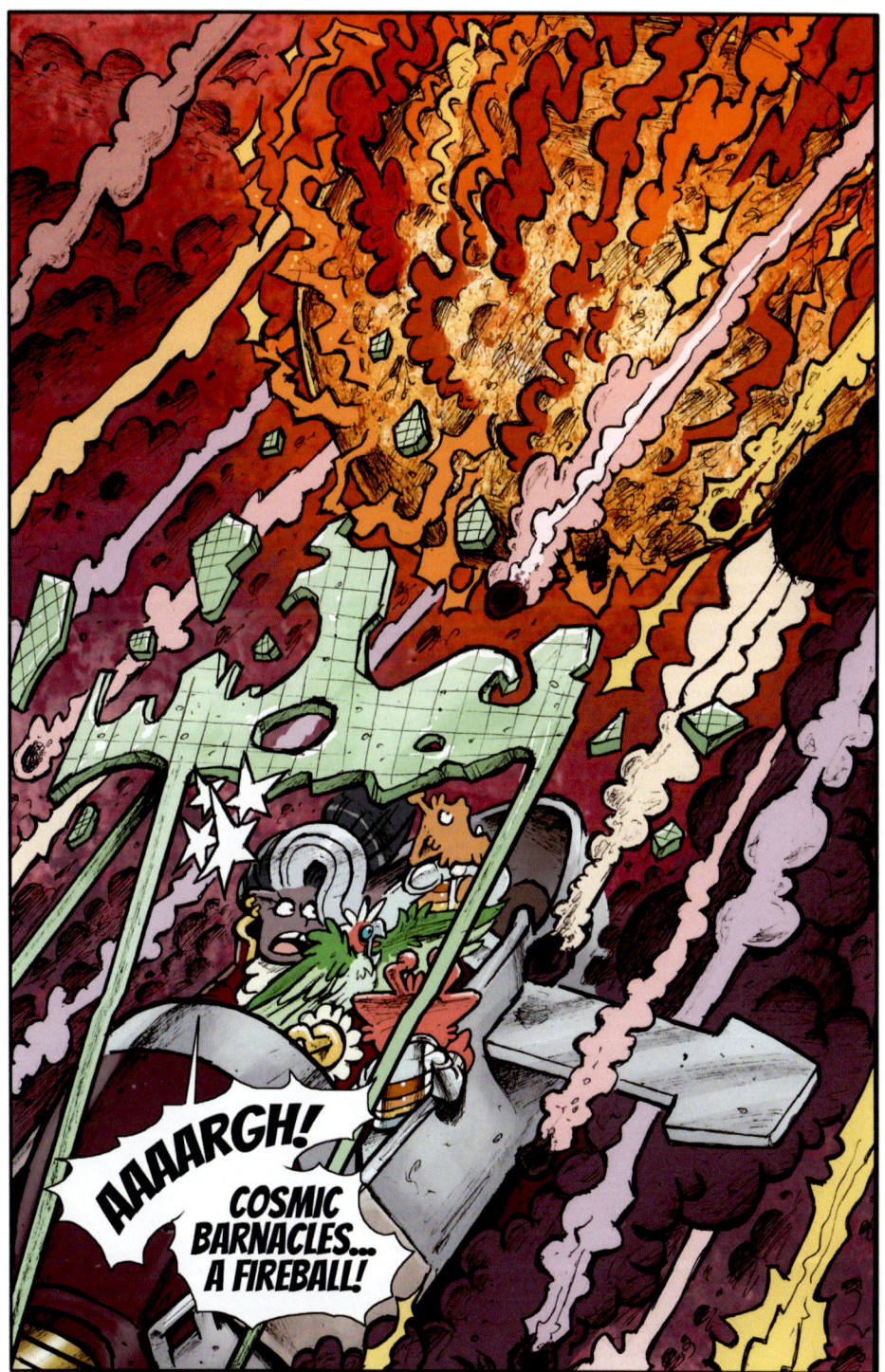

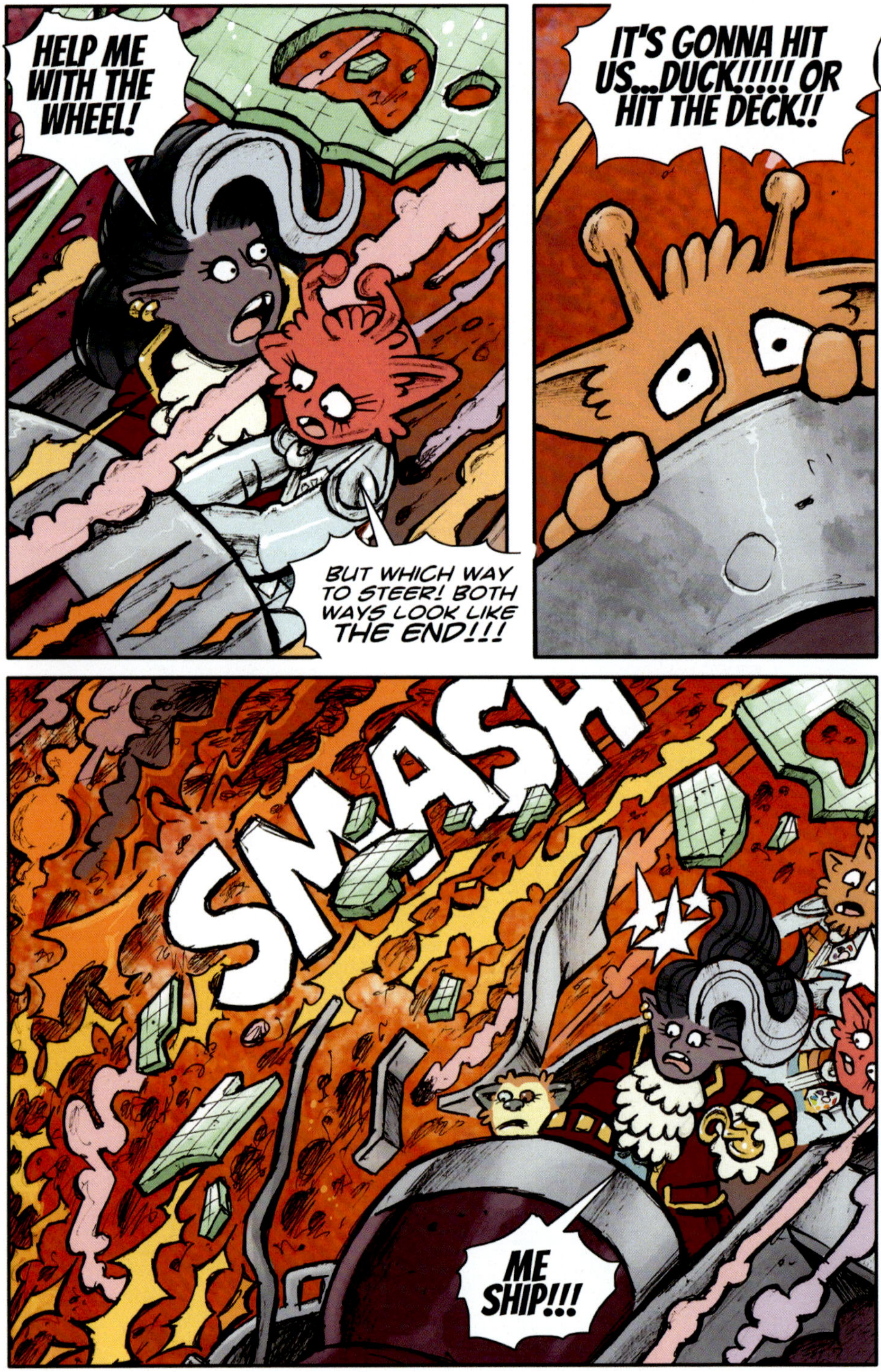

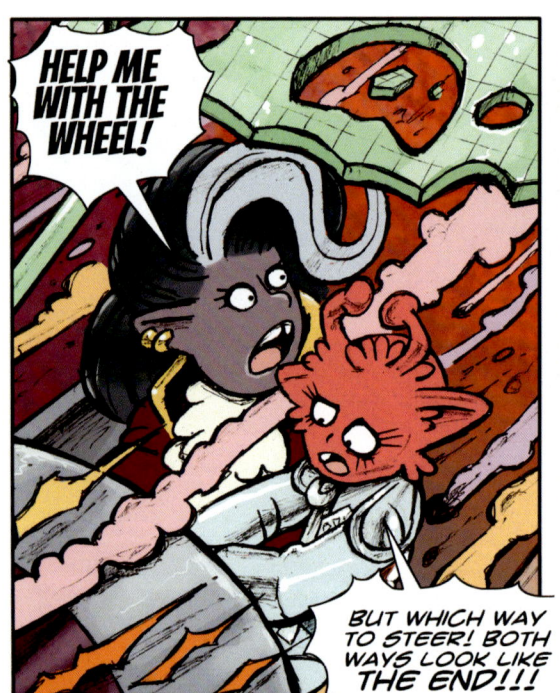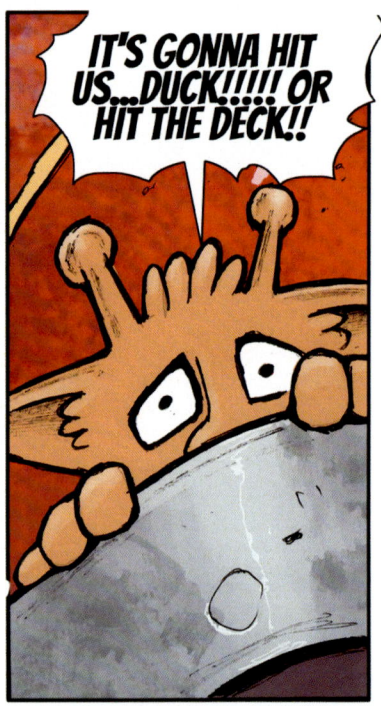

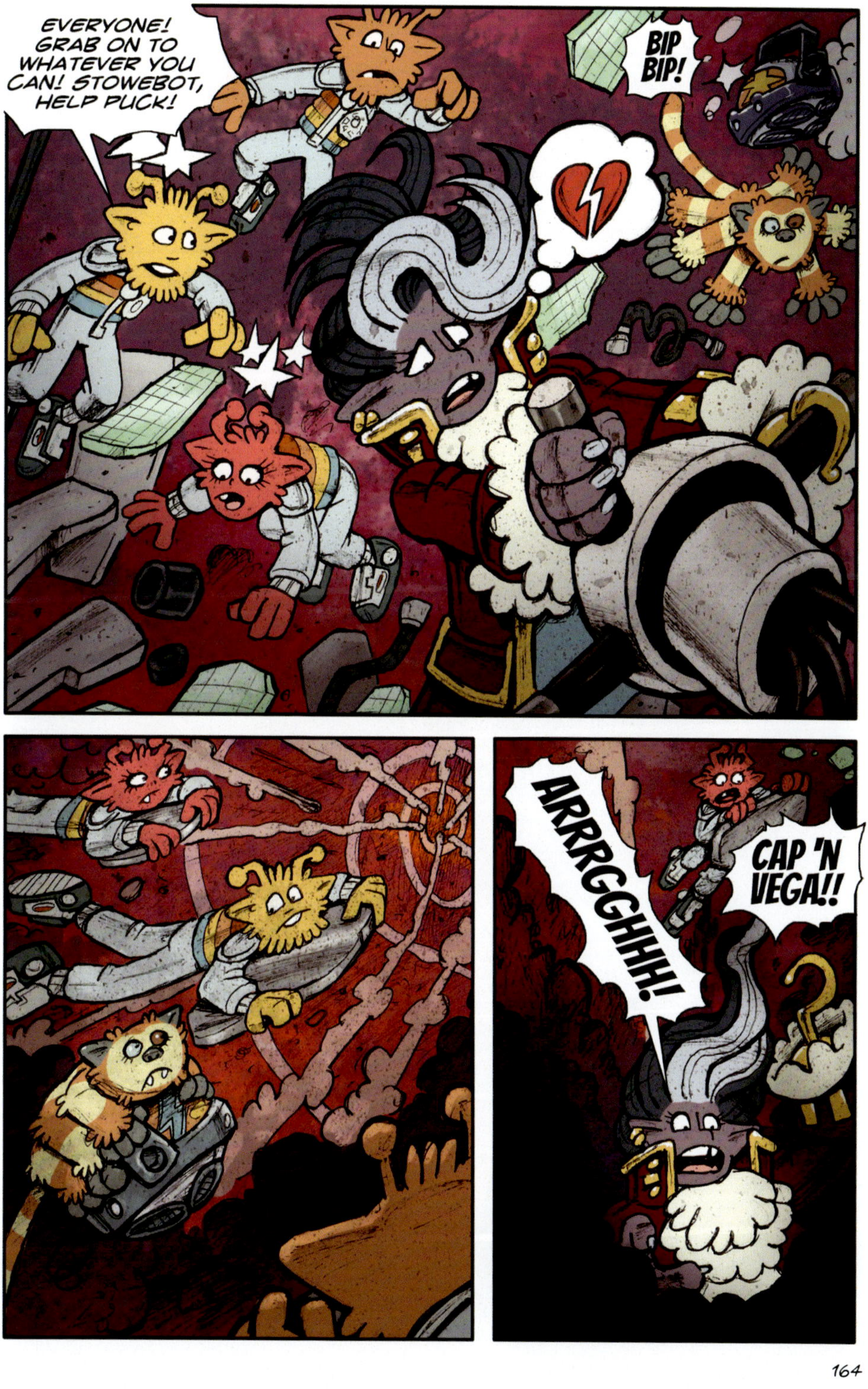

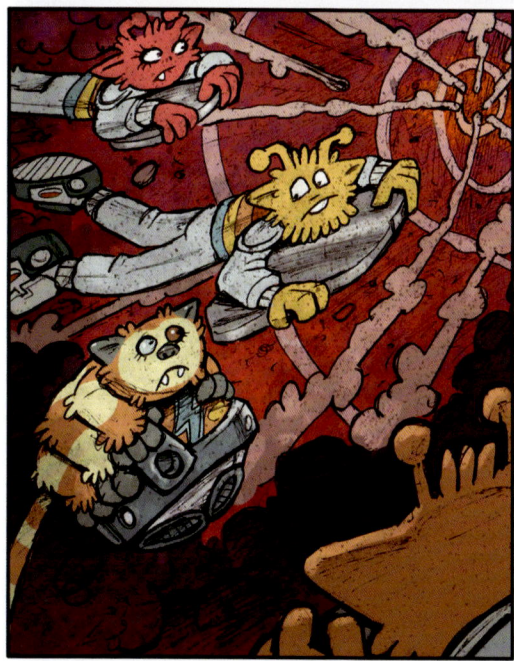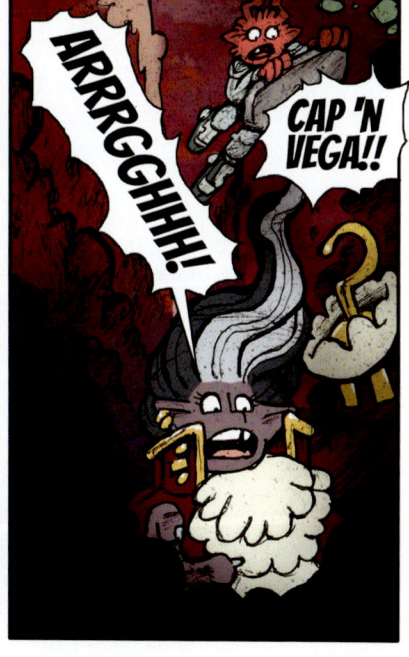

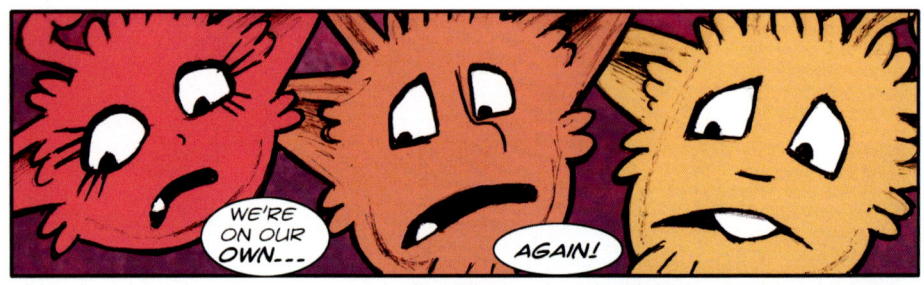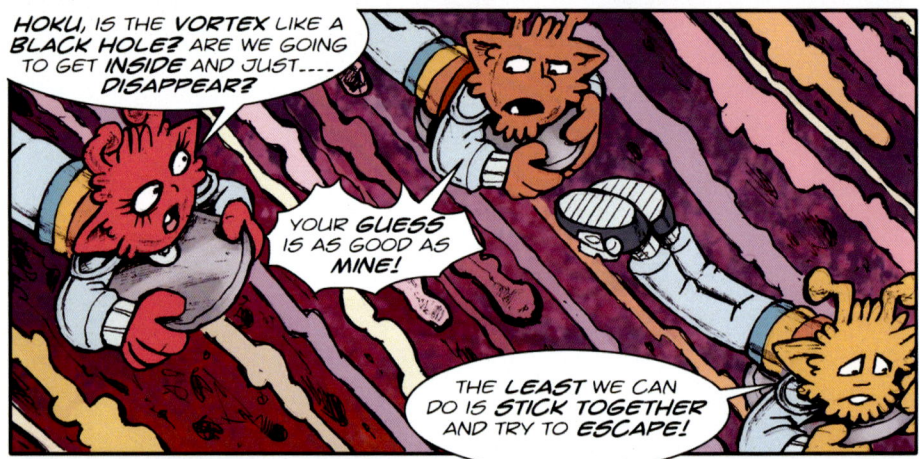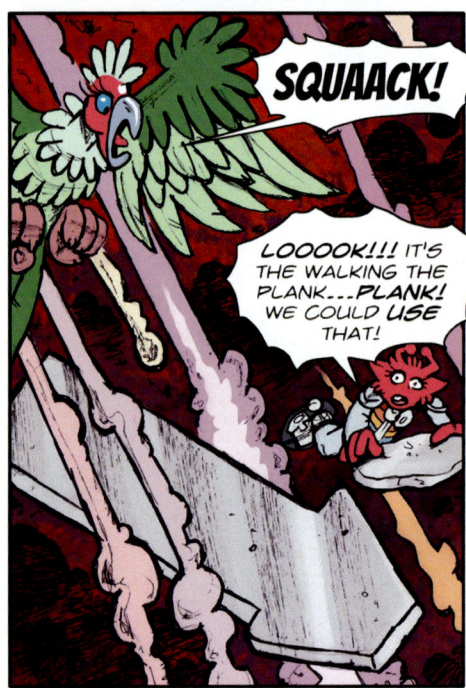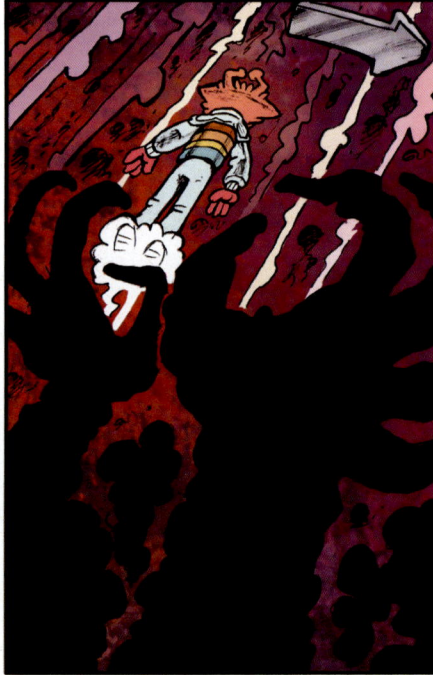

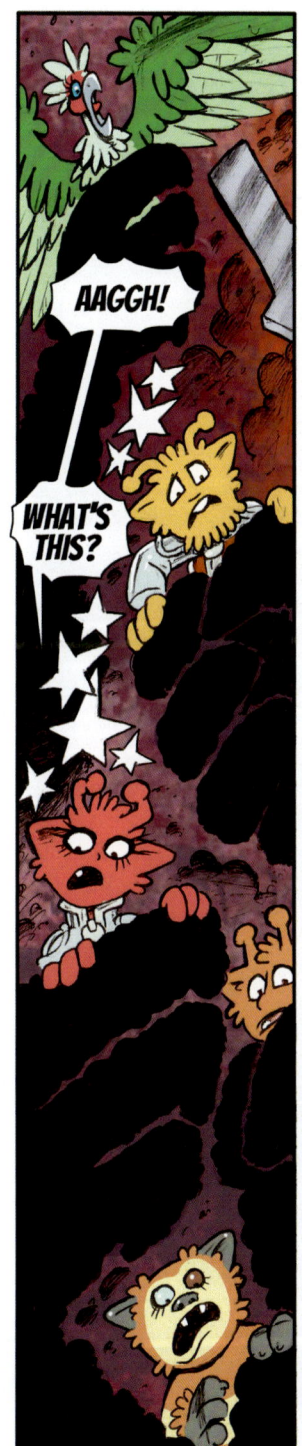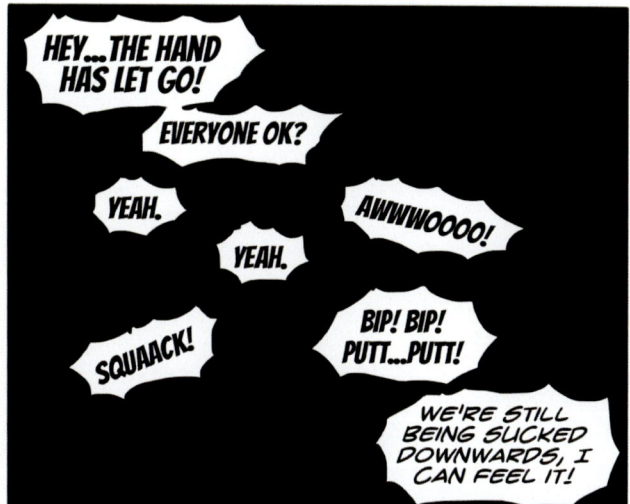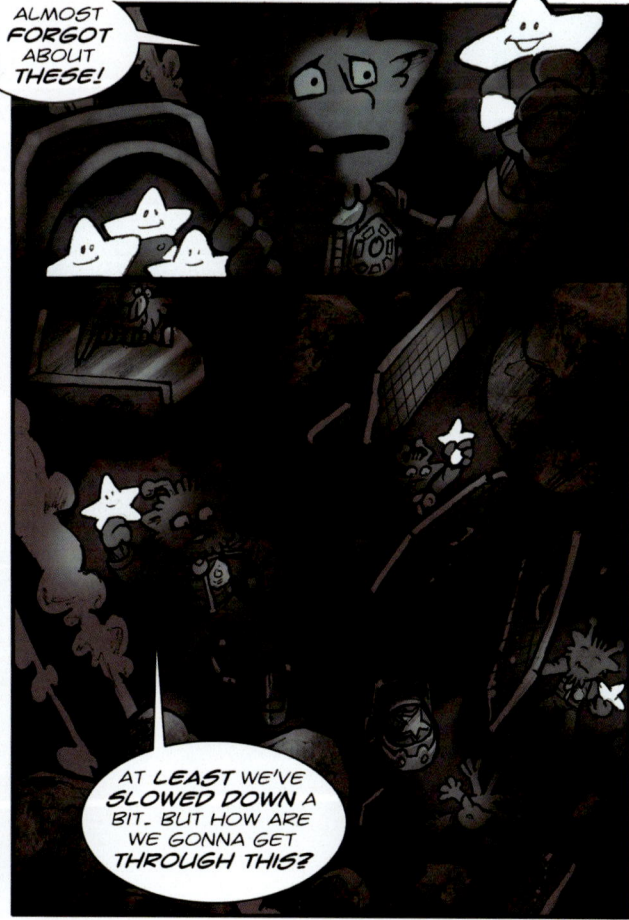

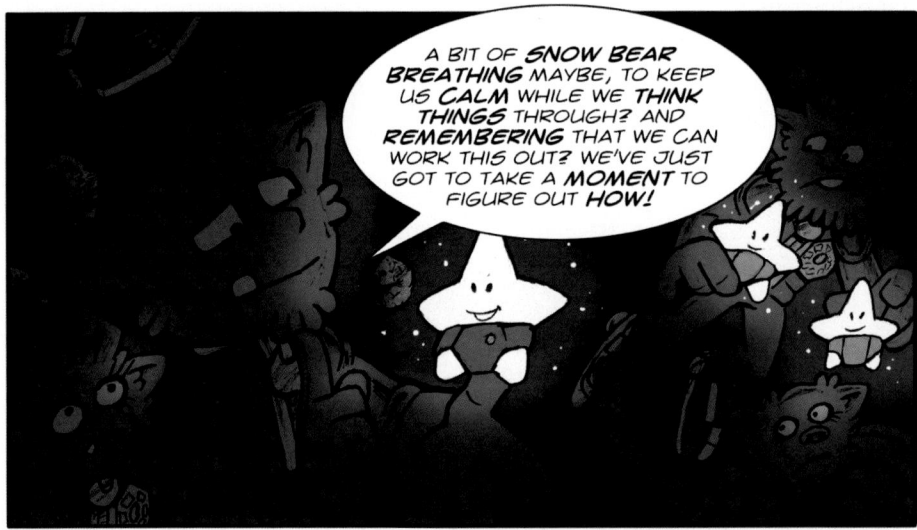
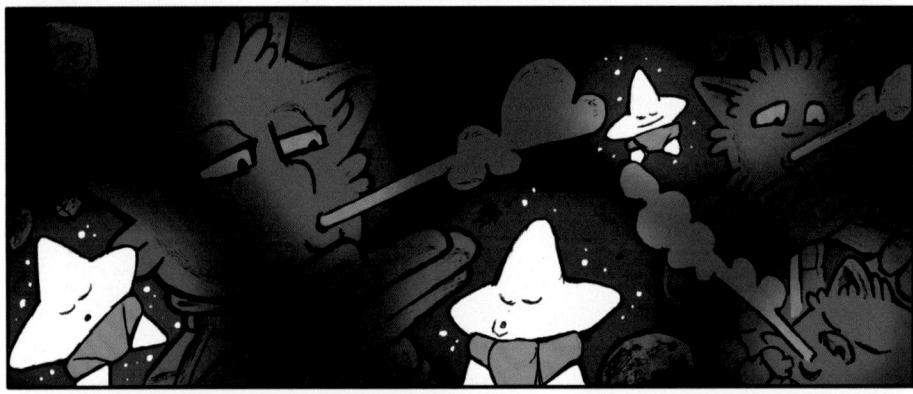
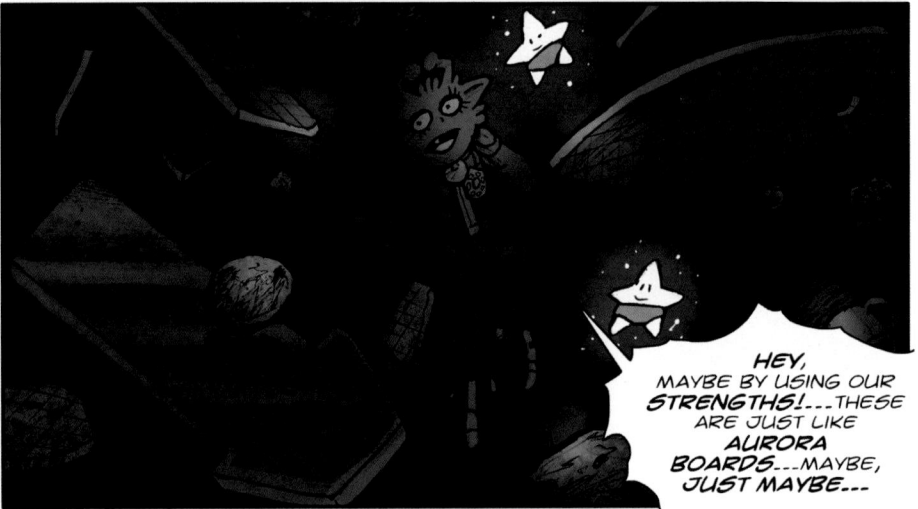

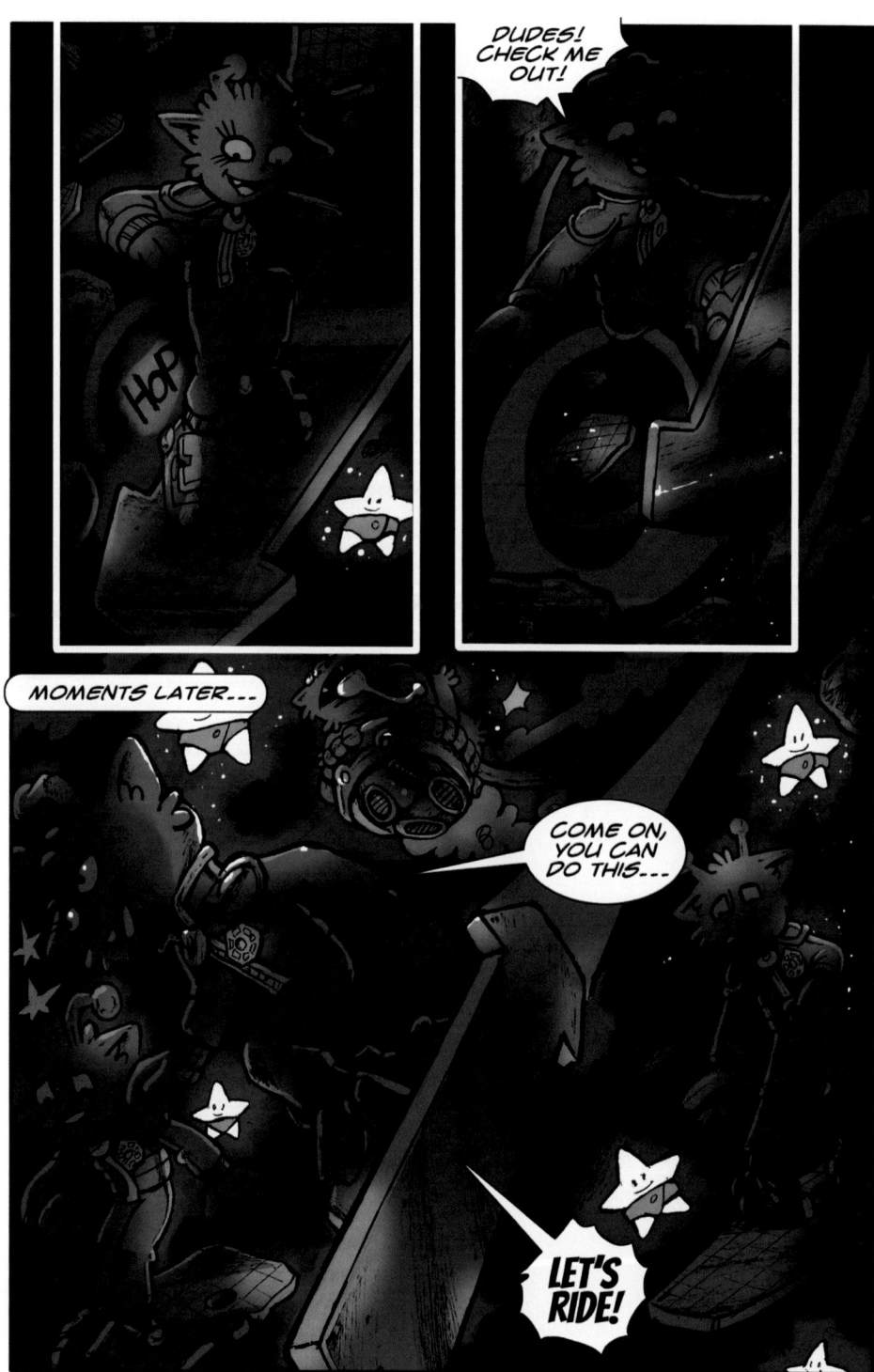

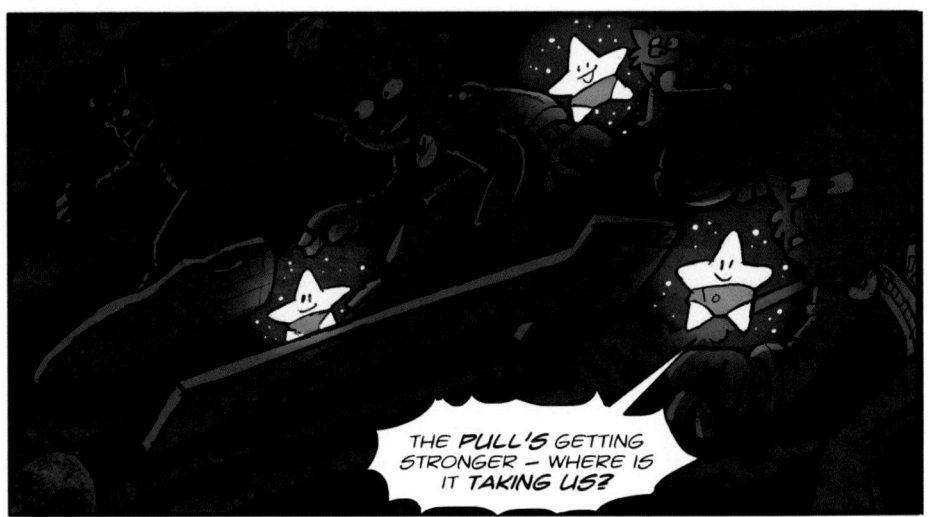

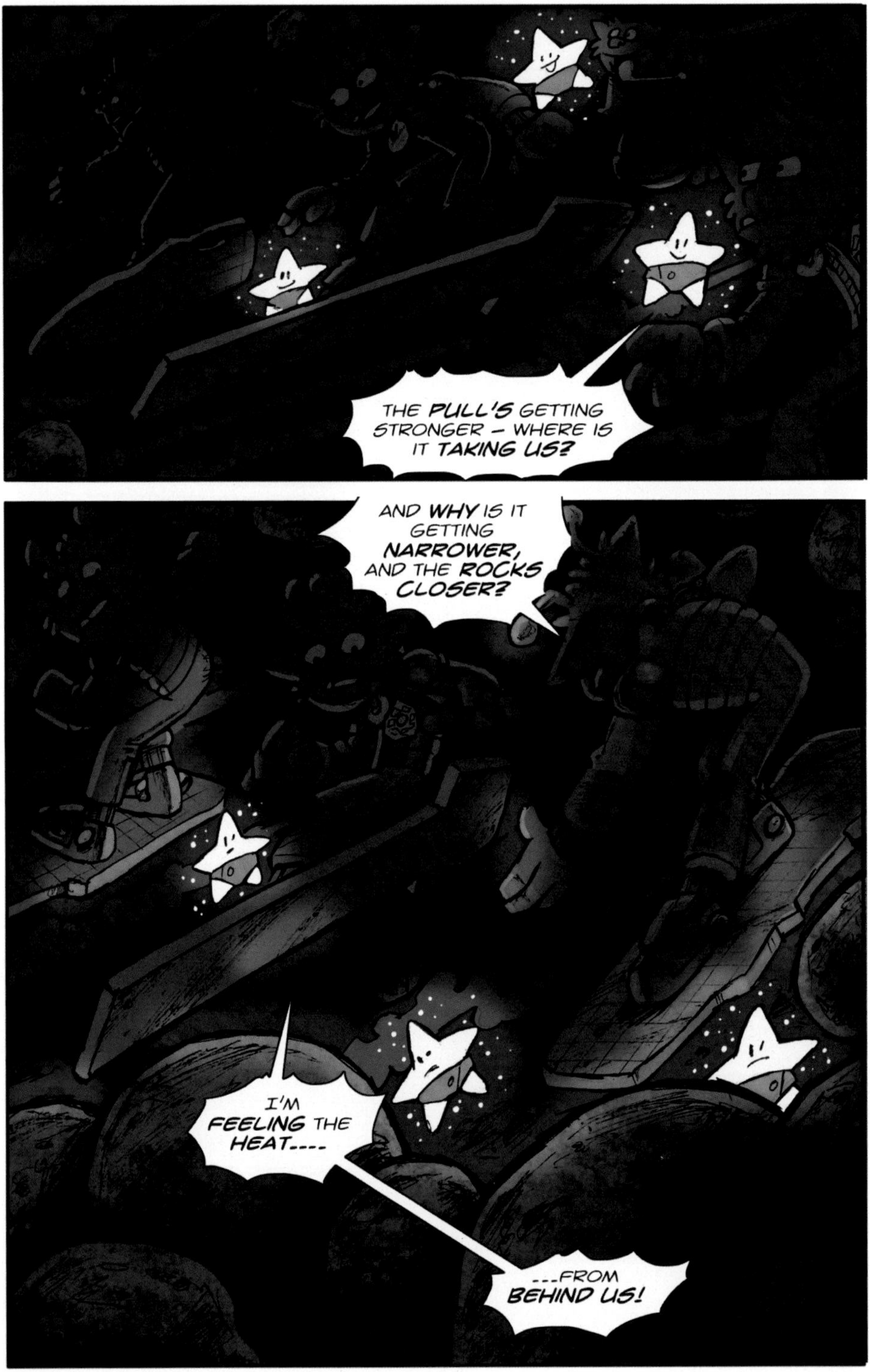

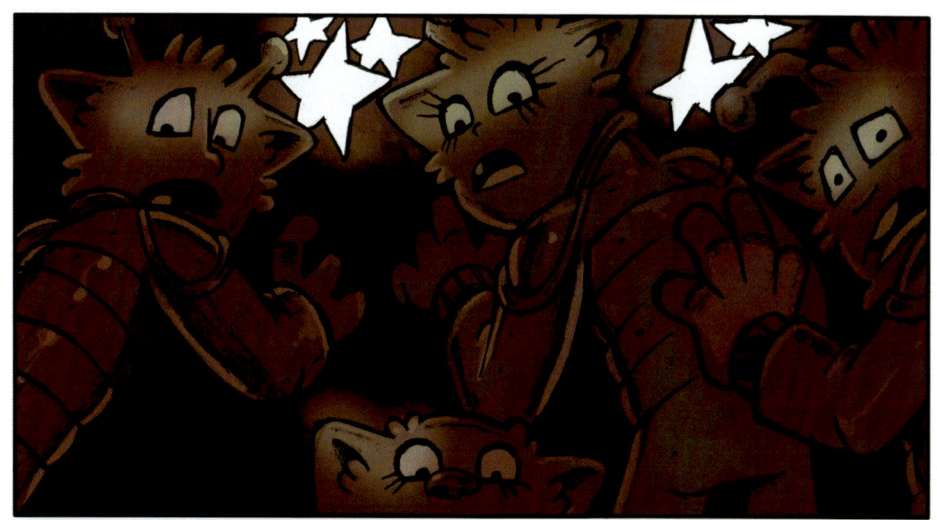

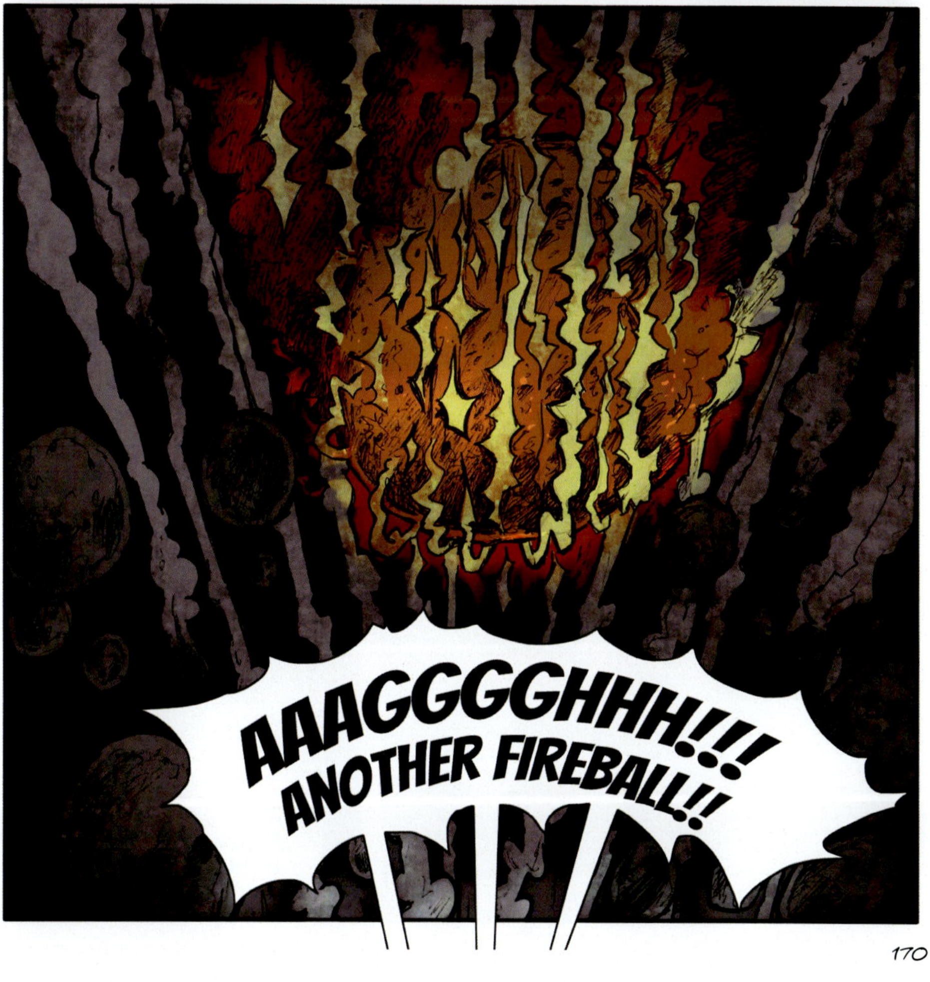

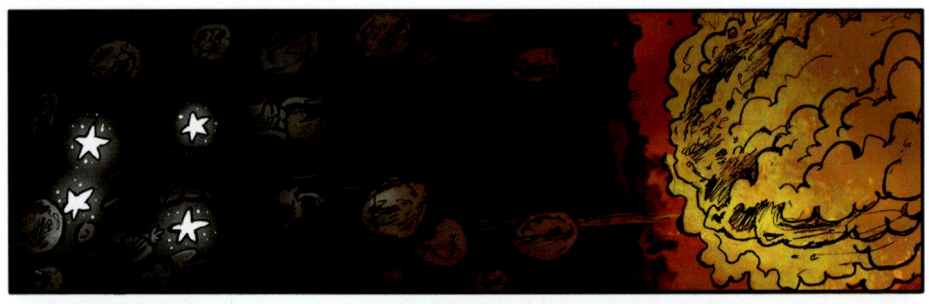

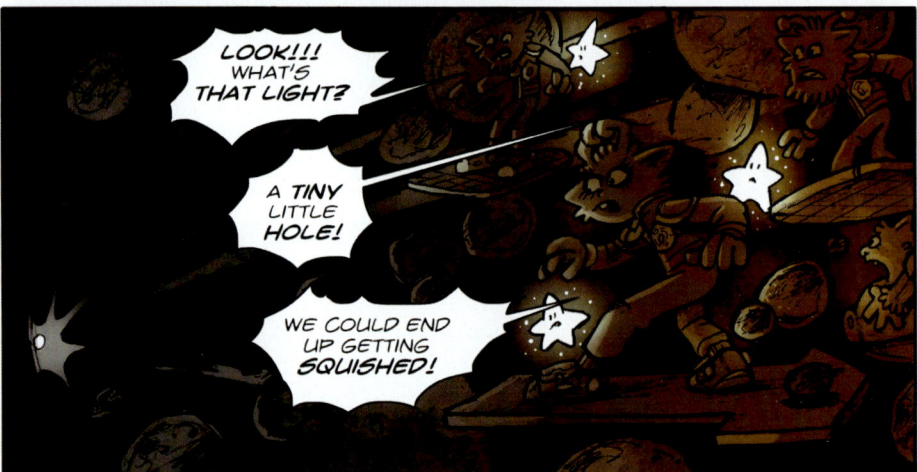

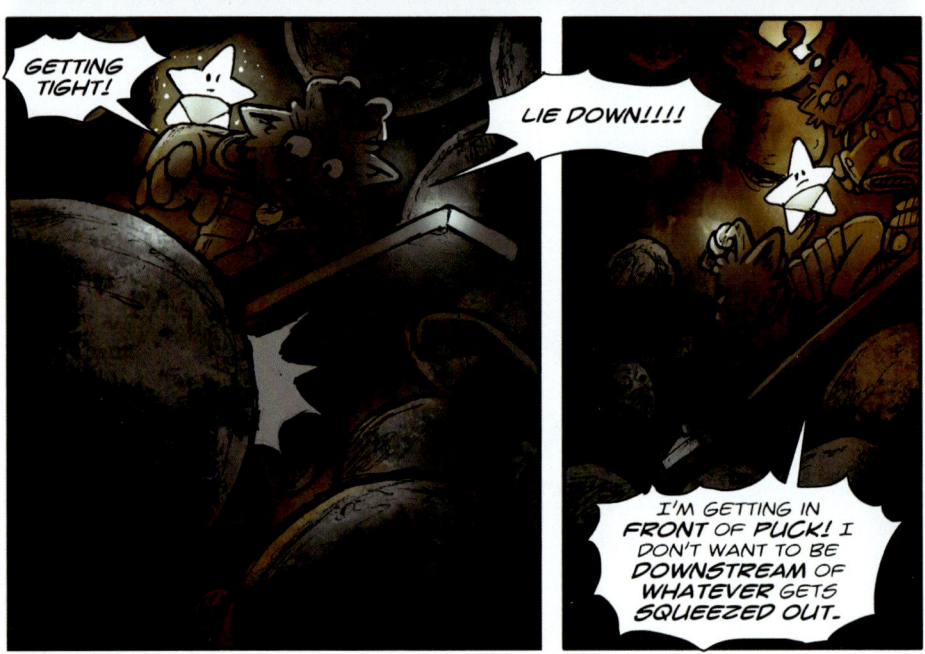

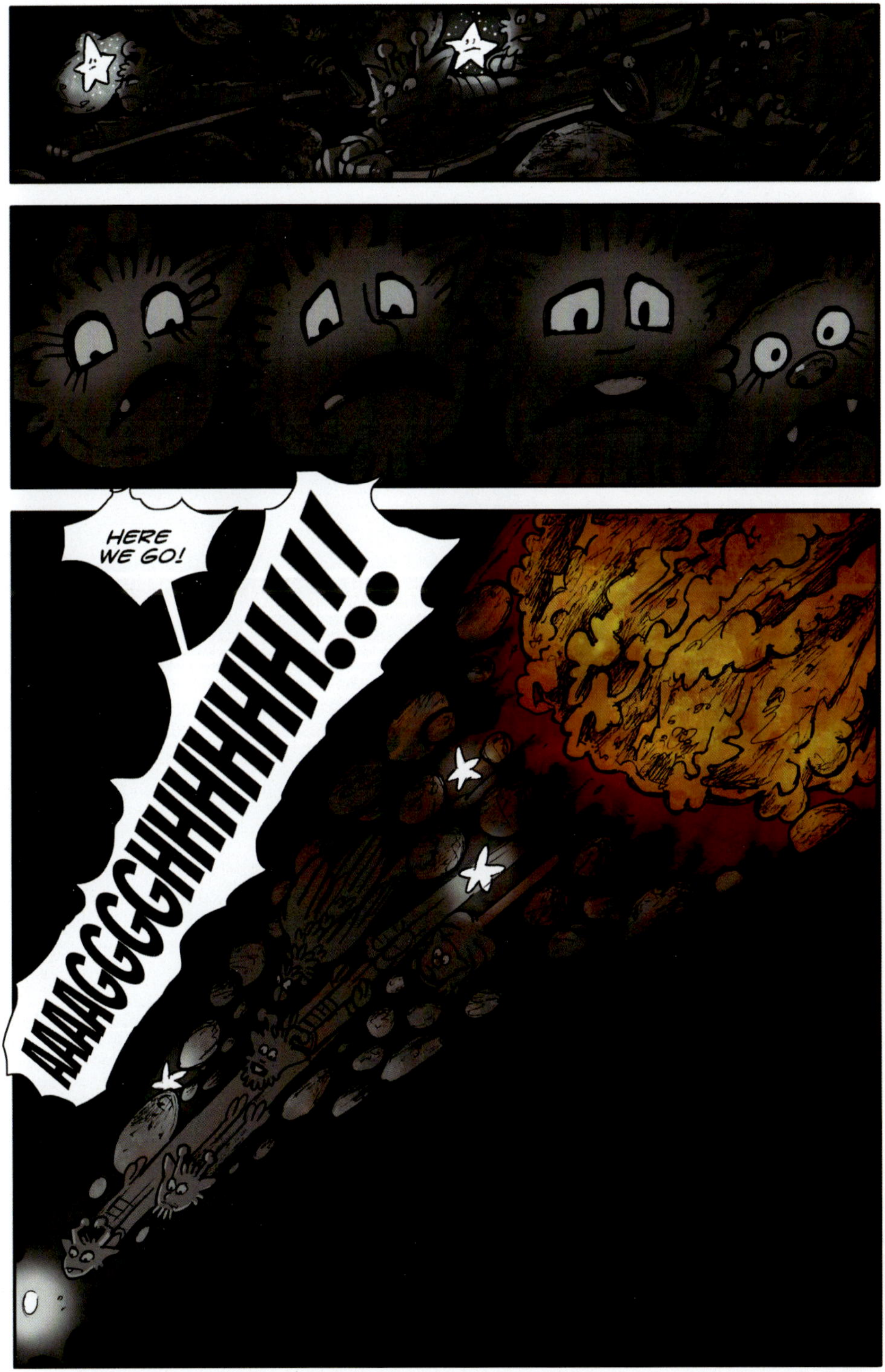

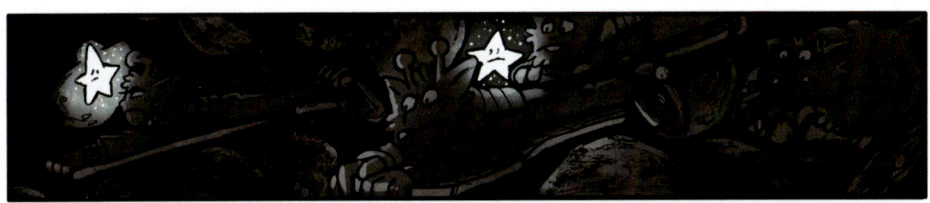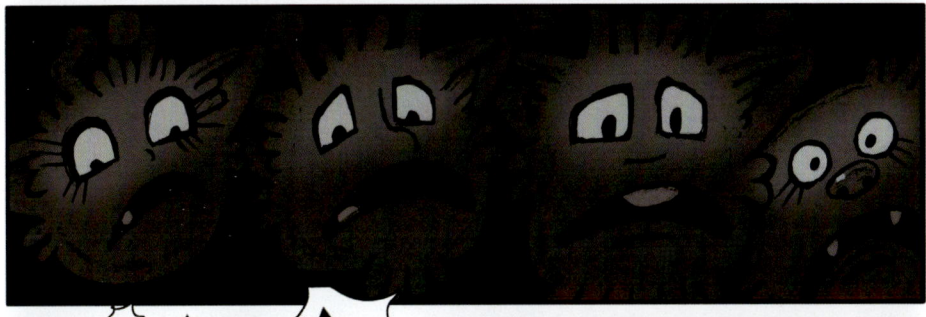

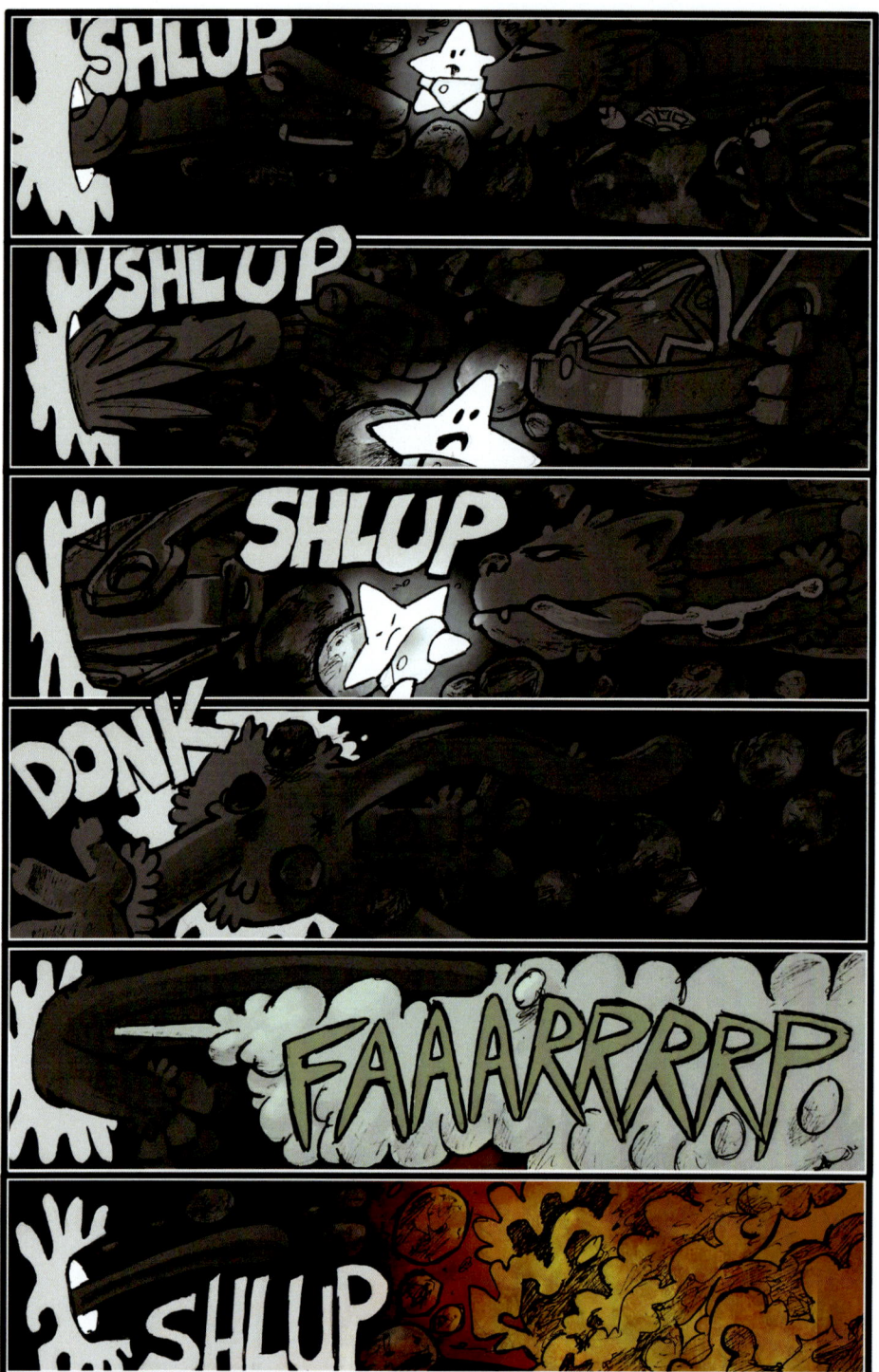

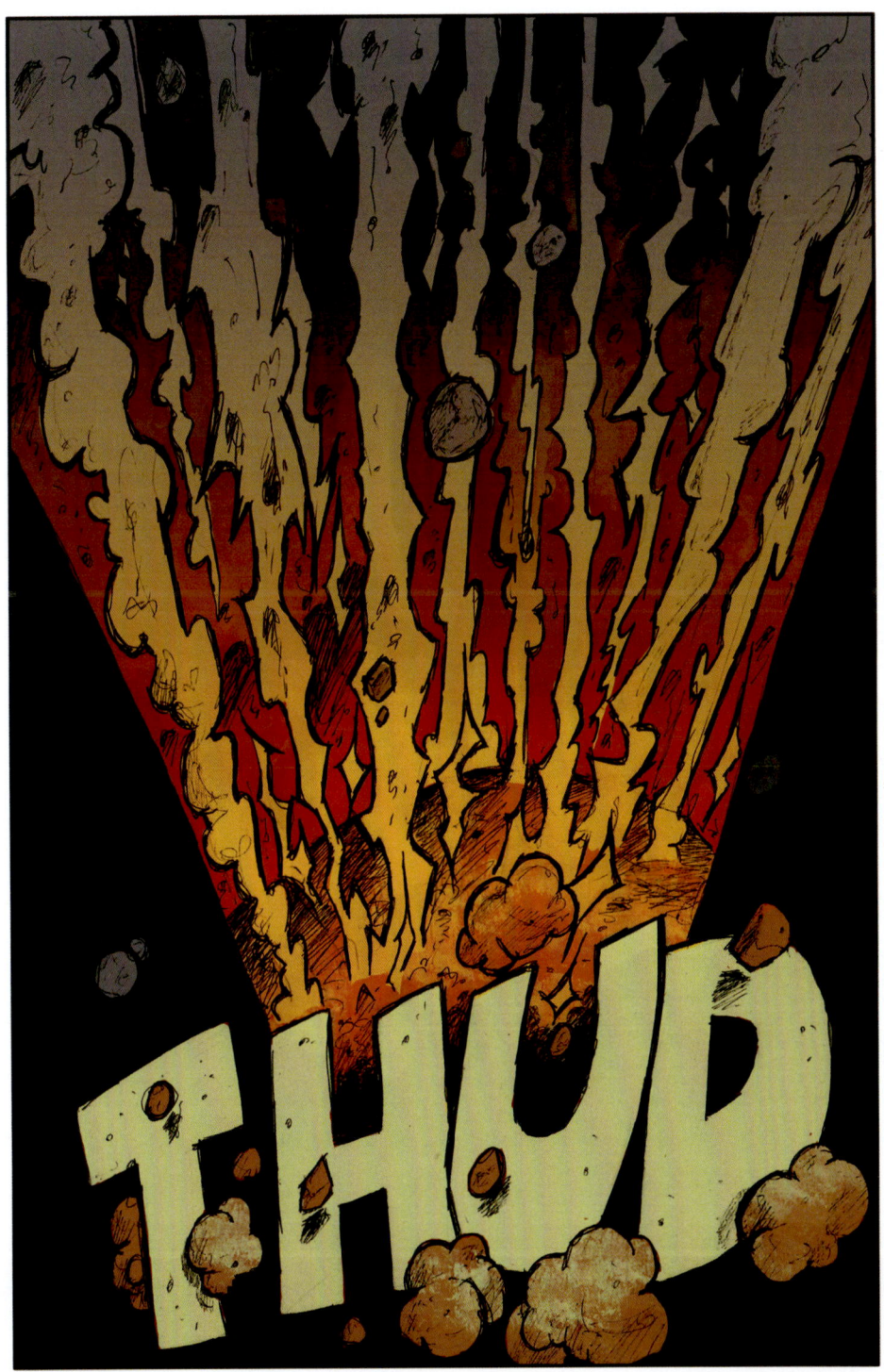

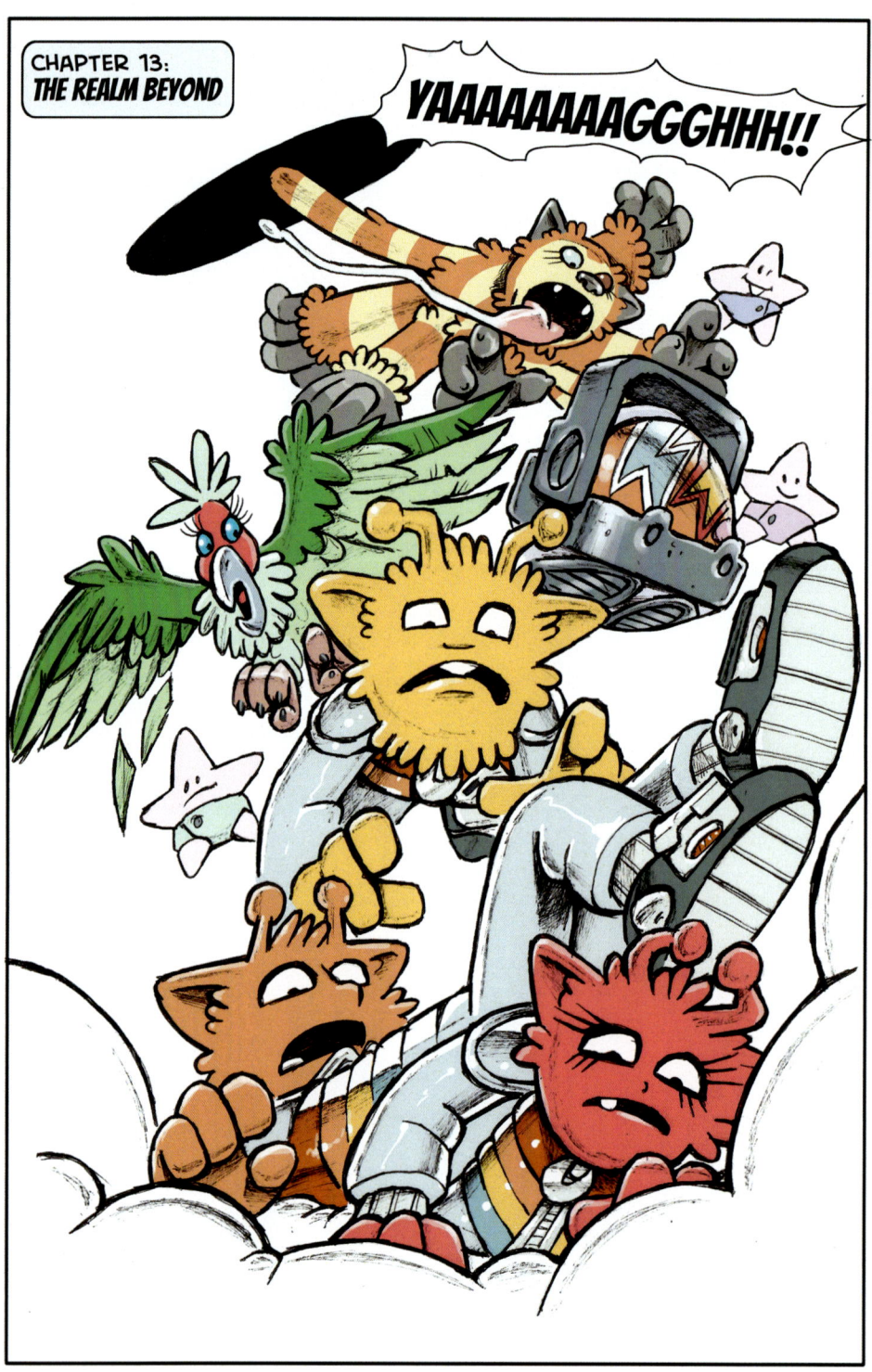

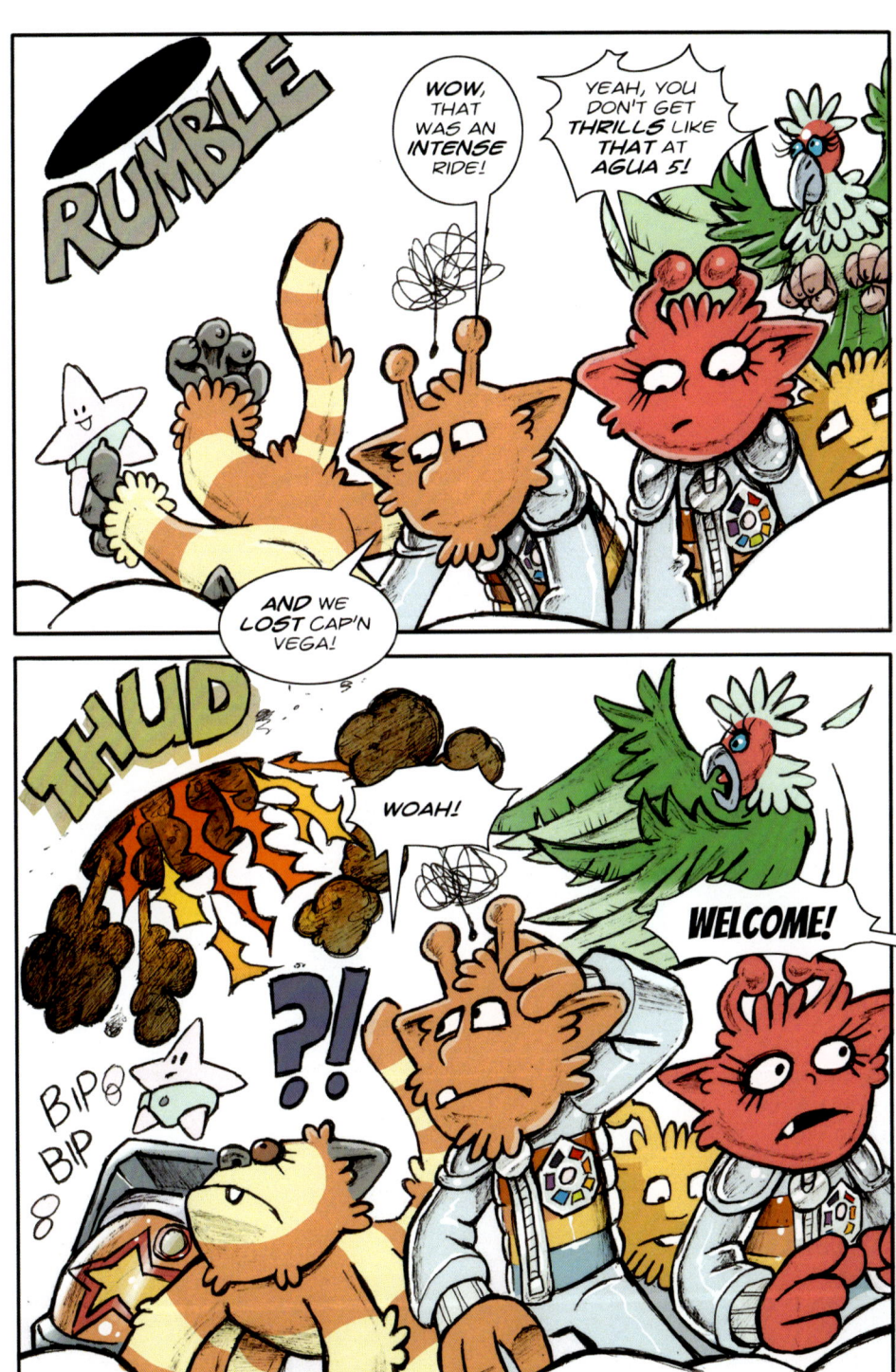

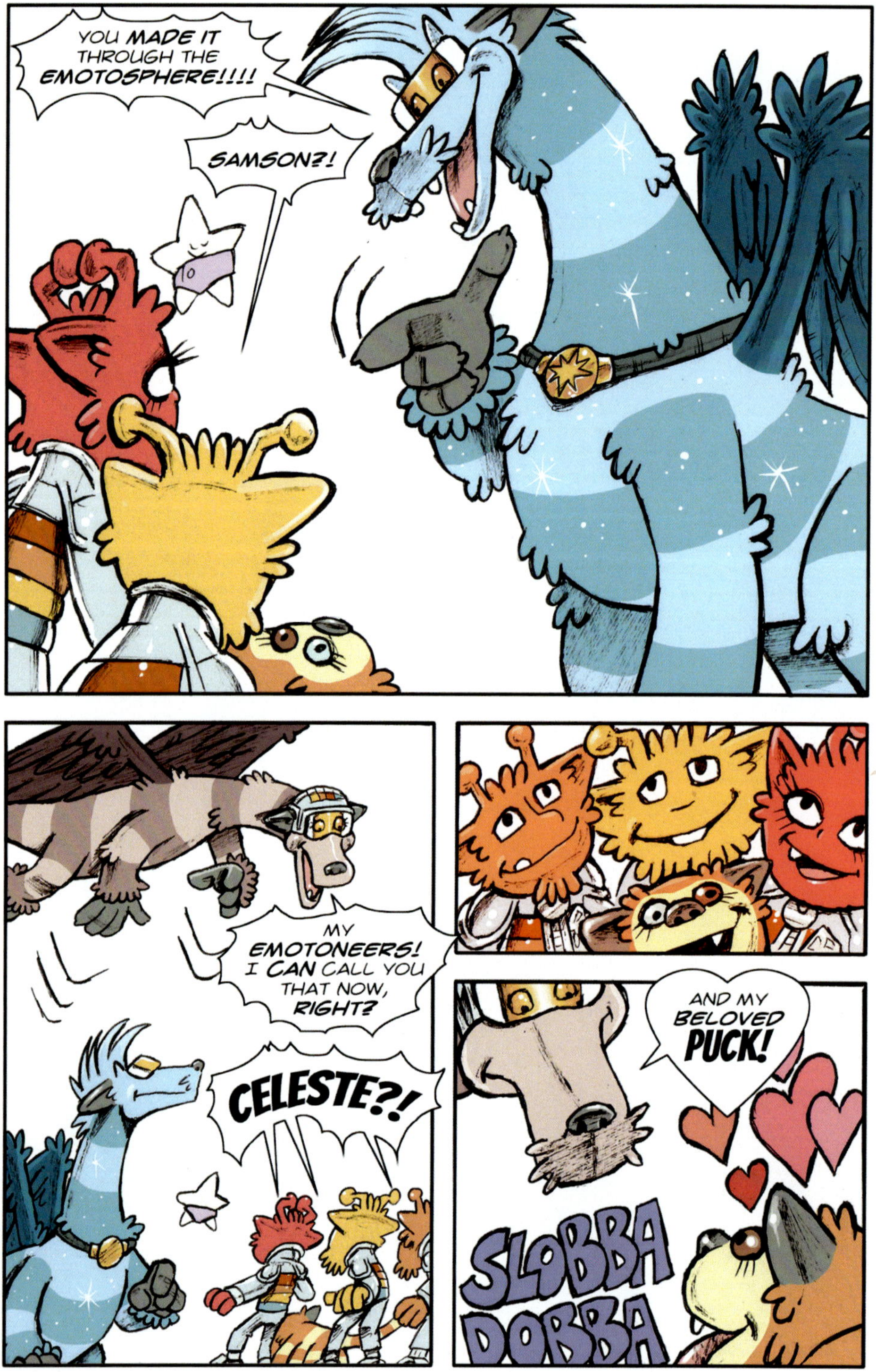

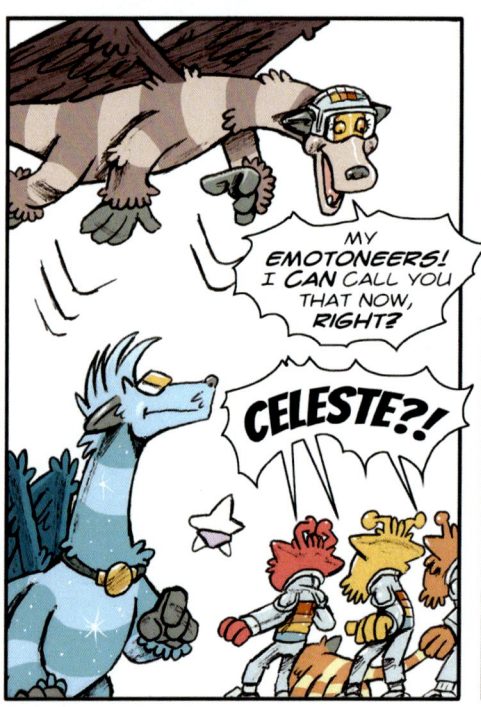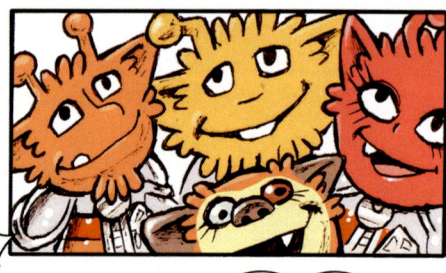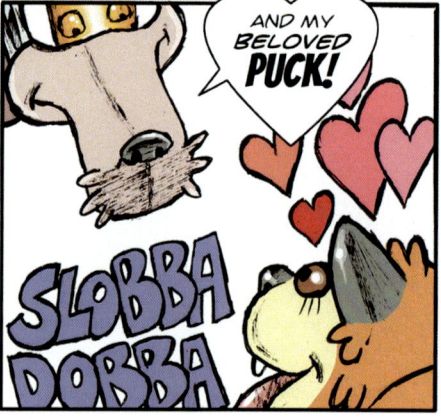

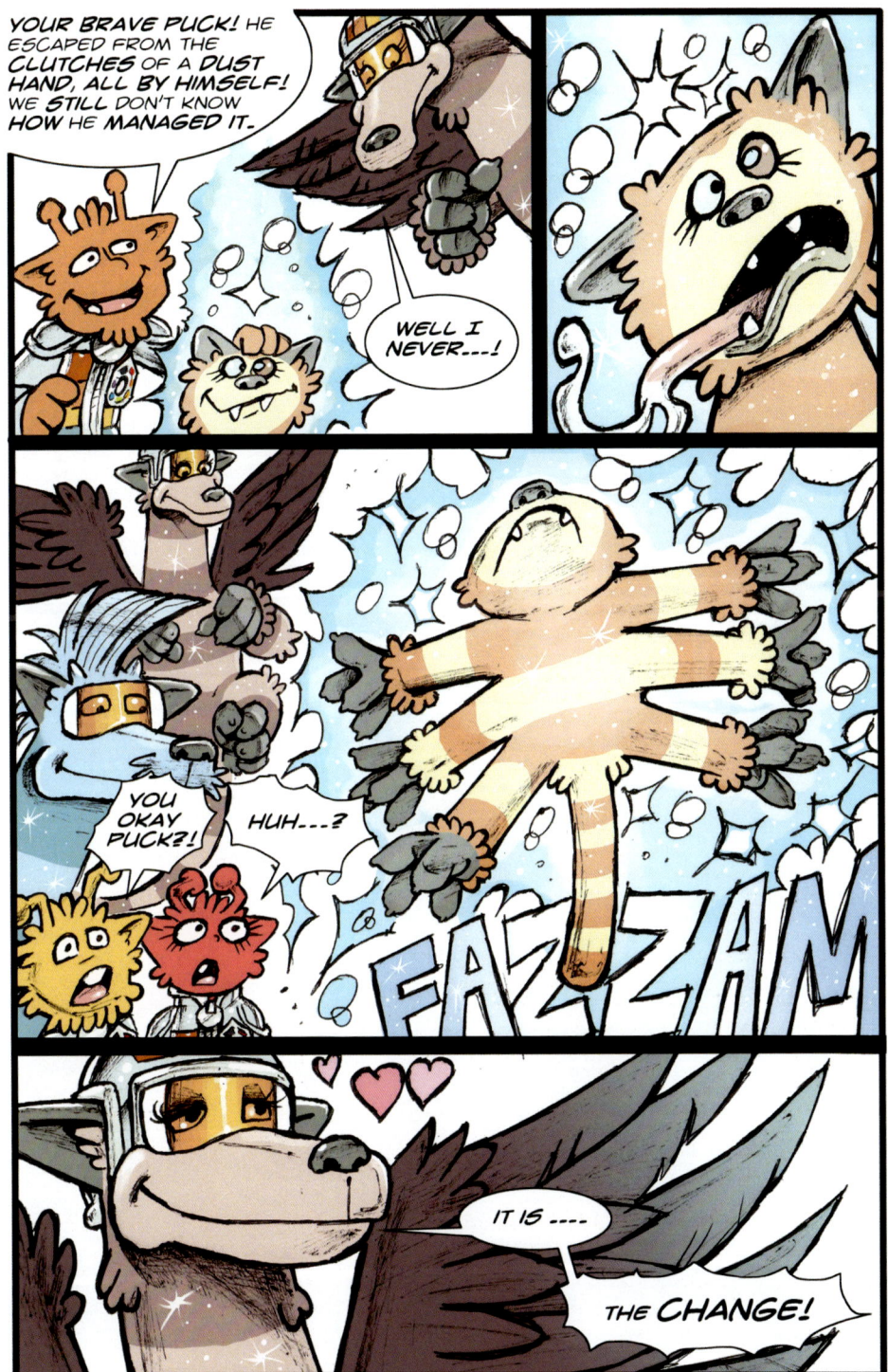

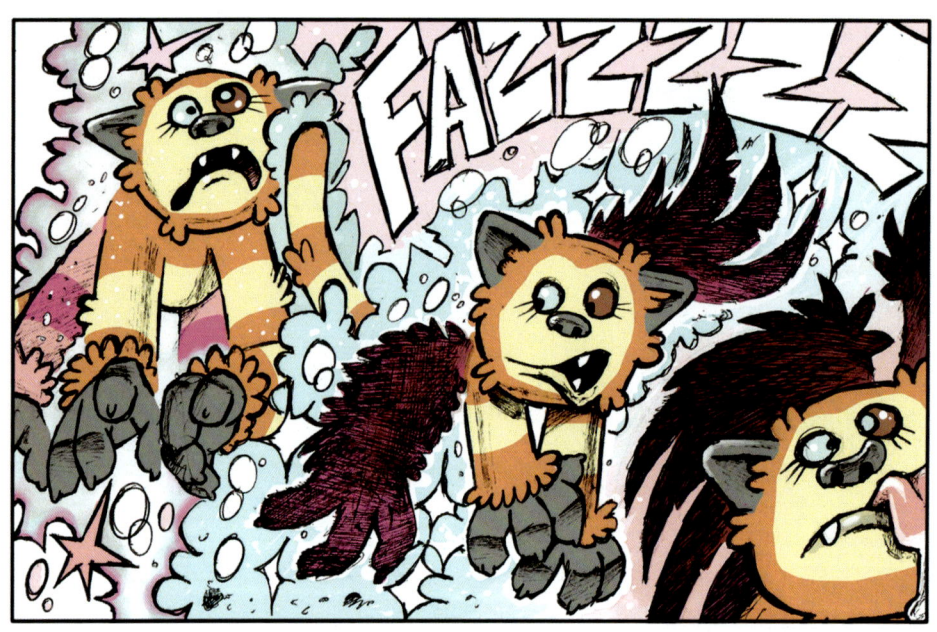
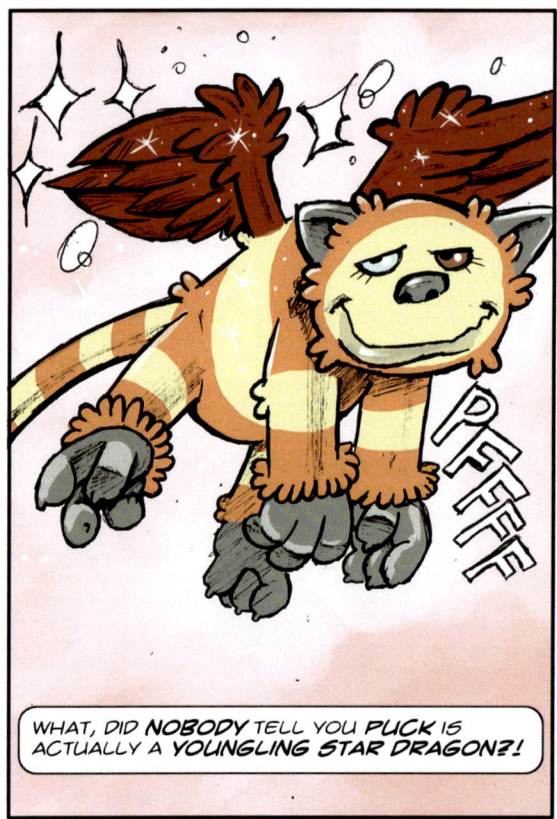
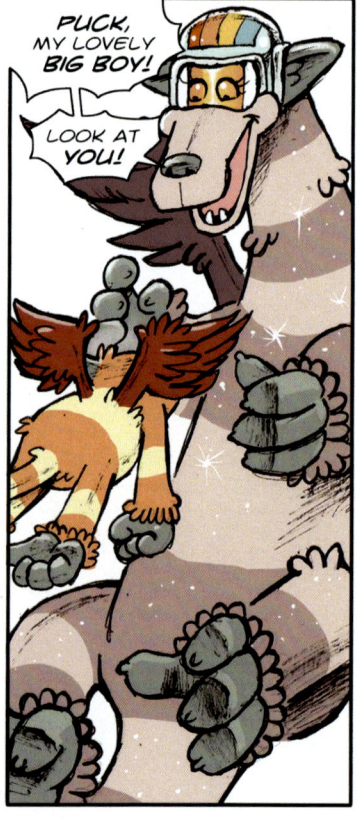

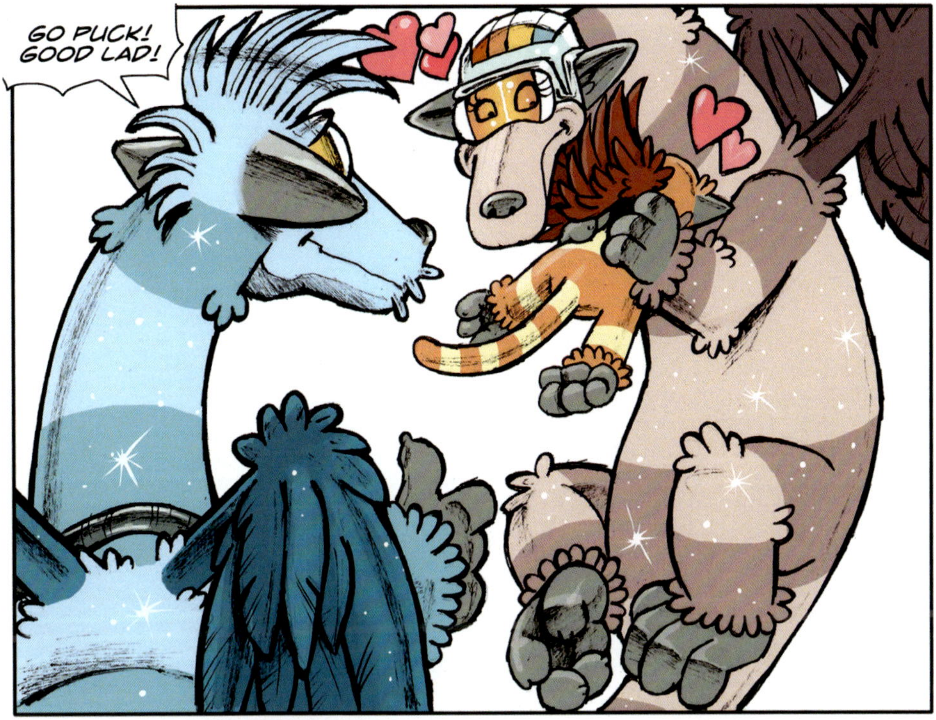

GO PUCK! GOOD LAD!

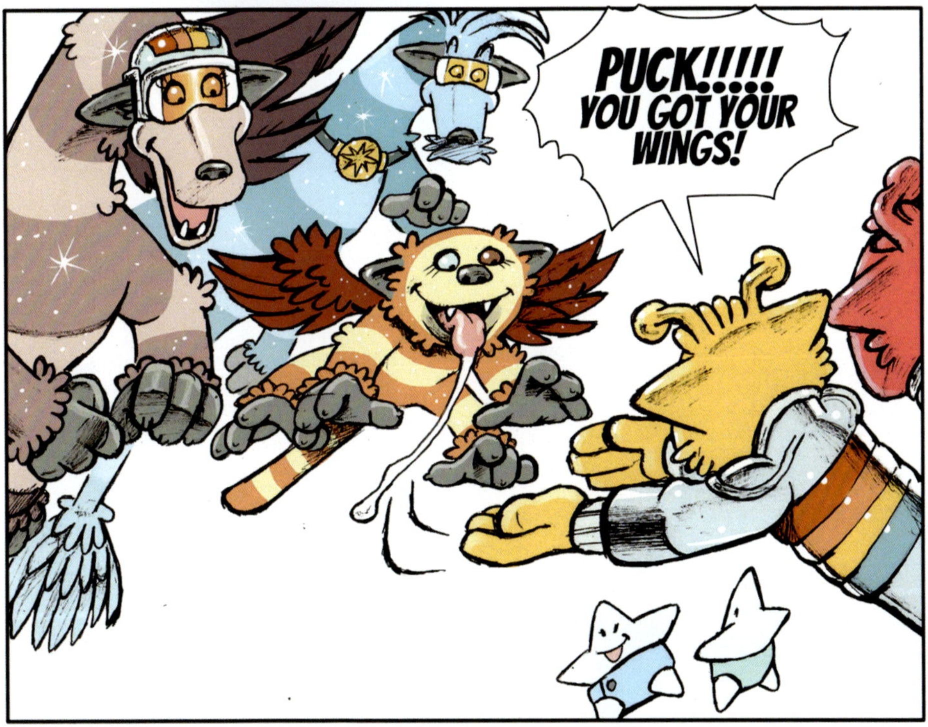

PUCK!!!!! YOU GOT YOUR WINGS!

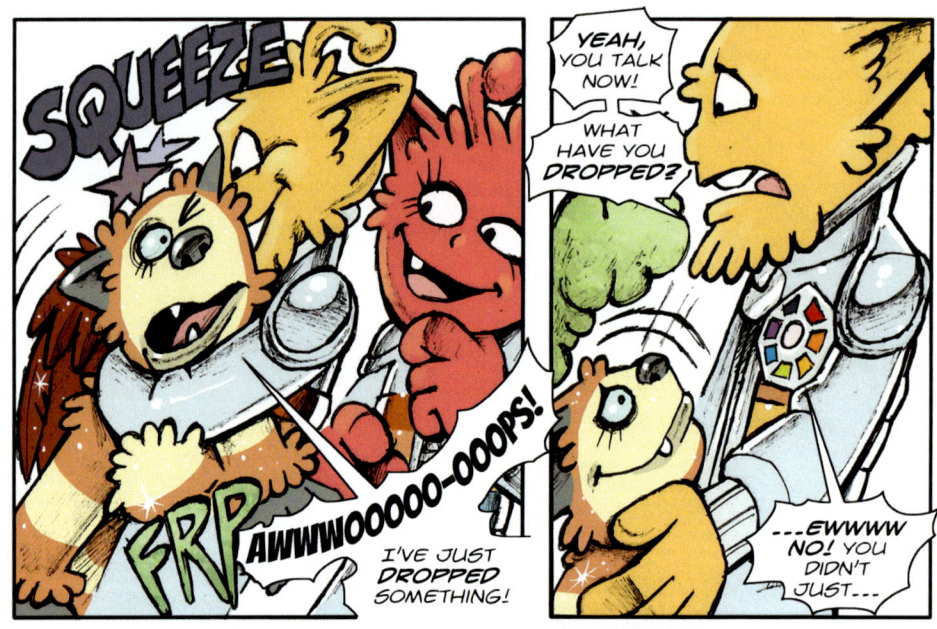

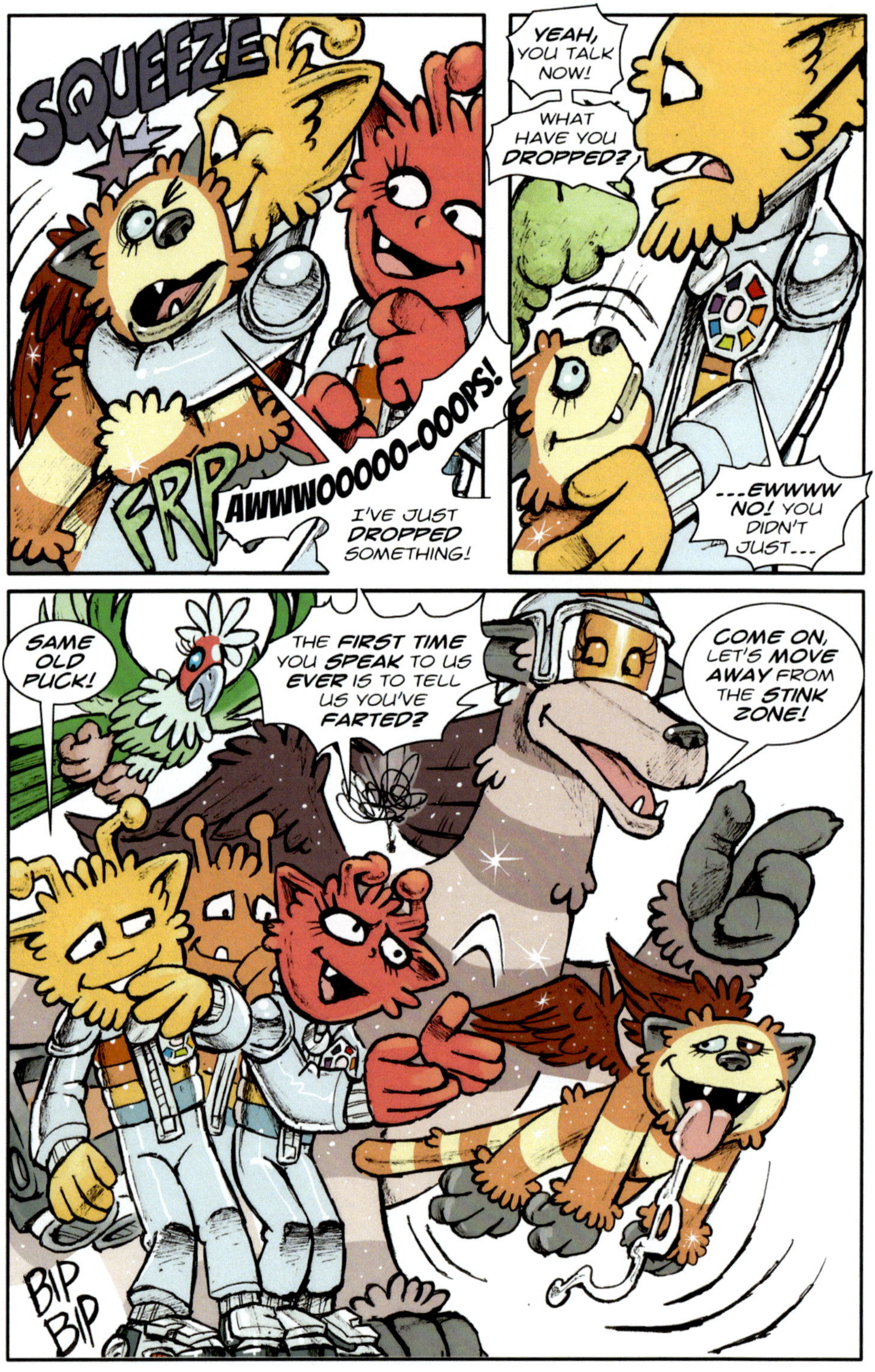

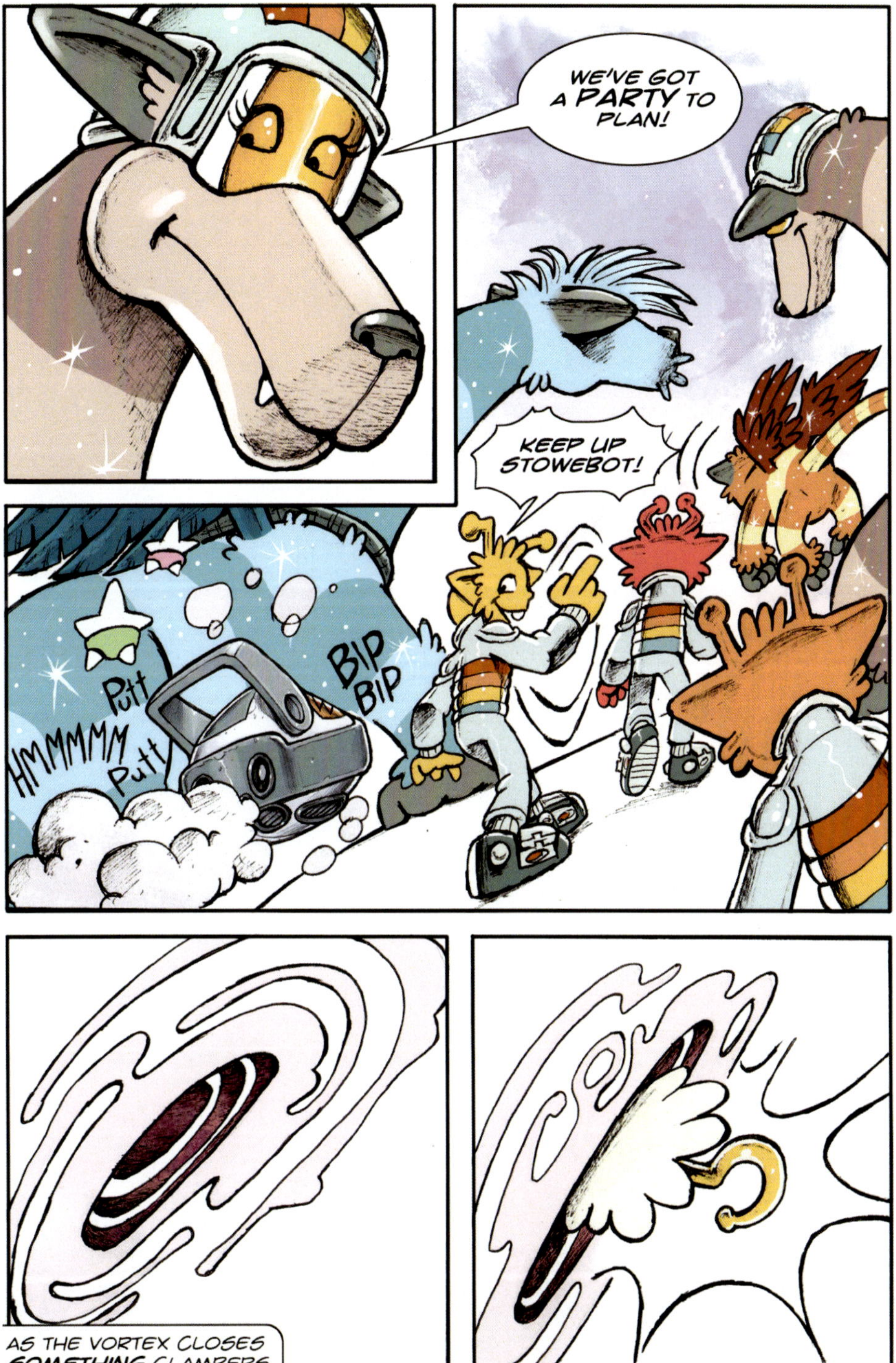

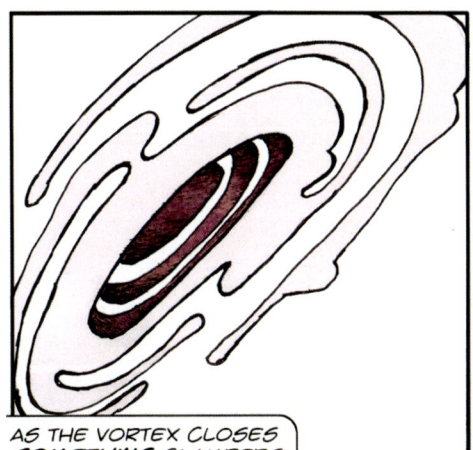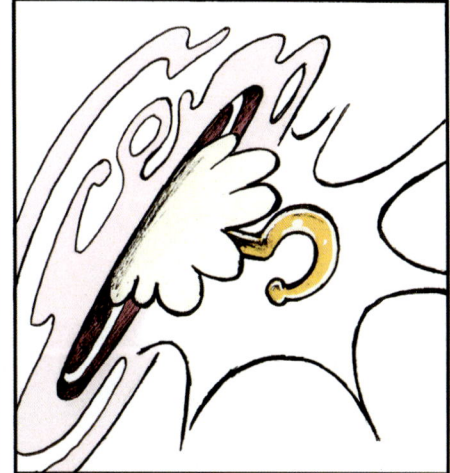

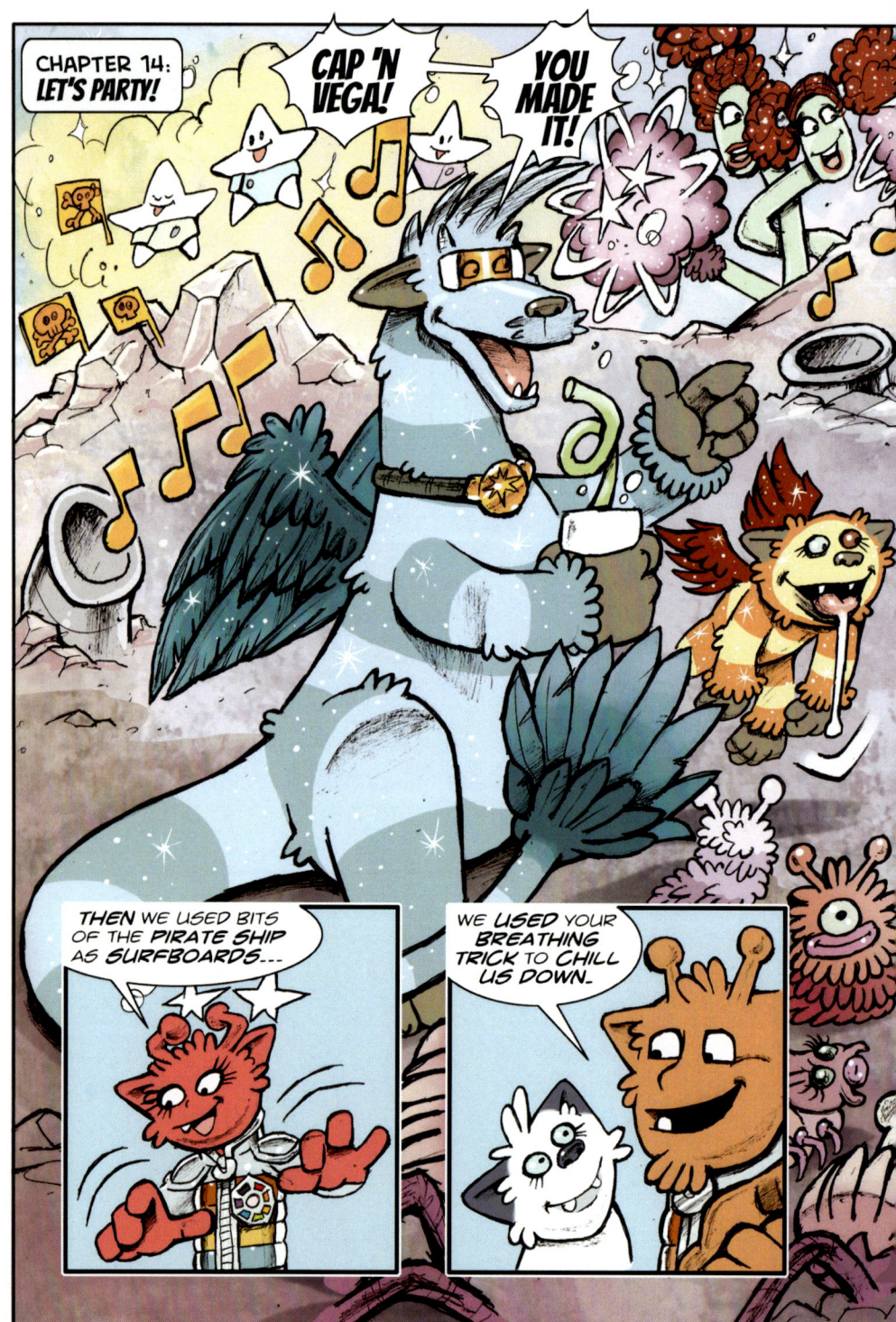

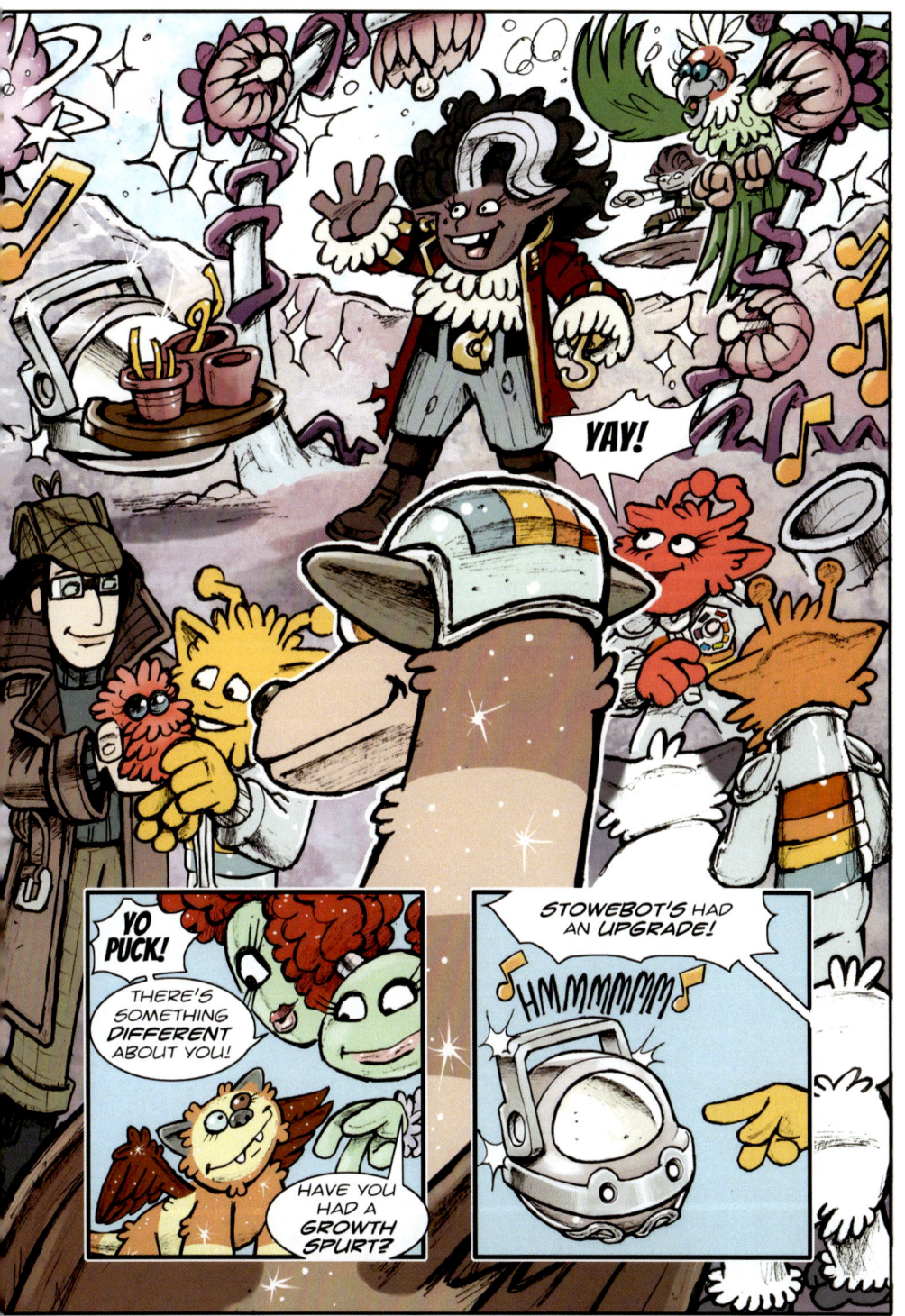

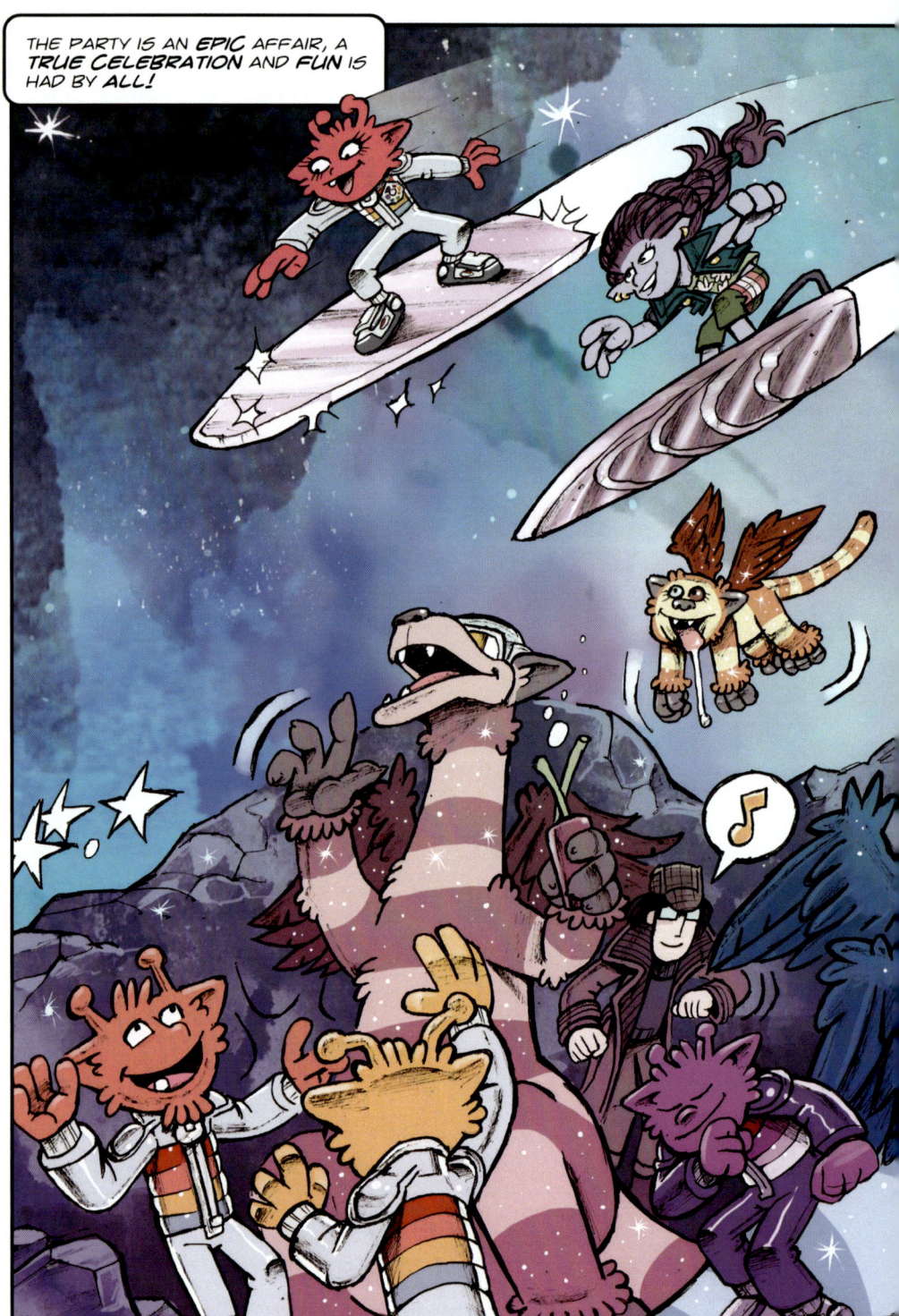

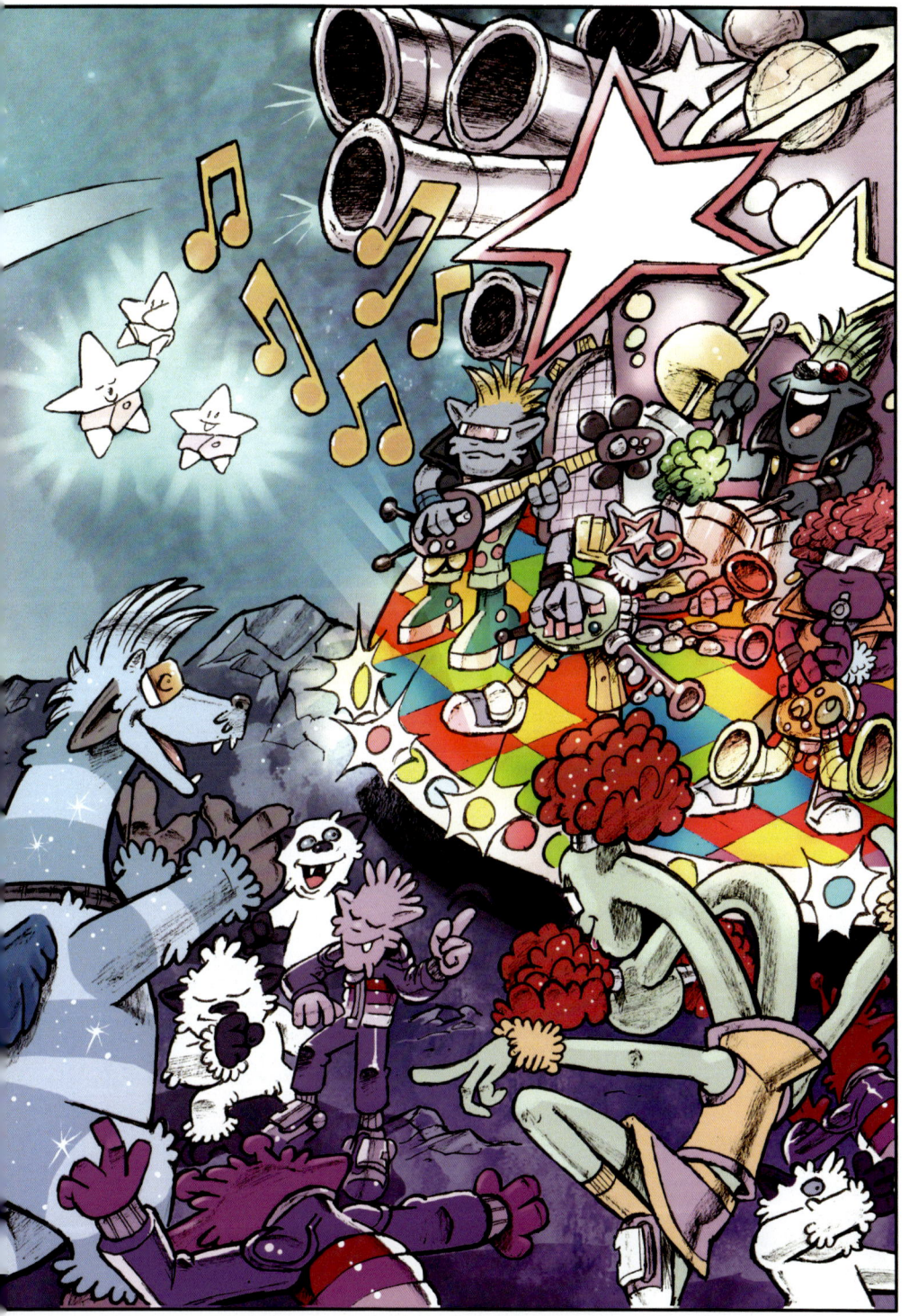

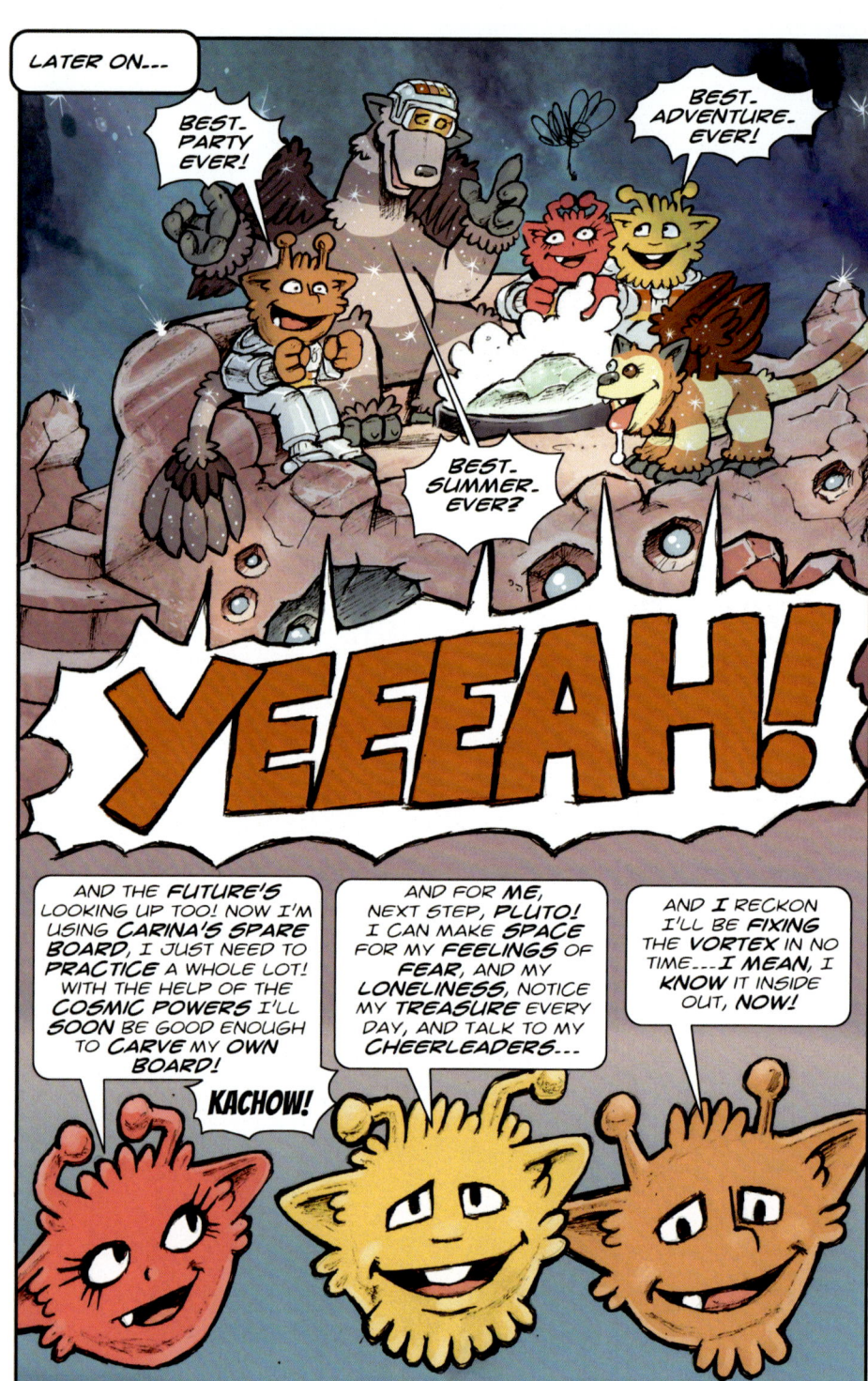

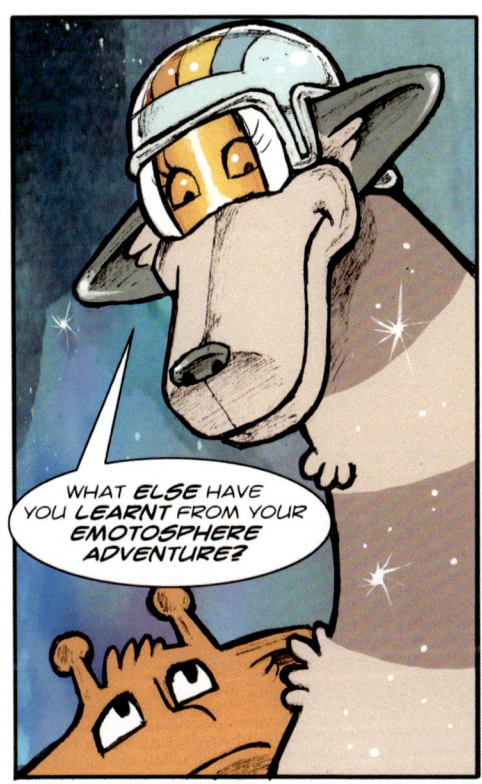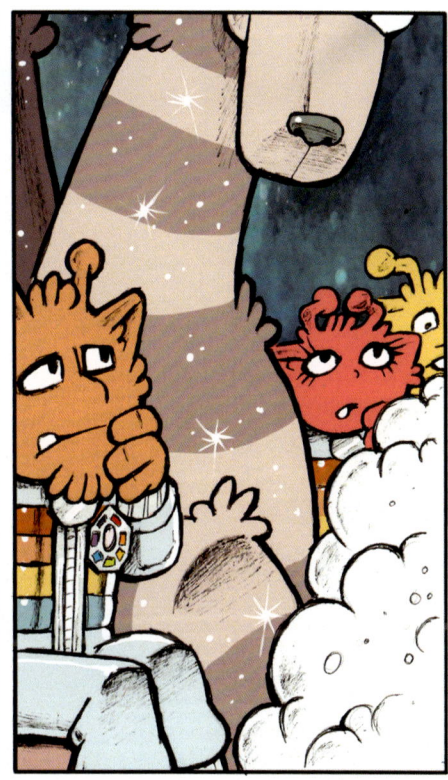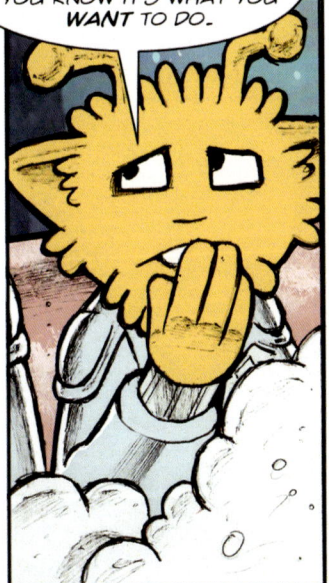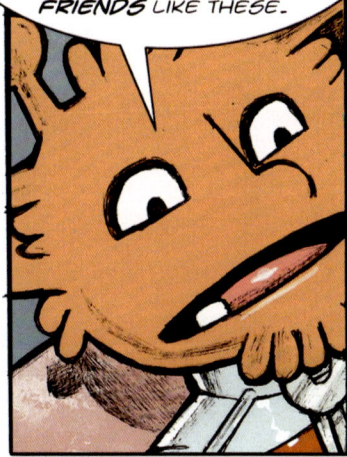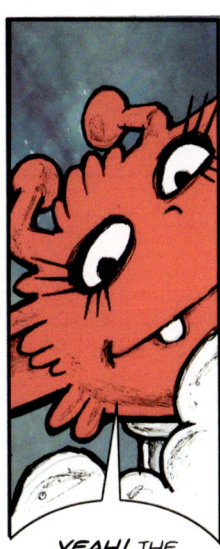

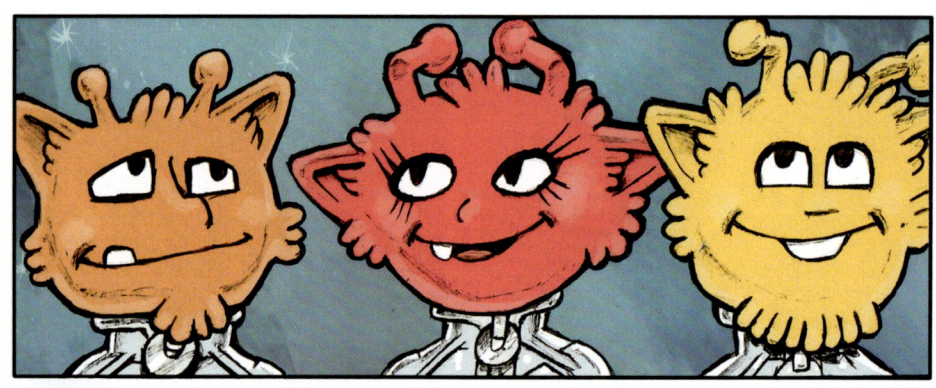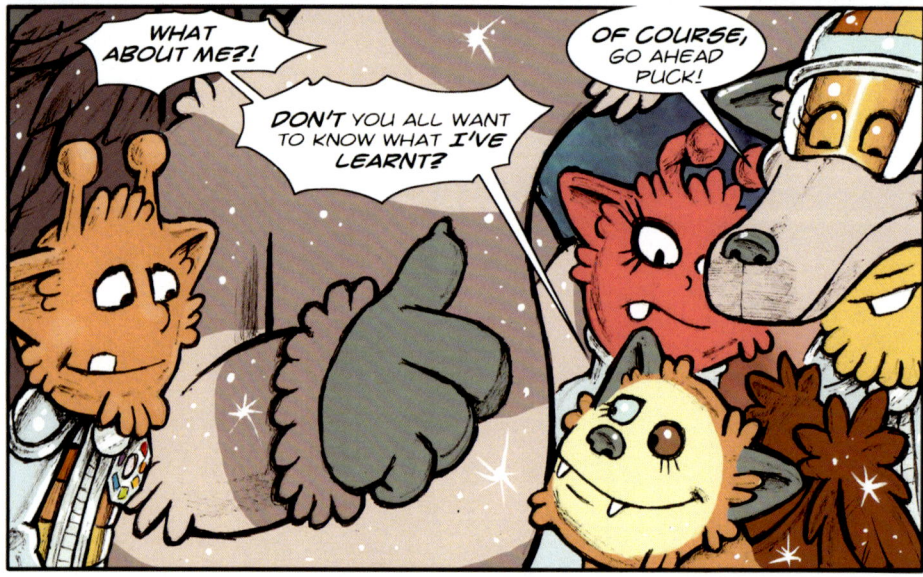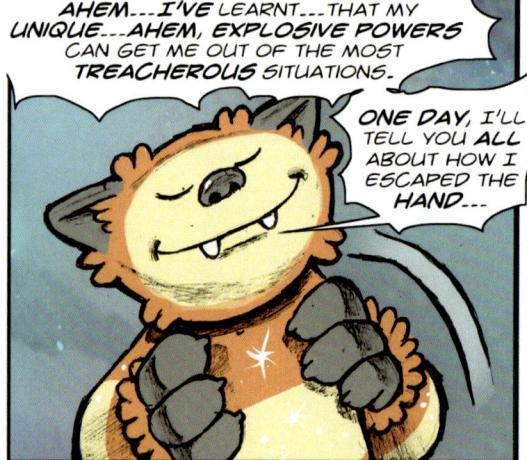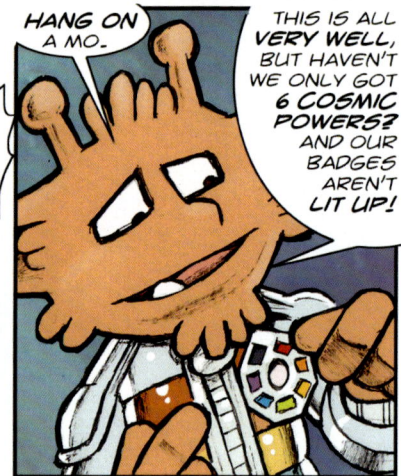

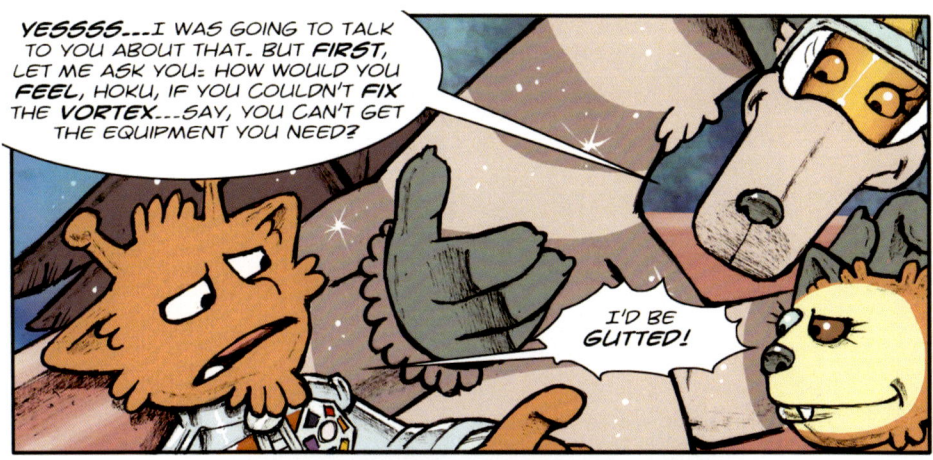
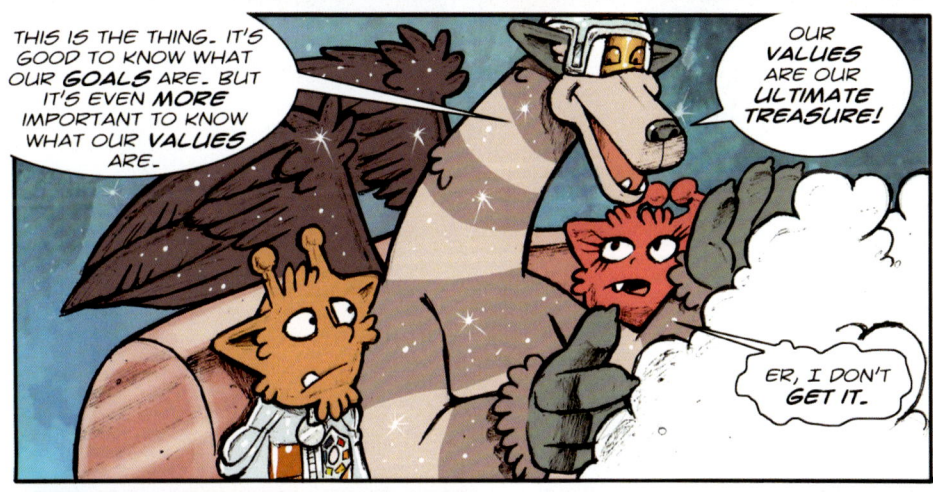
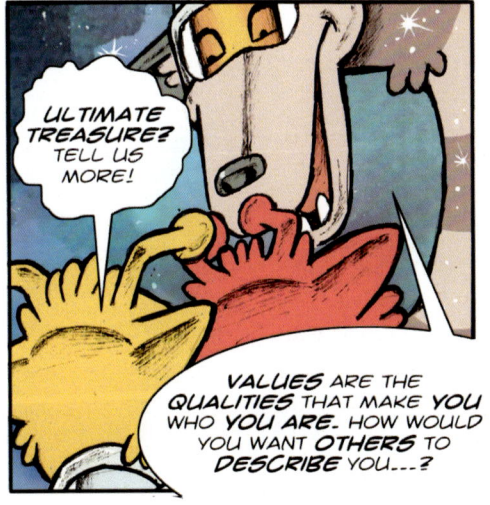
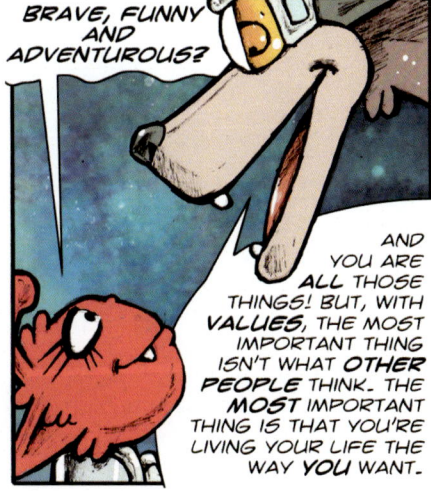

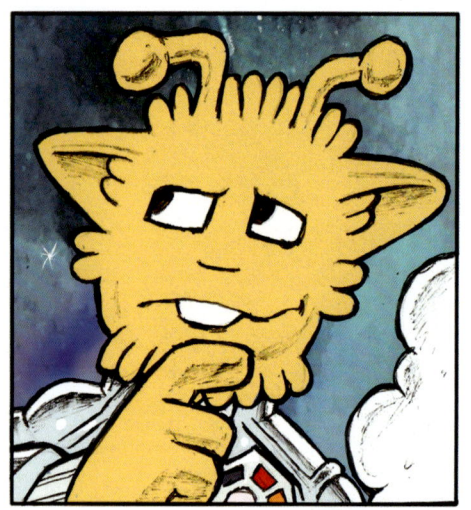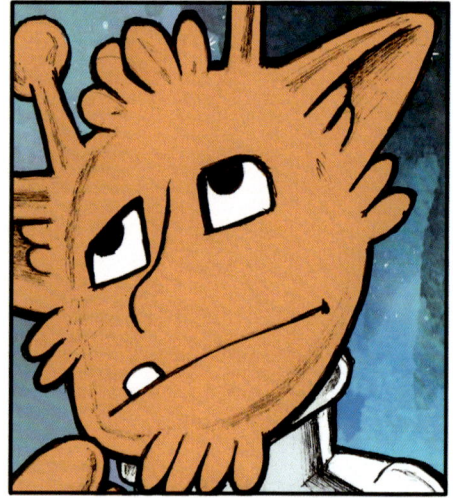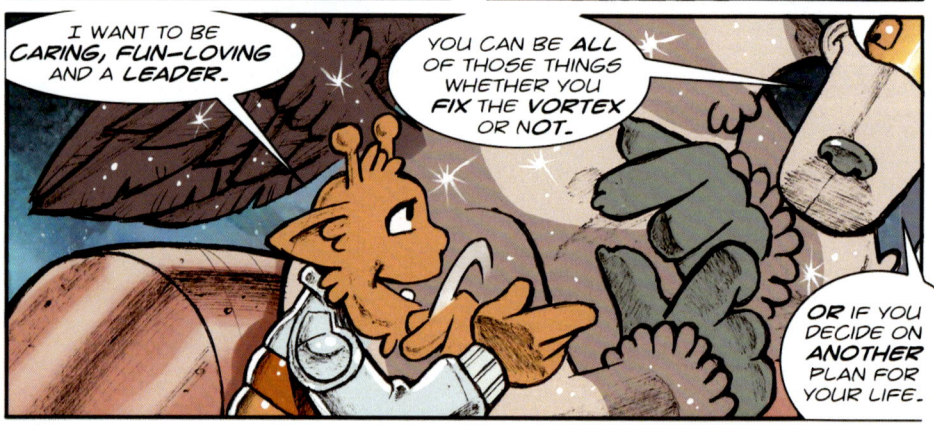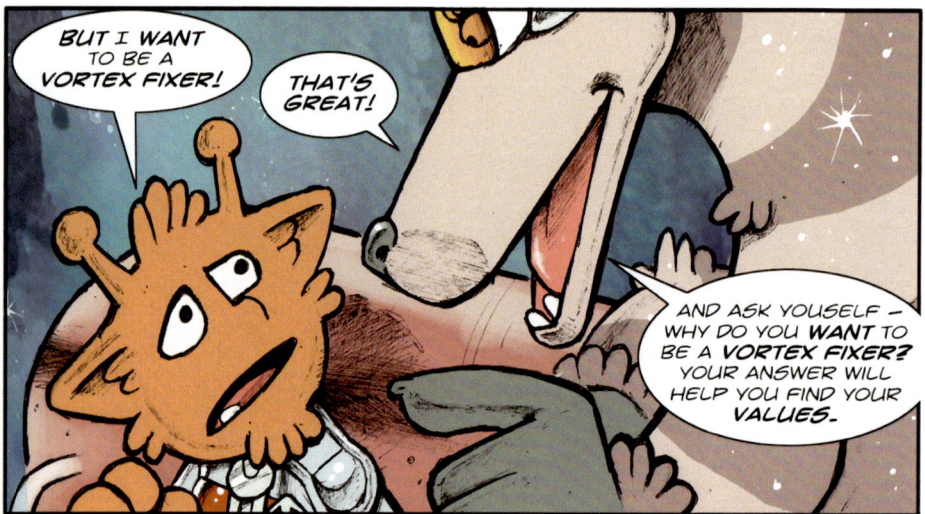

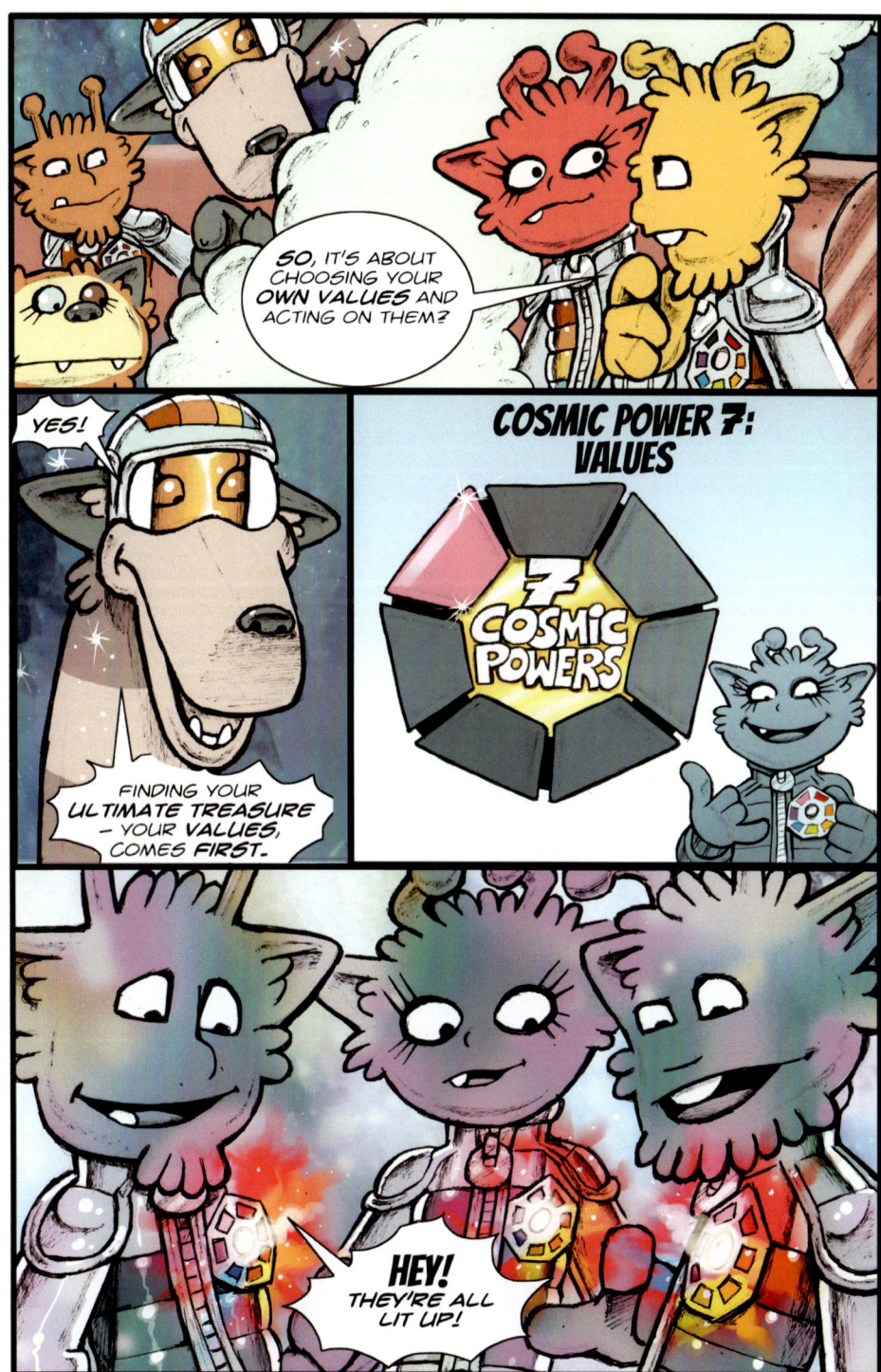

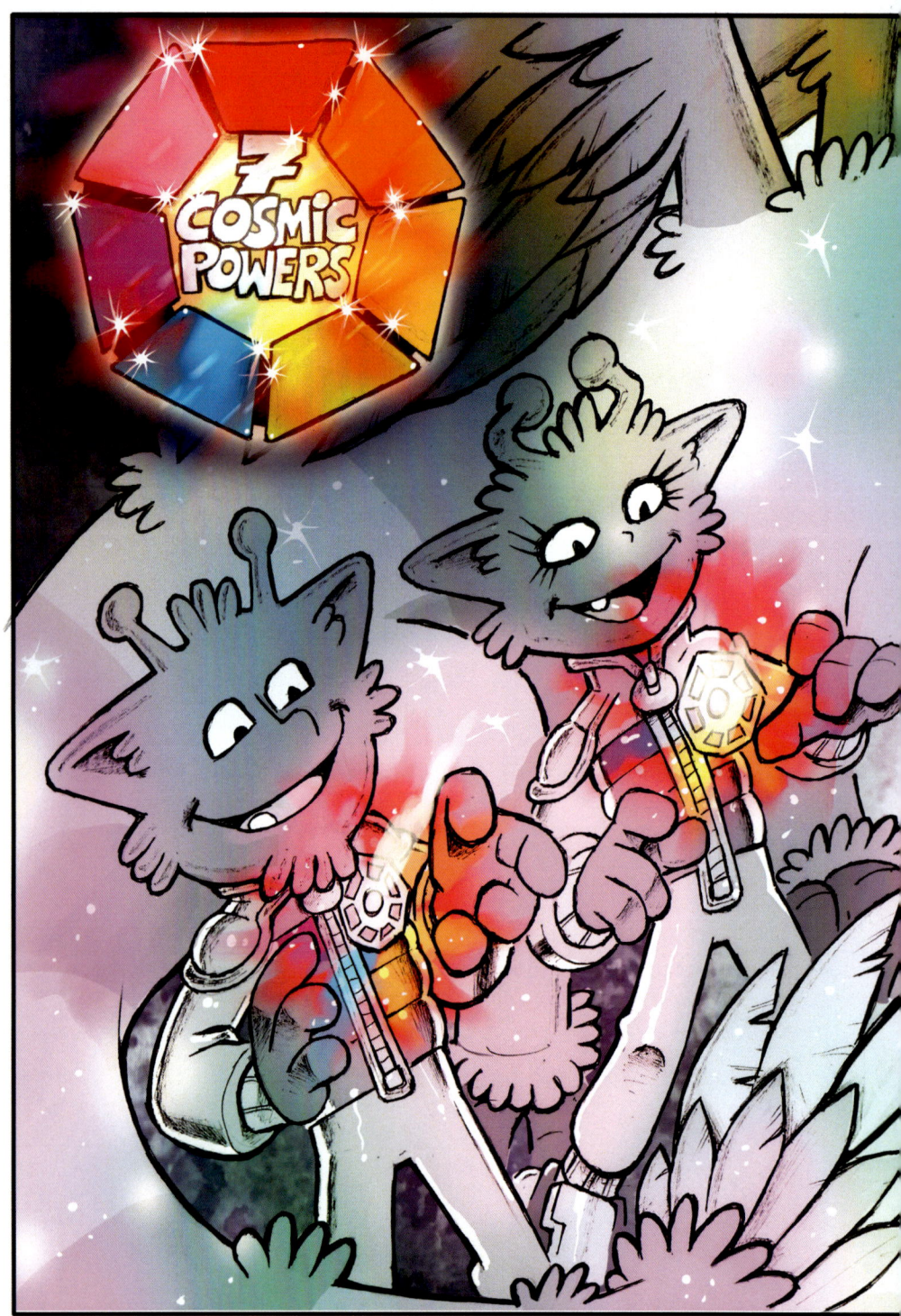

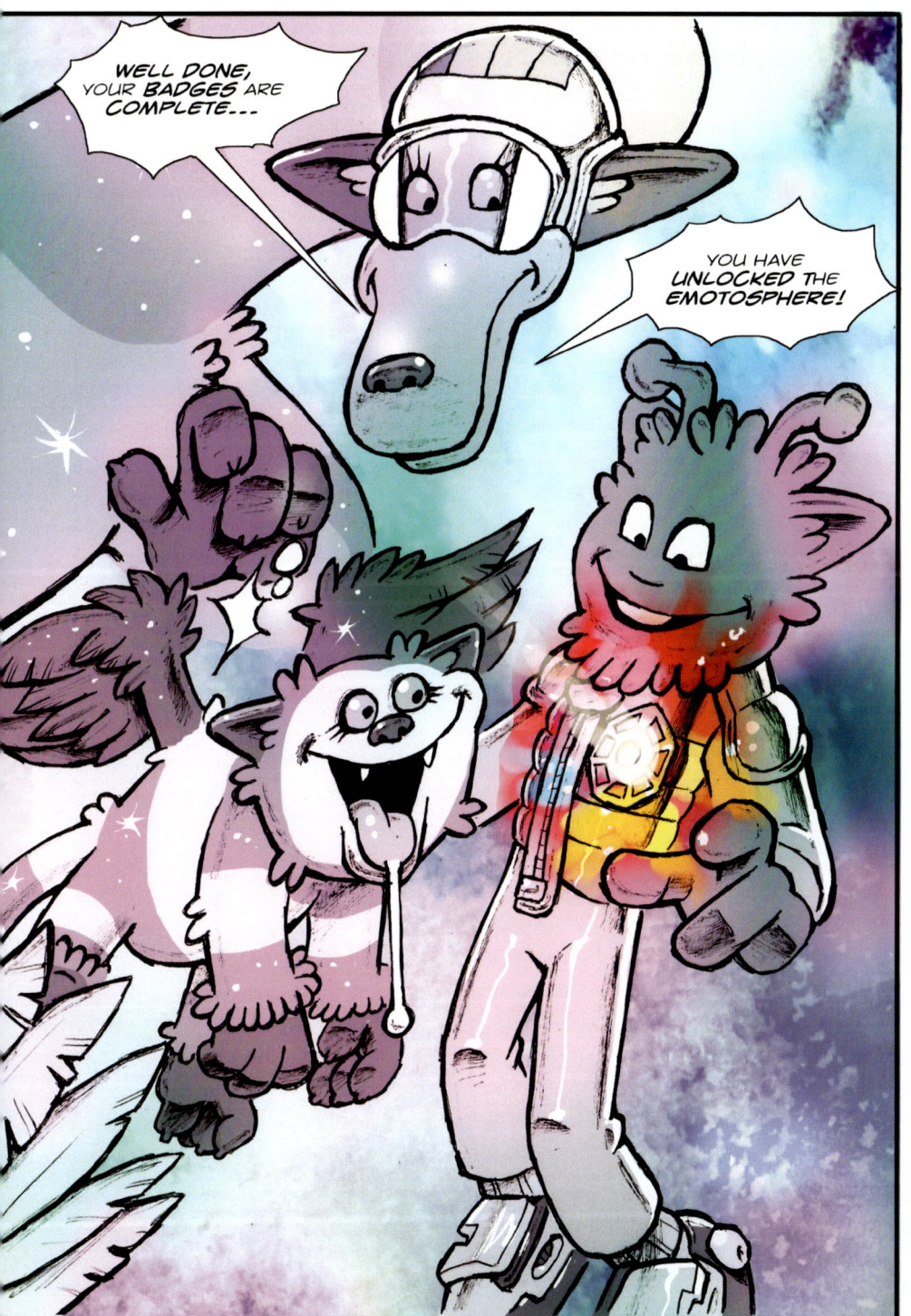

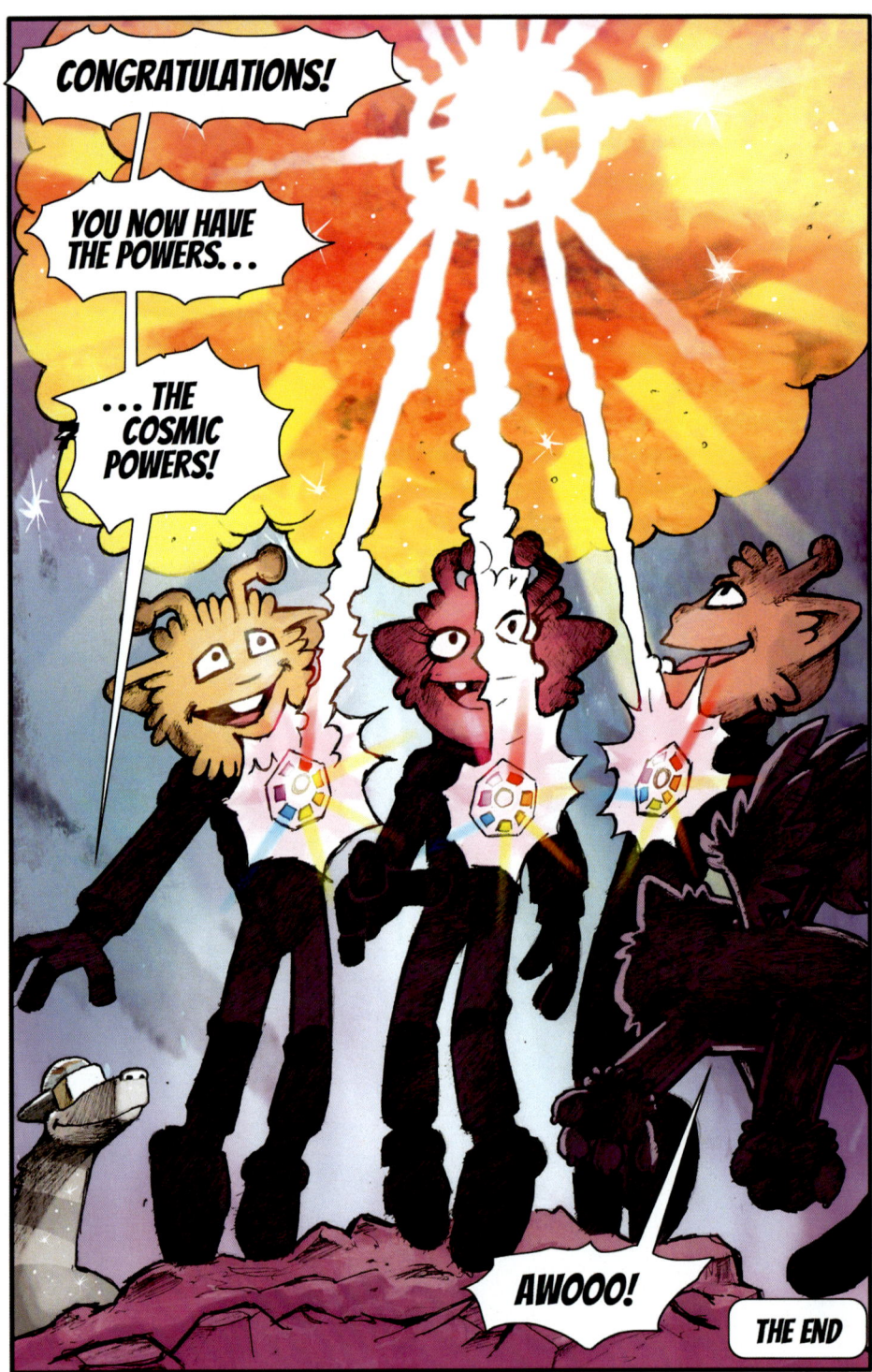

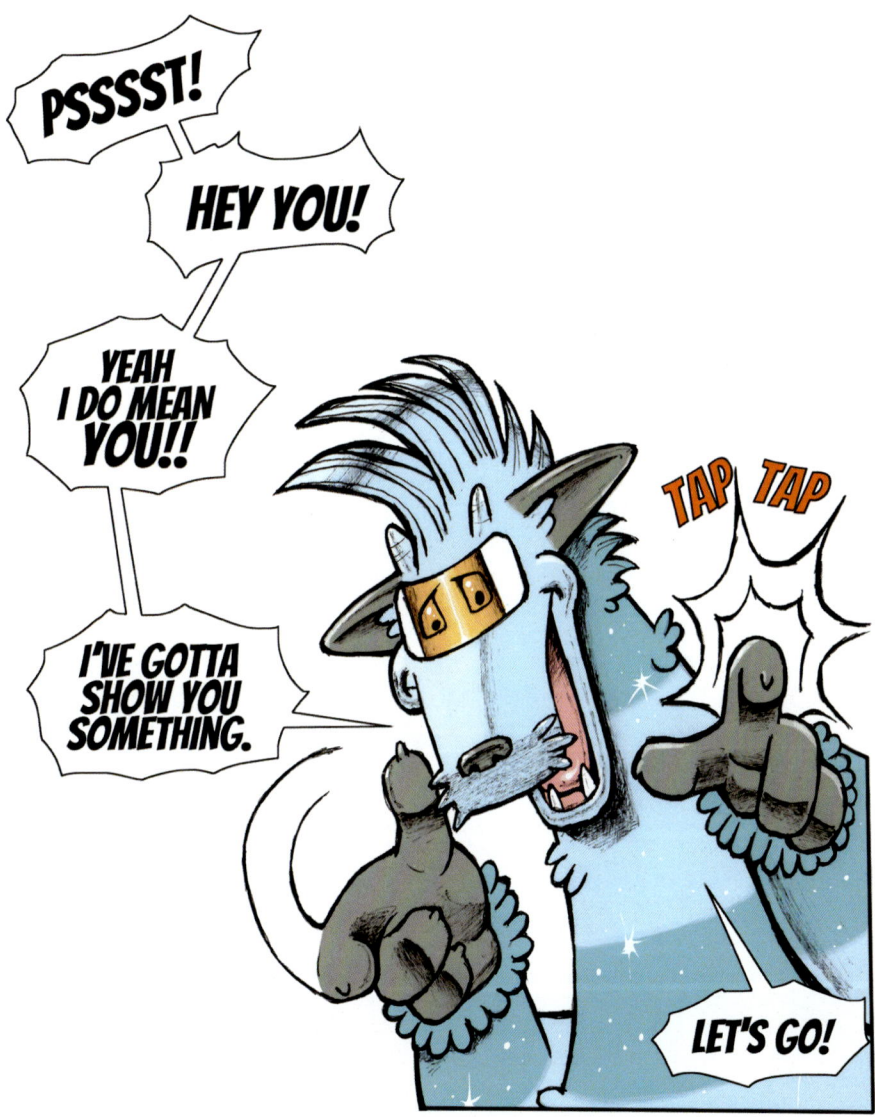

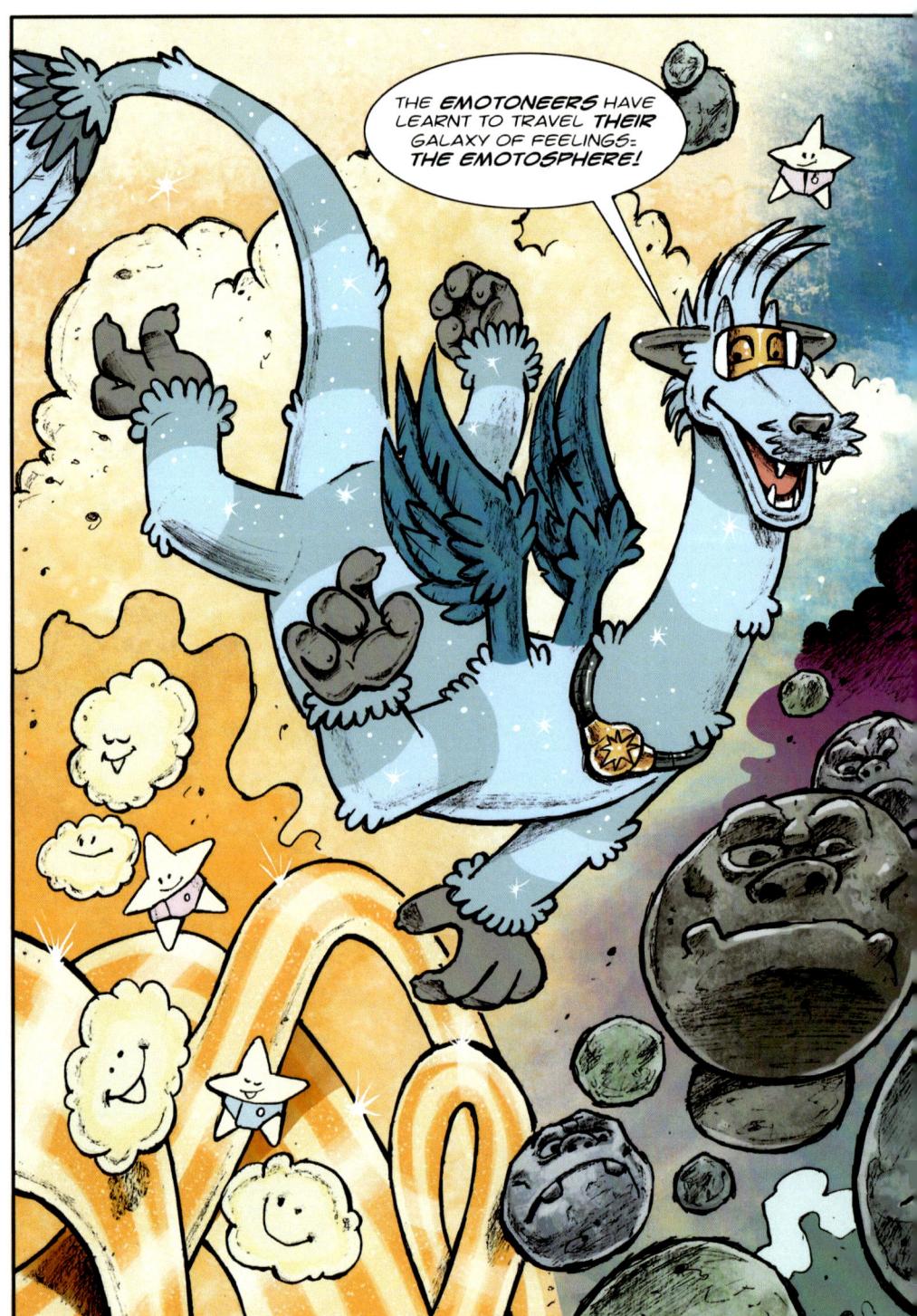

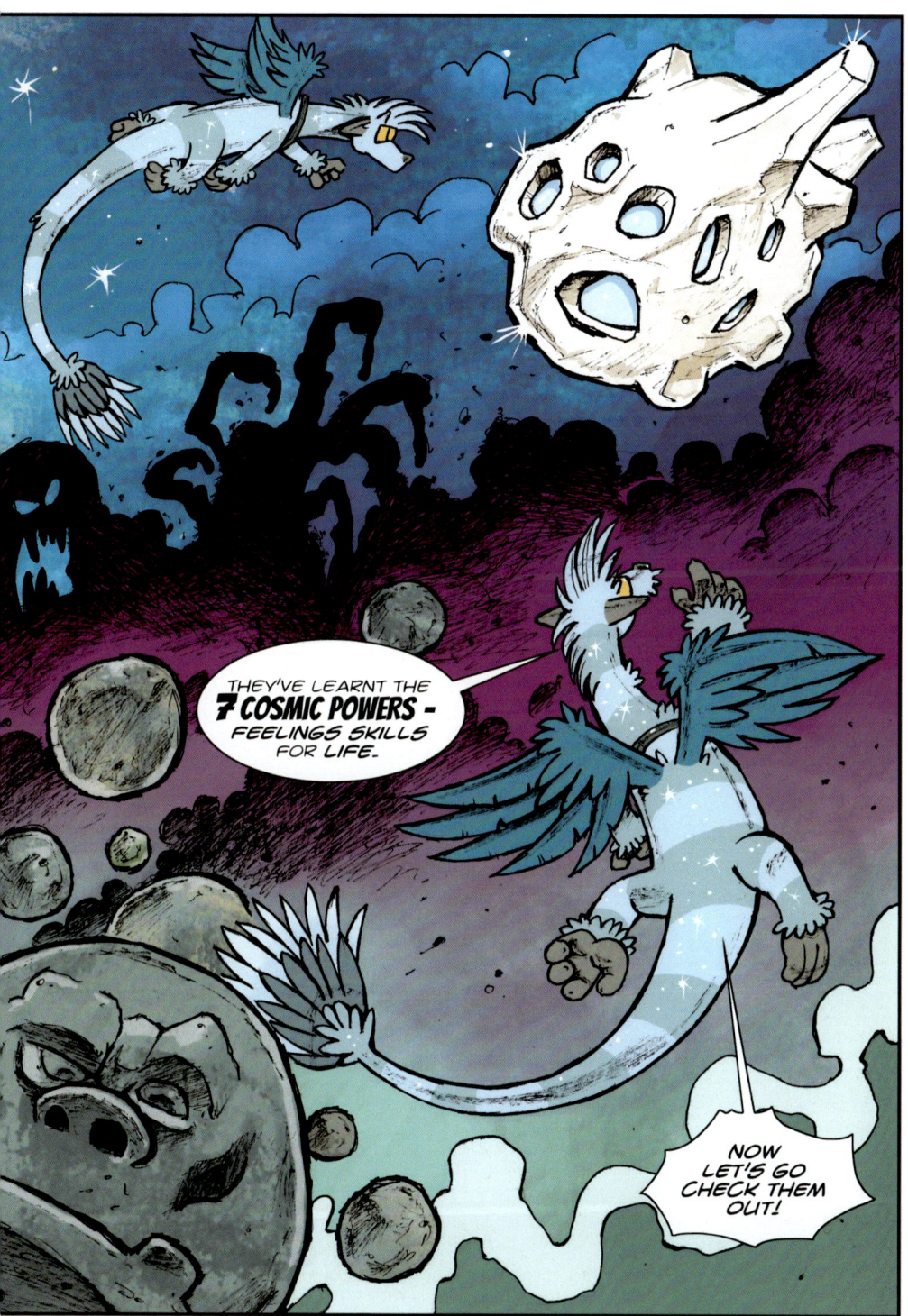

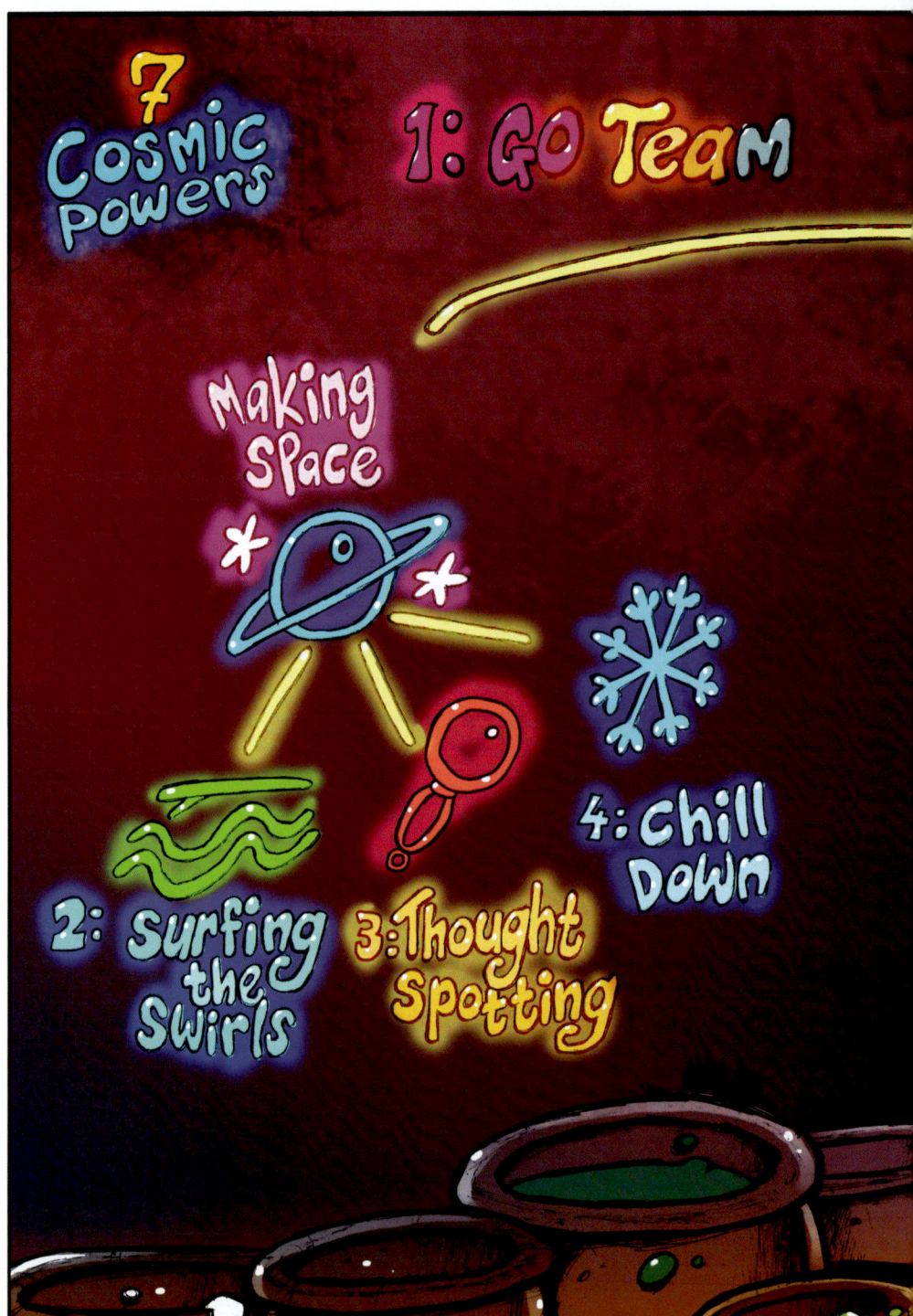

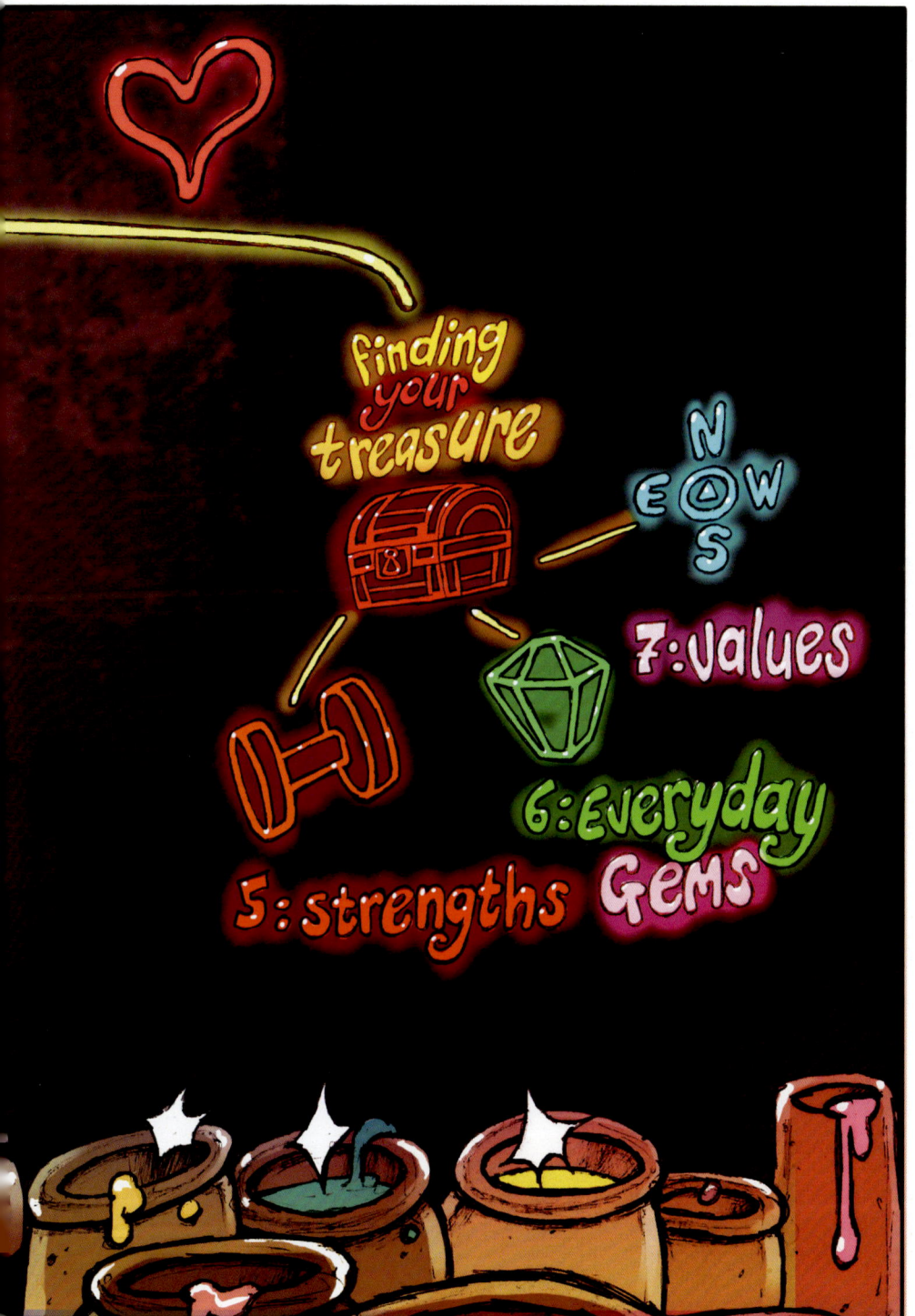

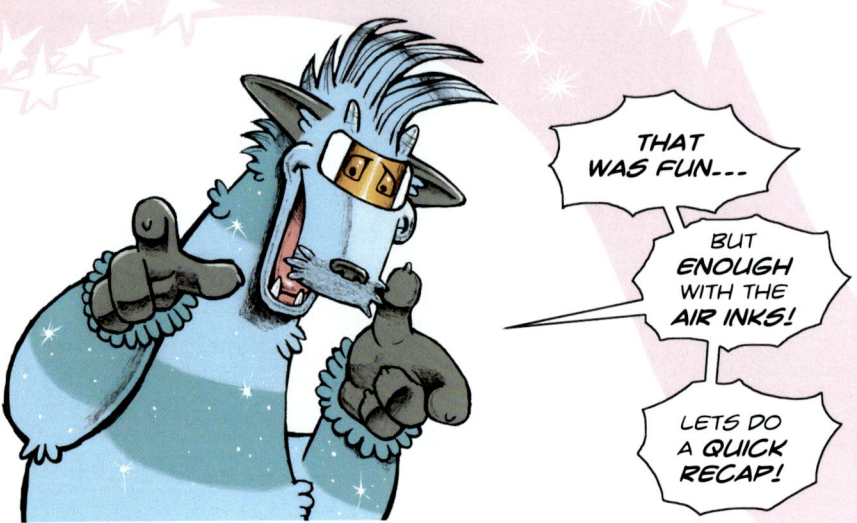

1: GO TEAM!

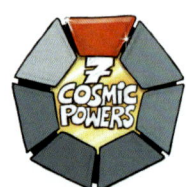

HAVING A STRONG TRUSTED TEAM AROUND YOU

2: SURFING THE SWIRLS

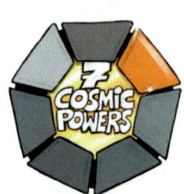

RIDING OUT THE UPS 'N DOWNS AND INS 'N OUTS OF YOUR EMOTIONS

3: THOUGHT SPOTTING

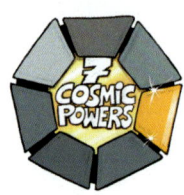

TAKING THE POWER OUT OF TRICKY THOUGHTS

HARD TO THINK OF SOMEONE ON YOUR TEAM?

WANT SOMEONE ELSE TO TALK TO ABOUT HOW YOU'RE FEELING?

GIVE THESE FOLKS A CALL—
CHILDLINE— 0800 1111
YOUNG MINDS— 0808 802 5544

(UK ONLY. IN OTHER COUNTRIES, ASK A DOCTOR WHO TO CALL)

4: CHILL DOWN

RELAX YOUR BODY AND YOUR EMOTIONS WILL FOLLOW

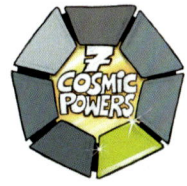

5: STRENGTHS

THE AWESOME STUFF YOU'RE INTO

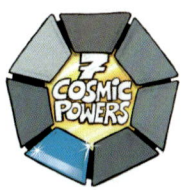

6: EVERYDAY GEMS

THE TREASURE IN YOUR LIFE EVERYDAY, WHEN YOU TAKE THE TIME TO LOOK

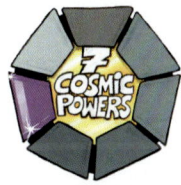

7: VALUES

THE QUALITIES THAT GUIDE YOUR LIFE AND MAKE IT YOUR OWN

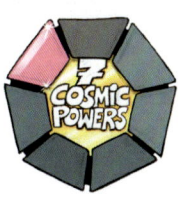

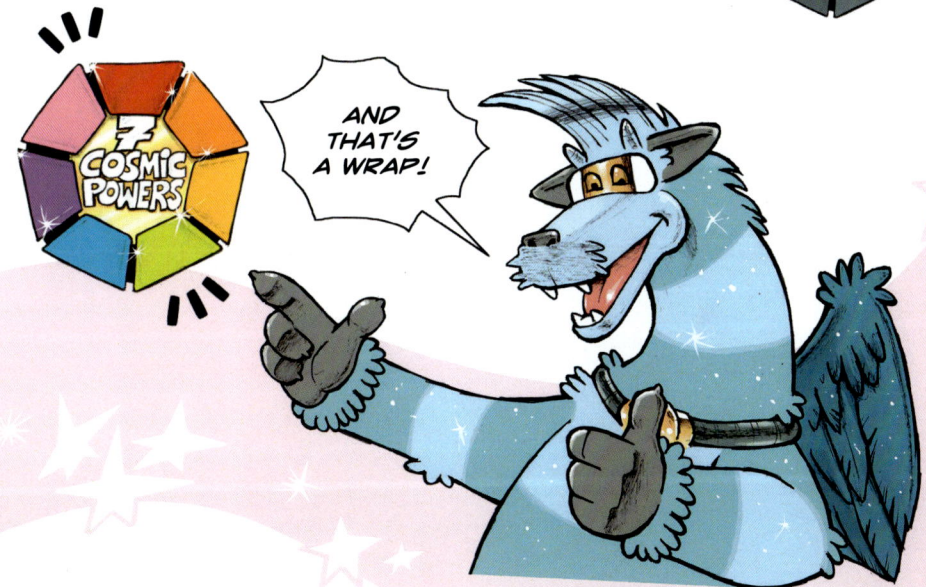

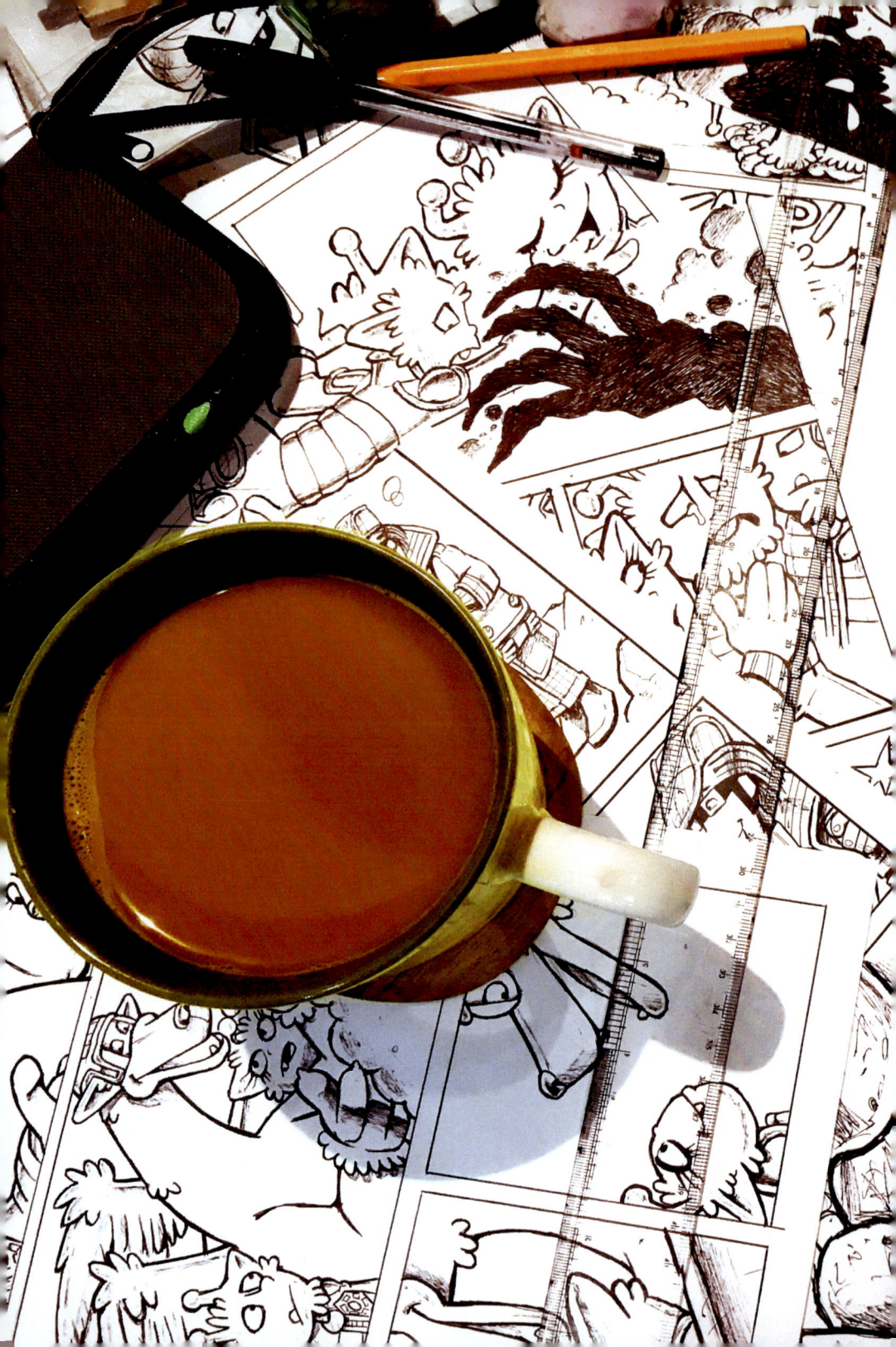